Challenging Concepts in Neurology

Titles in the Challenging Concepts in series

Anaesthesia (Edited by Dr Phoebe Syme, Dr Robert Jackson, and Professor Timothy Cook)

Cardiovascular Medicine (Edited by Dr Aung Myat, Dr Shouvik Haldar, and Professor Simon Redwood)

Emergency Medicine (Edited by Dr Sam Thenabadu, Dr Fleur Cantle, and Dr Chris Lacy)

Infectious Diseases and Clinical Microbiology (Edited by Dr Amber Arnold and Professor George E. Griffin)

Interventional Radiology (Edited by Dr Irfan Ahmed, Dr Miltiadis Krokidis, and Dr Tarun Sabharwal)

Neurology (Edited by Dr Krishna Chinthapalli, Dr Nadia Magdalinou, and Professor Nicholas Wood)

Neurosurgery (Edited by Mr Robin Bhatia and Mr Ian Sabin)

Obstetrics and Gynaecology (Edited by Dr Natasha Hezelgrave, Dr Danielle Abbott, and Professor Andrew H. Shennan)

Oncology (Edited by Dr Madhumita Bhattacharyya, Dr Sarah Payne, and Professor Iain McNeish)

Oral and Maxillofacial Surgery (Edited by Mr Matthew Idle and Group Captain Andrew Monaghan)

Respiratory Medicine (Edited by Dr Lucy Schomberg, Dr Elizabeth Sage, and Dr Nick Hart)

Challenging Concepts in Neurology

Cases with Expert Commentary

Edited by

Dr Krishna Chinthapalli

Clinical Research Fellow, UCL Institute of Neurology, London, UK; Neurology Specialty Registrar, St George's Hospital, London, UK

Dr Nadia Magdalinou

Clinical Research Fellow, UCL Institute of Neurology, London, UK; Neurology Specialty Registrar, St George's Hospital, London, UK

Professor Nicholas Wood

Galton Professor of Genetics UCL, Vice Dean for Research, UCL Faculty of Brain Sciences, UCL Institute of Neurology, London, UK; Honorary Consultant, National Hospital for Neurology and Neurosurgery, London, UK

Series editors

Dr Aung Myat BSc (Hons) MBBS MRCP

BHF Clinical Research Training Fellow, King's College London British Heart Foundation Centre of Research Excellence, Cardiovascular Division, St Thomas' Hospital, London, UK

Dr Shouvik Haldar MBBS MRCP

Electrophysiology Research Fellow & Cardiology SpR, Heart Rhythm Centre, NIHR Cardiovascular Biomedical Research Unit, Royal Brompton & Harefield NHS Foundation Trust, Imperial College London, London, UK

Professor Simon Redwood MD FRCP

Professor of Interventional Cardiology and Honorary Consultant Cardiologist, King's College London British Heart Foundation Centre of Research Excellence, Cardiovascular Division and Guy's and St Thomas' NHS Foundation Trust, St Thomas' Hospital, London, UK

OXFORD
UNIVERSITY PRESS

OXFORD
UNIVERSITY PRESS

Great Clarendon Street, Oxford, OX2 6DP,
United Kingdom

Oxford University Press is a department of the University of Oxford. It furthers the University's objective of excellence in research, scholarship, and education by publishing worldwide. Oxford is a registered trade mark of Oxford University Press in the UK and in certain other countries

Impression: 1

Published in the United States of America by Oxford University Press
198 Madison Avenue, New York, NY 10016, United States of America

British Library Cataloguing in Publication Data
Data available

Library of Congress Control Number: 2015947231

ISBN 978-0-19-966477-1

Printed in Great Britain by
Ashford Colour Press Ltd, Gosport, Hampshire

FOREWORD

The National Hospital Queen Square, as it is has been affectionately known by generations of neurologists, was founded in 1860 as the first hospital in the world to be devoted to neurological cases. Over the succeeding years, the Hospital became one of the most important centres of neurological training in the world. By the 1950s, doctors from 55 countries were attending the hospital's teaching rounds, and more than 1000 students annually attended the celebrated case demonstrations by the hospital's physicians. Such case-based learning has remained central to the hospital's teaching effort since its foundation, and this book reflects this distinguished tradition.

Prior to 1860, neurology was not a formed specialty. The approach to neurological diagnosis was to a large extent random, with no underpinning structure, process or method. It was in part due to the work of the hospital's physicians, notably Hughlings, Jackson, Gowers, Bastian, and Holmes, that a systematized method of clinical diagnosis was developed. This clinico-anatomical method involves a two-stage process, now adopted universally, and it remains at the heart of the process of diagnosis. In the first stage, the clinical history and examination signs are used by the physician to localize the site of pathology in the nervous system. In the second stage, the type of pathology (the etiology) is identified by features of the history such as the mode of onset of the neurological disorder, its tempo, progression, demography and clinical associations, and its clinical context.

Investigatory methods have become more sophisticated, especially in relation to neuropathology, biochemistry, neuroimaging and most recently molecular biology and clinical genetics and, as a result, diagnosis can now be much more refined. Although modern investigatory methods can be extremely powerful tools, and the precision and detail of etiological diagnosis have advanced massively in recent years, the importance of obtaining a careful history and conducting a careful examination remain at the core of neurological diagnosis. In contemporary neurology, the history still needs to be taken in detail, but with the doctor focusing on the important points, and the examination also needs to be meticulous, but again directed towards the systems which are most relevant. Investigations can then be targeted correctly to address the questions posed by the clinical evaluation. Nothing is more deprecated than casual history taking and aimless examination followed by unfocused investigation. For a long time neurology had suffered the reputation of being a solely diagnostic specialty with no treatment possible, but this too has completely changed. In recent years, a succession of effective therapies for what were previously untreatable conditions have been introduced into clinical practice, and these advanced investigatory and treatment options have changed the whole landscape of the specialty.

In this book, the modern approach to diagnosis and management is elegantly demonstrated though a series of 22 case histories. The salient history and the examination signs are given for each case, followed by targeted investigation resulting in successful diagnosis. Each case is then summarized and the modern management described. These case descriptions are model examples of how neurology should be practiced today.

The cases are carefully chosen. All are topics in which knowledge and treatment have significantly advanced in recent years, and many include diagnoses that frequently cause difficulty. Areas often ignored, such as uro-neurology, neuro-otology and neuro-rehabilitation, are also deliberately included.

Each chapter is written jointly by a trainee and a senior expert in the field. The trainees have all been through, or are going through, training at Queen Square and the senior doctors are acknowledged experts worldwide. A standard format has been adopted with very helpful 'learning points', 'clinical tips', 'expert comments', and a 'final word from the expert' added in each case. The case discussions include tables of differential diagnoses and lists of crucial references. There is useful guidance on such topics as when to do a lumber puncture and when to arrange complex genetic or immunological tests. The case studies in this book reflect the perspectives of both the trainee and the expert, are of uniformly very high quality, and are instructive and exceptionally well written.

The editors, Dr Krishna Chinthapalli and Professor Nick Wood are to be congratulated on bringing together an outstanding collection of cases, which demonstrate the art and the beauty of neurological diagnosis, and the contemporary advances in investigation and treatment. In medicine, case-based learning is a fundamental part of clinical apprenticeship, and this book exemplifies this method brilliantly. It should be mandatory reading for all aspiring neurological trainees, and can be read with pleasure and with profit by neurologists at every level.

Professor Simon Shorvon
UCL Institute of Neurology and National Hospital
for Neurology and Neurosurgery, Queen Square, London

CONTENTS

EXPERTS

Kailash P. Bhatia
Professor of Clinical Neurology, Sobell Department for Motor Neuroscience, UCL Institute of Neurology, London, UK; Honorary Consultant Neurologist, National Hospital for Neurology, Queen Square, London, UK

Adolfo M. Bronstein
Professor of Clinical Neuro-otology and Consultant Neurologist, Imperial College London, London, UK; Consultant Neurologist, National Hospital for Neurology and Neurosurgery, Queen Square, London, UK

Martin M. Brown
Professor of Stroke Medicine, Department of Brain Repair and Rehabilitation, Institute of Neurology, University College London, UK

Declan Chard
Senior Clinical Research Associate, NMR Research Unit, Queen Square Multiple Sclerosis Centre, UCL Institute of Neurology, UK; National Institute for Health Research (NIHR), University College London Hospitals, Biomedical Research Centre, UK

Mark J. Edwards
Senior Lecturer, Sobell Department for Motor Neuroscience, UCL Institute of Neurology, London, UK; Honorary Consultant Neurologist, National Hospital for Neurology, Queen Square, London, UK

Sofia H. Eriksson
Consultant Neurologist and Honorary Senior Lecturer, Department of Clinical and Experimental Epilepsy, National Hospital for Neurology and Neurosurgery, London, UK

Angela Gall
Consultant in Rehabilitation Medicine, London Spinal Cord Injury Centre, Royal National Orthopaedic Hospital, Stanmore, UK

Gavin Giovannoni
Professor of Neurology, Blizard Institute, Barts and the London School of Medicine and Dentistry, Queen Mary University London, UK; Royal London Hospital, UK

Henry Houlden
Professor of Neurology, Department of Molecular Neuroscience, Institute of Neurology and National Hospital for Neurology and Neurosurgery, Queen Square, London, UK

Dimitri M. Kullmann
Professor of Neurology, UCL Institute of Neurology, London, UK

Robin Lachmann
Consultant in Inherited Metabolic Disease, Charles Dent Metabolic Unit, National Hospital for Neurology and Neurosurgery, Queen Square, London, UK

Hadi Manji
Consultant Neurologist, National Hospital for Neurology and Neurosurgery, Queen Square, London, UK

Marco Mula
Consultant in Neurology and Epileptology, Department of Neurology, St George's Hospital, London, UK

Edel O'Toole
Professor of Molecular Dermatology and Honorary Consultant Dermatologist, Barts and the London School of Medicine and Dentistry, Queen Mary University London, UK; Royal London Hospital, Barts Health NHS Trust, London, UK

Jalesh N. Panicker
Consultant Neurologist, Department of Uro-Neurology, The National Hospital for Neurology and Neurosurgery and UCL Institute of Neurology, Queen Square, London, UK

Marios C. Papadopoulos
Professor of Neurosurgery, St. George's, University of London, London, UK

Gordon T. Plant
Consultant Neurologist and Neuro-Ophthalmologist, Moorfields Eye Hospital, London; National Hospital for Neurology and Neurosurgery, London; St Thomas' Hospital, London, UK

Paul Riordan-Eva
Consultant Ophthalmic Surgeon, King's College Hospital, London, UK

Martin N. Rossor
Professor of Clinical Neurology, Dementia Research Centre, UCL Institute of Neurology, Queen Square, London, UK

Laszlo K. Sztriha
Consultant Neurologist, King's College Hospital, London, UK

Chris Turner
Consultant Neurologist, MRC Centre for Neuromuscular Diseases, National Hospital for Neurology and Neurosurgery, Queen Square, London, UK

Daniel C. Walsh
Consultant Neurosurgeon, King's College Hospital, London, UK

Graham Warner
Consultant Neurologist, Department of Neurology, Royal Surrey County Hospital, Guildford, UK

CONTRIBUTORS

Sara Ajina
Wellcome Trust Clinical Research Training Fellow, FMRIB Centre, University of Oxford, UK

Krishna Chinthapalli
Clinical Research Fellow, UCL Institute of Neurology, London, UK; Neurology Specialty Registrar, St George's Hospital, London, UK

Suchitra Chinthapalli
Dermatology Specialist Registrar, Royal London Hospital, Barts Health NHS Trust, London, UK

Ruth Dobson
Clinical Research Fellow, Blizard Institute, Barts and the London School of Medicine and Dentistry, Queen Mary University London, UK; Royal London Hospital, UK

Karen M. Doherty
Department of Clinical Neurosciences, Royal Victoria Hospital, Belfast, UK

Diego Kaski
Neurology Registrar, National Hospital for Neurology and Neurosurgery, London, UK; Honorary Clinical Research Fellow, Imperial College London, London, UK

Fiona Kennedy
Clinical Research Fellow, Department of Brain Repair and Rehabilitation, Institute of Neurology, University College London, UK

Benedict D. Michael
NIHR Academic Clinical Lecturer, The Walton Centre NHS Foundation Trust and the Institute of Infection and Global Health, University of Liverpool, UK

Jan Novy
Neurologist, Department of Clinical Neurosciences, CHUV, University of Lausanne, Switzerland

David Paling
Consultant Neurologist, Department of Clinical Neurology, Royal Hallamshire Hospital, Sheffield Teaching Hospitals NHS Trust, Sheffield, UK; Department of Neuroscience, University of Sheffield, UK

Ross W. Paterson
Clinical Research Fellow, Institute of Neurology, Queen Square, University College London, UK

Dipa Raja Rayan
MRC Clinical Research Training Fellow, MRC Centre for Neuromuscular Diseases, UCL Institute of Neurology, London, UK

Ignacio Rubio-Agusti
Consultant Neurologist, Movement Disorders Unit, Hospital Universitario La Fe, Valencia, Spain

Natalie S. Ryan
Clinical Research Fellow, Dementia Research Centre, UCL Institute of Neurology, Queen Square, London, UK

Anna Sadnicka
Clinical Research Fellow, Sobell Department for Motor Neuroscience, UCL Institute of Neurology, London, UK; Honorary Registrar, National Hospital for Neurology, Queen Square, London, UK

Anish N. Shah
Consultant Ophthalmic Surgeon, Jersey General Hospital, Jersey, UK

Vino Siva
Specialist Registrar in Neurosurgery, South Thames/London Neurosurgical Training Programme, London, UK

Jennifer Spillane
Clinical Research Fellow, UCL Institute of Neurology, London, UK

William M. Stern
Neurology Registrar, South London Rotation, London, UK

David J. Stoeter
Intensive Care and Anaesthesiology Specialist Registrar, The Royal Liverpool University Hospital, Liverpool, UK

Jonathan D. Virgo
Medical Ophthalmology Specialist Registrar, Moorfields Eye Hospital, London; St Thomas' Hospital, London, UK

Umesh Vivekananda
Clinical Research Fellow, Department of Clinical and Experimental Epilepsy, UCL Institute of Neurology, London, UK

Joel S. Winston
Clinical Research Fellow, Wellcome Trust Centre for Neuroimaging, UCL, Queen Square, London, UK; Department of Clinical Neurophysiology, National Hospital for Neurology and Neurosurgery, London, UK

Sui Wong
Consultant Neurologist and Neuro-Ophthalmologist, Moorfields Eye Hospital, London; St Thomas' Hospital, London, UK

ABBREVIATIONS

3,4-DAP	3,4-diaminopyridine
A&E	accident and emergency department
ACE	angiotensin-converting enzyme
ACom	anterior communicating artery
AD	Alzheimer's disease, autonomic dysreflexia
ADC	apparent diffusion coefficient
ADEM	acute disseminated encephalomyelitis
ADPKD	autosomal dominant polycystic kidney disease
AED	anti-epileptic drug
AFO	ankle-foot orthosis
AGEP	acute generalized exanthematous pustulosis
ALS	amyotrophic lateral sclerosis (spinal muscular atrophy)
AMPA	α-amino-3-hydroxy-5-methyl-4-isoxazolepropionic acid
AMTS	Abbreviated Mental Test Score
ANA	antinuclear antibody
ANCA	antineutrophil cytoplasmic antibody
ANMDARE	anti-NMDA-receptor encephalitis
AQP4	aquaporin-4
ASIA	American Spinal Injuries Association
AT	antithrombotic treatment
ATLS	Advanced Trauma Life Support
AV	arteriovenous
AVM	arteriovenous malformation
BAO	basilar artery occlusion
bd	twice daily
BMI	body mass index
BPPV	benign paroxysmal positional vertigo
CAA	cerebral amyloid angiopathy
CADASIL	cerebral autosomal-dominant arteriopathy with subcortical infarcts and leucoencephalopathy
CBD	corticobasal degeneration
CCF	carotid cavernous fistula
CEMRA	contrast-enhanced magnetic resonance angiography
CI	confidence interval
CIDP	chronic inflammatory demyelinating polyneuropathy
CIS	clinically isolated syndrome
CISC	clean intermittent self-catheterization
CIT	cognitive impairment test
CJD	Creutzfeldt-Jakob disease
CK	creatine kinase
CMAP	compound muscle action potential
CMV	cytomegalovirus
CNS	central nervous system
CPAP	continuous positive airways pressure
CRION	chronic relapsing inflammatory optic neuropathy
CRP	C-reactive protein
CS	cavernous sinus
CSF	cerebrospinal fluid
CSW	cerebral salt wasting
CT	computed tomography
CTA	CT angiography
CTV	CT venogram/venography
CVST	cerebral venous sinus thrombosis
CXR	chest radiograph
DBN	downbeat nystagmus
DCI	delayed cerebral ischaemia
DIND	delayed ischaemic neurological deficit
DLB	dementia with Lewy bodies
DM	myotonic dystrophy (dystrophica myotonica)
DNAR	do not attempt resuscitation
DNET	dysembryoplastic neuroepithelial tumours
DRESS	drug rash with eosinophilia and systemic symptoms
DSA	digital subtraction angiography
DSD	dyssynergic distal sphincter
DVLA	Driving and Vehicle Licensing Agency
DWI	diffusion-weighted imaging
EBV	Epstein-Barr virus
ECA	external carotid artery
EDS	excessive daytime sleepiness
EDSS	Expanded Disability Status Scale
EEG	electroencephelogram
EMG	electromyography/myogram
ENA	extractable nuclear antigen
ENT	ear, nose, and throat

EOG	electro-oculogram
ERT	enzyme replacement therapy
ESR	erythrocyte sedimentation ratio
FAF	fundus autofluorescence
FAM	Functional Assessment Measure
FBC	full blood count
FDA	Food and Drug Administration
FDG	fluorodeoxyglucose
FDG-PET	fluorodeoxyglucose positron emission tomography
FES	functional electrical stimulation
FFA	fundus fluorescein angiography
FIM	Functional Independence Measure
FLAIR	fluid attenuation inversion recovery
FMD	fibromuscular dysplasia
Fol	folic acid
FSHD	facioscapulohumeral muscular dystrophy
GABA	γ-aminobutyric acid
GBS	Guillain-Barré syndrome
GCS	Glasgow coma scale/score
GP	general practitioner
GRE	gradient-recalled echo
H&E	haematoxylin-eosin
HASU	hyperacute stroke unit
HHV6	human herpes virus type 6
HIV	human immunodeficiency virus
HO	heterotopic ossification
HSV	herpes simplex virus
IA	intra-arterial
IBS	irritable bowel syndrome
ICA	internal carotid artery
ICD	implantable cardiac defibrillator
ICP	intracranial pressure
ICU	intensive care unit
IEM	inborn error of metabolism
IHCD-II	International Headache Classification-Secondary Headaches
IIH	idiopathic intracranial hypertension
IL-6	interleukin-6
IMA	internal maxillary artery
IPS	inferior petrosal sinus
ISNCSCI	International Standards for Neurological Classification after Spinal Cord Injury
ITU	intensive therapy unit
IV	intravenous
IVA	intra-arterial thrombosis
IVIG	intravenous immunoglobulin
IVT	intravenous thrombolysis
KAFO	knee-ankle-foot orthosis
LE	limbic encephalitis
LEMS	Lambert-Eaton myasthenic syndrome
LETM	longitudinally extensive transverse myelitis
LFT	liver function test
LGMD	limb girdle muscular dystrophy
LHON	Leber's hereditary optic neuropathy
LMWH	low molecular weight heparin
LP	lumbar puncture
LPS	lumbo-peritoneal shunt
LSD	lysosomal storage disorder
MAP	mean arterial pressure
MCA	middle cerebral artery
MCP	middle cerebellar peduncle
metHb	methaemoglobin
MG	myasthenia gravis
MHRA	Medicines and Healthcare Products Regulatory Agency
MIDD	maternally inherited diabetes and deafness
MMSE	Mini-Mental State Examination
MRA	magnetic resonance angiography
MRC	Medical Research Council
MRI	magnetic resonance imaging
MRS	Modified Rankin scale/score
MRV	magnetic resonance venography
MS	multiple sclerosis
MSA	multiple system atrophy
MSLT	multiple sleep latency testing
NBIA	neuronal brain iron accumulation
NG	nasogastric
NHS	National Health Service
NICU	neurological intensive care unit
NIHSS	National Institute of Health Stroke Scale
NIV	non-invasive ventilation
NK	natural killer
NMDA	*N*-methyl-D-aspartate
NMDAR	NMDA receptor
NMO	neuromyelitis optica
NRR	neuroretinal rim
NSAID	non-steroidal anti-inflammatory drugs
OCB	oligoclonal band, oral contraceptive pill
OCP	oral contraceptive (pill)
OCT	optical coherence tomography
OH	orthostatic hypertension
ONSF	optic nerve sheath fenestration

OR	odds ratio
OSA	obstructive sleep apnoea
oxyHb	oxyhaemoglobin
PBMC	peripheral blood mononuclear cell
PCA	posterior cerebral artery, posterior cortical atrophy
PCom	posterior communicating artery
PCR	polymerase chain reaction
PD	Parkinson's disease
PEEP	positive end expiratory pressure
PERM	progressive encephalomyelitis with rigidity
PET	positron emission tomography
PFO	patent foramen ovale
PICA	posterior inferior cerebellar artery
PLE	paraneoplastic limbic encephalitis
PLED	periodic lateralizing epileptiform discharge
PLEX	plasma exchange
PML	progressive multifocal leucoencephalopathy
PNET	primitive neuroepithelial tumours
PRIS	propofol infusion syndrome
prn	when necessary
PROMM	proximal myotonic myopathy
PTC	pseudotumour cerebri
PVR	post-void residual volume
QMS	Quantitative Myasthenia Score
RAPD	relative afferent pupillary defect
RBC	red blood cell
RBD	REM sleep behaviour disorder
RCT	randomized controlled trial
REM	rapid eye movement
RhF	rheumatoid factor
RNFL	retinal nerve fibre layer
RNS	repetitive nerve stimulation
SAH	subarachnoid haemorrhage
SCA	superior cerebellar artery
SCAR	serious cutaneous adverse reactions
SCI	spinal cord injury
SCIC	spinal cord injuries centre
SCIM	Spinal Cord Independence Measure
SCLC	small-cell lung cancer
SE	status epilepticus
SIADH	syndrome of inappropriate antidiuretic hormone
SJS	Stevens-Johnson syndrome
SLE	systemic lupus erythematosus
SMA	spinal muscular atrophy
SND	striatonigral degeneration
SNRI	serotonin-norepinephrine reuptake inhibitor
SOV	superior orbital vein
SPC	suprapubic catheter
SPECT	single photon emission computed tomography
SPS	stiff person syndrome
SSRI	selective serotonin reuptake inhibitor
SVP	spontaneous venous pulsation
SWI	susceptibility-weighted imaging
TAA	transient aura attack
TCD	transcranial Doppler
TCH	thunderclap headache
tds	three times daily
TED	thromboembolic disease
TEN	toxic epidermal necrolysis
TFT	thyroid function test
TIA	transient ischaemic attack
TOE	trans-oesophageal echocardiography
TOF	time-of-flight (MRI)
TORCH	toxoplasmosis, rubella, cytomegalovirus, and herpes simplex virus
TPMT	thiopurine methyltransferase
TSS	transverse sinus stenosis
TTE	trans-thoracic echocardiography
U&E	urea and electrolytes
UTI	urinary tract infection
VEP	visual evoked potential
VGCC	voltage-gated calcium channel
VGKC	voltage-gated potassium channel
VGKC-Abs	voltage-gated potassium-channel antibodies
VN	vestibular neuritis
VOR	vestibulo-ocular reflex
VPS	ventriculo-peritoneal shunt
VZV	varicella zoster virus
WAISR	Wechsler Adult Intelligence Scale-Revised
WBC	white blood cell
WCC	white cell count
WFNS	World Federation of Neurosurgical Societies

Table 0.1 Curriculum matrix

Book Chapters	1	2	3	4	5	6	7	8	9	10	11	12	13	14	15	16	17	18	19	20	21	22
1. General & Professional Content																						
1.1 History Taking	X	X	X	X	X	X	X	X	X	X	X	X	X	X	X	X	X	X	X	X	X	X
1.2 Neurological Examination	X	X	X	X	X	X	X	X	X	X	X	X	X	X	X	X	X	X	X	X	X	
1.4 Differential Diagnosis, Investigation & Management	X	X	X	X	X	X	X	X	X	X	X	X	X	X	X	X	X	X	X	X	X	X
1.10 Clinical Pharmacology of Neurological Disorders	X	X	X	X	X	X	X	X	X	X	X	X	X	X	X	X	X	X	X	X	X	X
2. Major Topics within Neurology Curriculum																						
2.1 Head Injury																						
2.2 Headache		X			X		X			X		X			X		X					
2.3 Disorders of Consciousness					X												X	X			X	
2.4 Disorders of Sleep					X				X		X									X		
2.5 Disorders of Higher Function &Behaviour			X		X				X			X				X	X	X				
2.6 Epilepsy & Loss of Consciousness					X										X	X	X				X	X
2.7 Cerebrovascular Disease							X			X					X			X				
2.8 Neurological Complications of Systemic Cancer														X			X				X	
2.9 Infections of Nervous System					X																	
2.10 CSF Disorders	X	X			X					X		X					X					
2.11 Demyelination &Vasculitis	X							X				X										
2.13 Parkinsonism & Related Disorders						X										X	X			X		
2.14 Motor Neuron Disease														X								
2.16 Disorders of the Visual System	X	X	X				X		X			X										
2.17 Disorders of the Cranial Nerves	X	X		X			X											X				
2.18 Disorders of the Spine, Spinal Cord, Roots & Spinal Injury	X											X		X					X			
2.19 Disorders of Peripheral Nerve													X	X								
2.20 Disorders of Autonomic Nervous System														X			X			X		
2.21 Disorders of Muscle									X				X	X								
3. Allied Topics within Neurology Curriculum																						
3.1 Clinical Neurophysiology			X		X	X			X		X		X	X	X		X				X	
3.2 Neuroendocrinology									X				X								X	
3.3 Neurogenetics						X			X				X			X						X
3.4 Neurointensive Care							X							X								
3.5 Neuro-otology				X									X									
3.7 Neuropathology												X			X							
3.8 Neuropsychiatry																X				X		
3.9 Neuropsychology			X						X							X						
3.10 Neuroradiology	X	X	X		X		X		X	X		X	X		X	X	X	X	X	X	X	
3.11 Neurorehabilitation	X																		X			
3.12 Neurosurgery		X								X									X			
3.13 Neurourology								X											X	X		

CASE

1 Becoming blind in one eye

Ruth Dobson

Expert commentary Gavin Giovannoni

Case history

A 29-year-old woman presented with a two-day history of visual loss affecting the left eye. This was associated with moderately severe left-sided retro-orbital pain, which was worse on eye movement. She had no significant past medical history, was not on any medication, and denied the consumption of excessive alcohol or illicit drugs. There was no family history of note.

On examination her visual acuity was reduced to counting fingers on the left and 6/6 on the right. Colour vision testing was not possible on the left because of reduced visual acuity, but was normal on the right. She had a somewhat sluggish direct pupillary reflex on the left and a left-sided relative afferent pupillary defect (RAPD). No abnormalities were identified on fundoscopy. Her eye movements were normal, but provoked left-sided retro-orbital pain. There was no diplopia. The remainder of her cranial nerve examination was normal. Neurological examination revealed no abnormality of tone, power, reflexes, or sensation in the upper or lower limbs. Systemic examination was unremarkable.

Investigations at this time included routine blood tests (full blood count, urea and electrolytes, thyroid function, and inflammatory markers), all of which were normal or negative. A gadolinium-enhanced MRI scan of the brain revealed gadolinium enhancement of the left optic nerve in keeping with optic neuritis (Figure 1.1), but no T2 hyperintensities were seen within the brain parenchyma. Given the severity of her visual loss, genetic testing for Leber's hereditary optic neuropathy (LHON) was performed and this was negative for the three most common mutations associated with this disease.

A diagnosis of optic neuritis was made. She was treated with a three-day course of intravenous methylprednisolone at a dose of 1g per day. Her visual function stabilized and her pain settled. Her visual acuity improved to 6/60 on day three. She was advised that her vision would continue to improve without the need for further treatment. On review two months later her visual acuity had improved further to 6/12, and she had a residual RAPD.

Four months later she re-presented with a subacute history of weakness and sensory disturbance affecting her trunk and lower limbs associated with back pain. She reported numbness ascending from her feet to her upper trunk over the two days prior to presentation. She had noticed numbness of her hands and forearms on the day of presentation. On getting out of bed that morning she had also experienced significant leg weakness and had fallen. The fall had prompted her to seek medical attention. She was not aware of any significant arm weakness. She had not passed urine on the day of presentation, and had not opened her bowels for two days. She

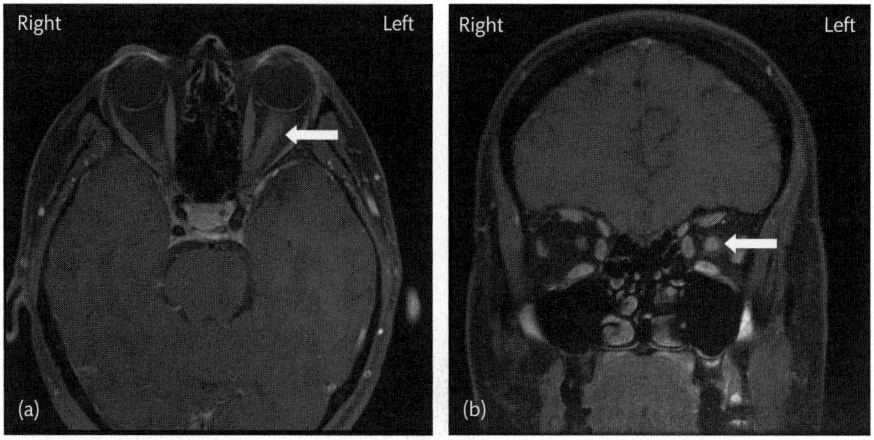

Figure 1.1 (a) Axial T1 fat-saturated image showing gadolinium enhancement in the left optic nerve. (b) Coronal T1 fat-saturated image showing gadolinium enhancement in the left optic nerve.

described some interscapular back pain, and had developed symptoms consistent with Lhermitte's syndrome (paraesthesia radiating down her upper and lower limbs on forward flexion of the neck). She complained of excessive hiccupping, which had woken her on the morning of admission.

On examination she had left optic atrophy consistent with her previous episode of optic neuritis. Cranial nerve examination was otherwise unremarkable. She had increased tone in both lower limbs. Tone was normal in both upper limbs, although she had bilateral pronator drift of her outstretched arms. She had mild bilateral weakness (MRC grade 4) of flexion and extension at the elbow and fingers. She had symmetrical pyramidal weakness of both lower limbs of MRC grade 3 at the hip and knee joints and MRC grade 2 at the ankles and feet. Her reflexes were pathologically brisk in all four limbs, and she had a right crossed adductor reflex. Plantar responses were bilaterally extensor. She had reduced sensation to all modalities in the upper and lower limbs, extending to the shoulders. There was reduced vibration sense to the elbow joint bilaterally in the upper limbs. She was in urinary retention.

Full blood count, urea and electrolytes, and inflammatory markers were unremarkable. Anti-nuclear antibodies were weakly positive, but anti-double-stranded DNA, anti-Ro, anti-La, antiphospholipid, anti-centromere, and anti-Scl-70 antibodies were negative. Anti-aquaporin-4 antibodies (NMO-IgG) were strongly positive. There was a CSF pleocytosis, with 75×10^6 leucocytes/L (80 per cent neutrophils). CSF protein and glucose were normal. There were no oligoclonal bands unique to the CSF.

An MRI showed a longitudinally extensive area of signal change throughout the cervical and thoracic spinal cord, extending into the brainstem (Figure 1.2).

She was treated with three days of methylprednisolone at a dose of 1g/day. Her hiccups were treated with a low dose of haloperidol, with a partial response. However, she continued to deteriorate, and five days following presentation she had power of 2/5 throughout her lower limbs and 3/5 in her upper limbs. Therefore the decision was taken to offer her rescue therapy with plasma exchange (PLEX). She responded well to five cycles of plasmapheresis, with some improvement in upper limb power and resolution of the troublesome hiccups before the end of the course of PLEX.

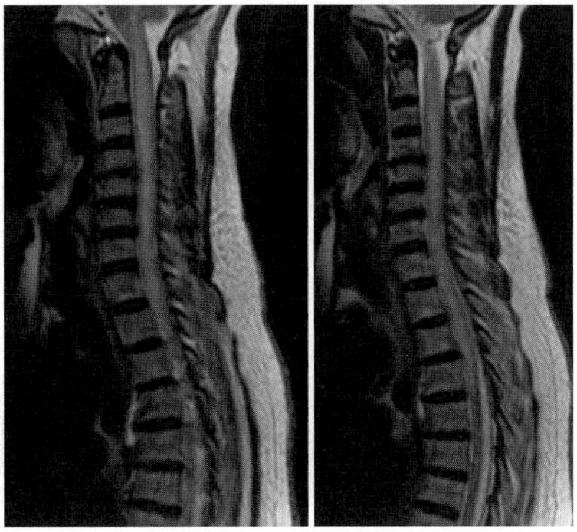

Figure 1.2 Sagittal T2-weighted MRI images of a longitudinally extensive cervical cord lesion.

After completing PLEX the decision was taken for long-term immunotherapy with azathioprine at a target dose of 2.5mg/kg. Her thiopurine methyltransferase (TPMT) level was tested prior to commencing azathioprine. Oral prednisolone was continued whilst the azathioprine dose was titrated to the target dose, and she did not have any further relapses of either transverse myelitis or optic neuritis. The oral prednisolone was then slowly weaned down and stopped.

The patient was discharged to a neurorehabilitation facility for further physical rehabilitation. She had residual visual impairment in the left eye and a spastic paraparesis, such that she required a walking stick to mobilize for distances greater than 20m. She required baclofen to treat painful lower limb spasms, and she developed troublesome sensory symptoms in the lower limbs which responded well to treatment with amitriptyline and gabapentin.

Expert comment

If this patient was tested for anti-aquaporin-4 antibodies at initial presentation and found to be positive, she would probably have been started on an immunomodulatory treatment that may have prevented her from having a further attack. Now that anti-AQP4 antibody assays are widely available, I would advocate routine testing for anti-APQ4 antibodies in patients presenting with recurrent or bilateral optic neuritis, poor recovery from unilateral isolated optic neuritis, longitudinally extensive transverse myelitis (LETM), or unexplained acute brainstem or hypothalamic syndromes with appropriate changes on imaging. Routine screening for anti-APQ4 antibodies, at presentation, in patients presenting with isolated unilateral optic neuritis, with features compatible with multiple-sclerosis-like demyelination on MRI, is not recommended as the vast majority of these cases will be anti-AQP4 seronegative.

Clinical tip Longitudinally extensive transverse myelitis

Longitudinally extensive transverse myelitis (involving three or more vertebral segments) is highly suggestive of NMO. This may extend into the brainstem, causing clinical features such as refractory hiccups, dysarthria, dysphagia, or respiratory compromise. If a patient has transverse myelitis extending in this way, they must be monitored extremely closely for these complications, and supportive treatment, such as NG feeding and/or ITU admission for ventilatory support, offered early.

Clinical tip Severe optic neuritis

The presence of severe optic neuritis, which progresses to near-total or total visual loss suggests an underlying cause such as NMO or Leber's hereditary optic neuropathy (LHON). Although optic neuritis associated with these conditions may improve with corticosteroids, longer-term treatment and prognosis is significantly worse than for idiopathic optic neuritis or optic neuritis associated with multiple sclerosis.

Discussion

Neuromyelitis optica (NMO), or Devic's disease as it is also known, is a clinically defined, severe demyelinating disease affecting the optic nerves and spinal cord. Whilst it was previously thought of as a subtype of multiple sclerosis (so-called optico-spinal MS), the discovery of the anti-aquaporin-4 antibody (NMO-IgG) together with an improved understanding of the underlying pathological processes heralded its classification as a separate entity.

Box 1.1 Revised diagnostic criteria for neuromyelitis optica [4]

Definite NMO:

- Optic neuritis
- **Acute myelitis**
- **At least two of three supporting criteria**
  - Contiguous spinal cord MRI lesion extending over ≥3 vertebral segments
  - **Brain MRI not meeting diagnostic criteria for multiple sclerosis**
  - NMO-IgG seropositive status

Diagnostic criteria for NMO were first suggested in 1999, and revised in 2006 (Box 1.1). Although early descriptions of the disease were of simultaneous (or near-simultaneous) bilateral optic neuritis and/or transverse myelitis, it has now been realized that there are disease relapses in up to 90 per cent of patients, with clinical attacks separated by months or even years. It remains a severe disorder, and within five years of disease onset more than 50 per cent patients are blind in one or both eyes or require ambulatory assistance [1].

NMO is more common in females than in males (ratio 9:1). The age of onset ranges from childhood to adulthood, with the median being 39 years [2]. Unlike multiple sclerosis, the prevalence is higher in Asian populations, where NMO accounts for up to half of all central nervous system (CNS) demyelinating illnesses. However, most people with NMO in the developed world are Caucasian [2].

Clinical features and investigative findings

The cardinal features of NMO are longitudinally extensive transverse myelitis and severe optic neuritis. The transverse myelitis typically spans at least three vertebral segments in a central symmetrical position within the spinal cord, and hence clinical symptoms and signs tend to be symmetrical. Transverse myelitis may extend into the brainstem, with resulting nausea, hiccups, and even dysarthria, dysphagia, or respiratory compromise. Signs suggestive of hypothalamic involvement, such as hypothermia, hypersomnolence, and SIADH have been described, although these are rare (Table 1.1).

Optic neuritis associated with NMO tends to be severe, often resulting in almost complete visual loss during the acute phase. Patients typically complain of progressive visual loss and colour desaturation over a period of a couple of days, associated with retro-orbital pain on eye movement. Optic nerve enhancement typical of optic neuritis may be seen on MRI, and visual evoked potentials (VEPs) show a characteristic increased latency, or even absence, consistent with optic neuritis (see Figure 1.3 and Table 1.2).

Table 1.1 Differential diagnosis of transverse myelitis

Transverse myelitis associated with neuromyelitis optica	• May occur in association with optic neuritis • Longitudinally extensive T2 MRI lesion extending over at least three vertebral segments • Symmetrical signal change on MRI • NMO-IgG seropositive • Prominent CSF pleocytosis (>50×10^6 leukocytes/L), predominantly neutrophils • Oligoclonal band negative (in ~80% cases) • MRI brain does not meet diagnostic criteria for MS (either normal or with lesion distribution typical for NMO: hypothalamic, callosal, periventricular, or brainstem)
Transverse myelitis associated with multiple sclerosis	• Other neurological deficits (optic neuritis, brainstem syndrome, cortical motor or sensory defecits) may also occur • Asymmetrical T2 signal change on MRI rarely exceeding twovertebral segments in length • CSF may show mild pleocytosis (<50×10^6 leukocytes/L), predominantly neutrophils • Unmatched oligoclonal bands in CSF • MRI meets diagnostic criteria for MS
Transverse myelitis associated with systemic autoimmune disease	• May be associated with systemic features of autoimmune disease, such as rash or arthritis, either contemporaneously or patients may report previous symptoms • Serological tests for autoimmune disease may be positive • Other investigations may indicate diagnosis
Anterior spinal artery occlusion	• Abrupt onset • Anterior spinal cord syndrome (paraparesis, loss of pain and temperature sensation with relative preservation of vibration sense and proprioception) • May have vascular risk factors (hypertension, diabetes, smoking) or risk factors for peripheral vascular embolic events • MRI shows thin linear lesion on T2 restricted to the anterior two-thirds of the spinal cord with changes on DWI
Arteriovenous malformation or fistula	• Typically gradually progressive 'stepwise'deterioration • Combined upper and lower motor neuron deficit • MRI shows long, possibly patchy, area of T2 signal change with areas of gadolinium enhancement • Tortuous vessels may be seen on cord surface • Spinal angiography confirms diagnosis
Radiation myelopathy	• Clinical history of radiotherapy with field including spinal cord • Progressive myelopathy with cord atrophy (rarely, there may be a subacute presentation) • MRI shows cord atrophy with T2 signal change;additional change seen in adjacent vertebrae in chronic cases
B12/folate deficiency	• May have clinical history of untreated pernicious anaemia, malnutrition, or gastric/bariatric surgery(rarely, associated with nitric oxide inhalational abuse) • Clinical history of painless weakness with loss of sensation • Low serum B12, macrocytic anaemia, elevated serum homocysteine • MRI spine shows long T2 lesion in dorsal columns and/or corticospinal tracts
Copper deficiency	• History of malnutrition or gastric/bariatric surgery • Low serum copper • MRI spine shows long T2 lesion in dorsal columns and/or corticospinal tracts

Data from *N Engl J Med*, 363(6), Frohman EM, Wingerchuk DM, Clinical practice. Transverse myelitis, pp. 564–72, © 2010, with permission from Massachusetts Medical Society.

Approximately 80 per cent patients with NMO have a relapsing course, as opposed to the monophasic illness initially described. Recovery from attacks is generally poor, and disability secondary to repeated relapses rapidly accumulates. Although the initial disability tends to be more severe in the monophasic subgroup, the relapsing subgroup have a worse prognosis in the long term.

CSF examination typically shows a leucocytosis (often $>50\times10^6$/L), consisting mostly of neutrophils. CSF protein may be raised, and CSF glucose is typically normal. In contrast with multiple sclerosis, intrathecal unmatched oligoclonal bands (IgG unique to the CSF) are not usually present.

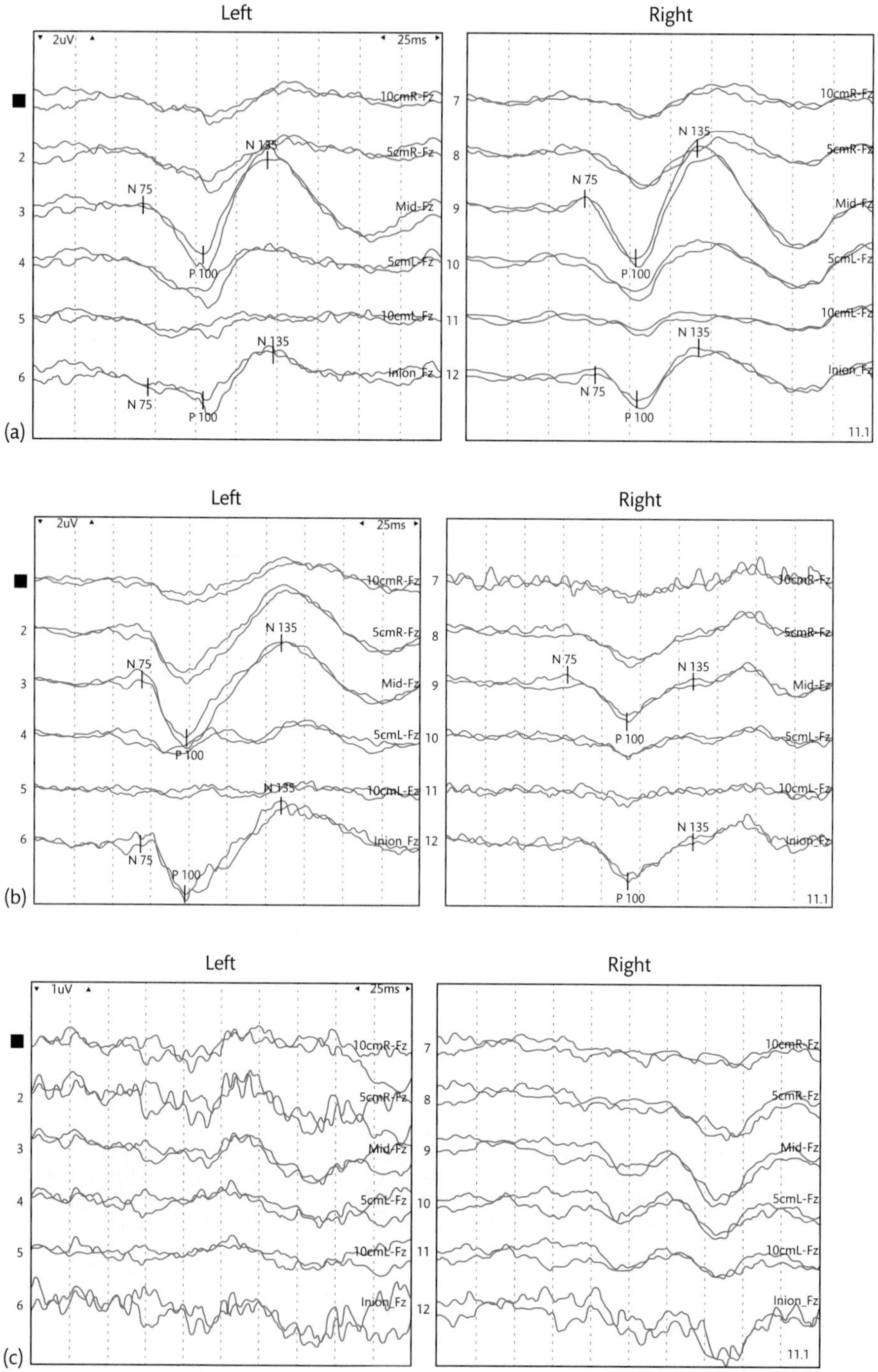

Figure 1.3 Normal, abnormal, and absent visual evoked potentials: (a) normal P100 latencies of 104msec on the right and 105msec on the left; (b) a delayed VEP on the right, with P100 latencies of 116msec on the right and 98.5msec on the left; (c) bilaterally absent VEPs, with no waveform seen. Note that the gain has been increased in this recording.

Images courtesy of Richard Pottinger, Royal London Hospital.

Table 1.2 Differential diagnosis of optic neuropathy

Optic neuritis associated with NMO	• Painful visual loss, with or without papillitis • Often severe • Can be unilateral or bilateral (simultaneous or consecutive) • Associated with transverse myelitis • Good response to intravenous steroid therapy • MRI shows optic nerve enhancement but no other features in keeping with MS
Optic neuritis associated with multiple sclerosis	• Painful visual loss/colour desaturation with or without papillitis • Variable severity • Most commonly unilateral, although other eye may be affected during a later relapse • Associated with other clinical features suggestive of MS • MRI may show optic nerve enhancement in addition to lesions meeting the diagnostic criteria for MS
Leber hereditary optic neuropathy	• Severe, bilateral, and sequential painless visual loss, mainly affecting the central visual field • Males predominantly affected (80–90%) • Mitochondrial DNA mutation; three common mutations implicated in >90% cases with testing commercially available
Optic neuritis associated with other inflammatory disorders	• Variable severity • May be bilateral or relapsing • May have peripheral stigmata of underlying systemic inflammatory disease (SLE, Sjögren's, sarcoidosis, Behçet's) • CRION is a rare idiopathic disorder with severe relapsing optic neuropathy that may progress to blindness
Infectious causes of optic neuropathy	• Tuberculosis • Syphilis • Lyme disease • Viral/para-infections
Toxic/nutritional optic neuropathy	• Nutritional optic neuropathies appear to be exacerbated by tobacco • Toxins implicated in causing optic neuropathy include carbon monoxide, methanol, ethylene glycol, and tobacco • Drugs that have been associated with optic neuropathies include ethambutol, isoniazid, amiodarone, linezolid, methotrexate, sildenafi,l and infliximab
Non-arteritic ischaemic optic neuropathy	• Painless visual loss in older patients, typical age >50 years • Coexistent vascular risk factors (hypertension, diabetes, smoking, hypercholesterolaemia) • Fundoscopy often normal
Arteritic ischaemic optic neuropathy	• Painless visual loss, typical age >70 years • Papillitis on fundoscopy • Patients may have a clinical history in keeping with polymyalgia rheumatica or temporal arteritis • Immediate high-dose corticosteroids may prevent further visual loss

Expert comment

It is important to note that this patient did not have local synthesis of oligoclonal IgG antibodies in their CSF, which is typical of NMO but is rarely found in association with optic neuritis compatible with demyelination (CIS) or MS. If this patient had had a lumbar puncture as part of her work-up for the initial episode of optic neuritis the lack of oligoclonal bands (OCBs) might have prompted anti-APQ4 antibody testing and hence the early initiation of long-term immunosuppressive therapy. I cannot stress enough how valuable the negative predictive value of CSF analysis is in patients presenting with clinically isolated syndromes (CISs) associated with MS; lack of OCBs should always prompt you to think of alternative diagnoses.

Since the discovery of NMO-IgG or anti-AQP4 antibodies the clinical phenotypes associated with these antibodies has spread. NMO-IgG or anti-AQP4 positivity, but not necessarily fulfilling diagnostic criteria for NMO, includes bilateral and/or recurrent optic neuritis, chronic relapsing inflammatory optic neuropathy (CRION), relapsing LETM, and acute brainstem and hypothalamic syndromes associated with abnormal imaging. NMO-IgG/anti-AQP4 seropositivity is also associated with other systemic autoimmune diseases, most notably Sjögren's syndrome, systemic lupus erythematosus (SLE), and myasthenia gravis. Optic neuritis and transverse myelitis occurring in association with these disorders is usually associated with anti-AQP4 seropositivity.

Over a third of patients with NMO either have symptoms consistent with a separate autoimmune disorder, or have other circulating antibodies in addition to the anti-aquaporin-4 antibody. The most frequent coexisting disorders are SLE, myasthenia gravis, Sjögren's syndrome, and thyroid autoimmunity. It must be noted that both SLE and Sjögren's syndrome can themselves cause transverse myelitis and optic neuritis, so care must be exercised when diagnosing NMO in patients with these pre-existing conditions.

MRI findings

As stated above, LETM is a hallmark of NMO, forming part of the diagnostic criteria. In contrast, MRI of the brain is typically normal at disease onset (apart from optic nerve enhancement during acute optic neuritis). If T2-weighted hyperintensities are present, they tend to be non-specific in appearance, and not consistent with a diagnosis of multiple sclerosis.

However, over time, up to 60 per cent of sufferers develop clinically silent lesions seen on T2-weighted MRI scans [2]. Approximately 10 per cent of patients develop lesions that meet the diagnostic criteria for multiple sclerosis. Typical sites for lesions in NMO include periventricular areas, the hypothalamus, and the periaqueductal brainstem. It is thought that this lesion distribution reflects areas that are particularly enriched with aquaporin-4 in the brain.

> **Learning point** Anti-aquaporin 4 antibodies
>
> The discovery of the anti-aquaporin-4 antibody extended the clinical phenotype of NMO considerably. It now forms part of the diagnostic criteria, and is present in 75–90 per cent of patients. The AQP4 water channel is seen throughout the CNS, but is most abundant in the optic nerves and spinal cord, thus accounting for the clinical phenotype seen in NMO. Although antibody pathogenicity has not been conclusively proven, the circumstantial evidence is overwhelming.

Aquaporin-4 antibody and immunopathology

The anti-aquaporin-4 antibody is present in 75–90 per cent patients with NMO. This antibody, which binds to the aquaporin-4 (AQP4) water channel, is thought to be pathogenic, although direct evidence for pathogenicity is lacking. AQP4 is a cell-membrane-based water channel, which is constitutively expressed in the principal collecting ducts of the kidney and the brain, where it is the most abundant water channel in the CNS. Whilst the anti-AQP4 antibody binds avidly to the distal collecting tubules in the kidney, renal function is typically normal in NMO. This is thought to reflect the relatively minor contribution of AQP4 to water homeostasis in the nephron [1].

Within the CNS AQP4 channels are most abundant in the optic nerves and spinal cord [2], thus providing circumstantial but convincing evidence linking the anti-AQP4 antibody to NMO. Furthermore, the titre of anti-AQP4 is seen to rise in the context of NMO relapses. However, cases of NMO patients who meet the clinical criteria for diagnosis, yet are seronegative for the anti-AQP4 antibody, do exist [3]. Given the rarity of this condition, it is not clear whether the clinical picture in this group differs significantly from those with seropositive NMO.

> **Learning point** Histology of neuromyelitis optica
>
> One important difference between NMO and MS is the histological appearance of lesions. In NMO there is perivascular IgG deposition with associated complement activation, loss of the AQP4 water channel, and necrosis with eosinophils and neutrophils. In MS, perivascular inflammation can also be seen, with infiltration of lymphocytes, activated macrophages, and microglia. In MS lesions there is prominent demyelination, with macrophages containing myelindebris seen in acute lesions.

Within CNS lesions there is loss of the AQP4 receptor and immune complex deposition around blood vessels. There is extensive demyelination and necrosis, with eosinophils and neutrophils in the inflammatory infiltrate [2].

Treatment

High-dose intravenous corticosteroid therapy is the first-line treatment for an acute attack of NMO. The majority of patients respond to this; however, plasma exchange and/or cyclophosphamide have been used in those patients who have severe disease (either sight-threatening optic neuritis or cervical myelitis with a risk of neurogenic respiratory compromise) and who are refractory to steroids.

Expert comment

Once the diagnosis was made the patient was appropriately treated. However, for acute attacks, the more severe cases of NMO may require plasma exchange to hasten recovery. Unfortunately, clinical trials have yet to be performed to establish the most appropriate treatment to prevent relapses in NMO and seropositive anti-AQP4 related disorders. However, several case series support the use of long-term immunosuppressive therapy. I currently favour induction therapy with corticosteroids followed by maintenance therapy with azathioprine or mycophenolate mofetil.

Rituximab (anti-CD20) therapy has emerged as an (off-license) alternative because of its relative ease of use and dosing schedule. In my personal experience rituximab needs to be combined with a therapy that targets T cells (e.g. azathioprine, mycophenolate, or ciclosporin). I have observed several severe relapses in patients with NMO treated on rituximab monotherapy. Finally, several case reports have recently been published showing some benefit of tocilizumab which interrupts interleukin-6 (IL-6) signalling by targeting the IL-6 receptor.

In the longer term, maintenance (steroid-sparing) therapy is recommended. To date, no large-scale randomized control trials have been performed in NMO. There is no evidence to support the use of interferon-beta as a disease-modifying therapy in NMO, and some have suggested that it may cause clinical deterioration [3]. Instead, azathioprine (at a dose of 2.5mg/kg/day) is commonly used, with methotrexate as an alternative. Thiopurine methyltransferase (TPMT) levels should be checked prior to starting azathioprine because of the risk of bone marrow suppression in people with certain TPMT gene polymorphisms. Patients usually require steroid cover whilst immunosuppressive therapy is being titrated up [3].

Given that NMO is presumed to be an antibody-mediated disease, trials have been performed using the anti-CD20 monoclonal antibody rituximab. However, to date these have been small and often open-label trials, at least in part due to the infrequency and severity of the illness. Other immunosuppressive agents, such as ciclosporin and mycophenolate, may be used in refractory cases, and whether there is a place in therapy for newer anti-CD20 monoclonal antibodies, such as ocrelizumab and ofatumumab, remains to be seen.

Final word from the expert

Following the discovery of the anti-AQP4 antibody, the clinical spectrum of NMO has expanded from a monophasic illness to a severe relapsing demyelinating disease. It is now recognized as a distinct entity from multiple sclerosis.

I would like to reiterate the comment above that interferon-beta therapy has no role to play in treating anti-AQP4-related disorders; several case studies suggest that it has the potential to exacerbate NMO. Unfortunately, there is no evidence at present to help one decide how long to continue with immunosuppressive or immunomodulatory therapy. Hopefully, evidence will emerge from the long-term follow-up of well-defined cohorts of patients to indicate whether or not NMO-anti-APQ4 seroreversion can be used as a guide to withdrawing immunosuppressive therapy.

References

1. Mata S, Lolli F. Neuromyelitis optica: an update. *J Neurol Sci* 2011;303(1–2): 13–21.
2. Wingerchuk DM, Lennon VA, Lucchinetti CF, et al. The spectrum of neuromyelitis optica. *Lancet Neurol* 2007; 6(9): 805–15.
3. Matthews LA, Baig F, Palace J, Turner MR. The borderland of neuromyelitis optica. *Pract Neurol* 2009; **9**(6): 335–40.
4. Wingerchuk DM, Lennon VA, Pittock SJ,Lucchinetti CF, Weinshenker BG. Revised diagnostic criteria for neuromyelitis optica. *Neurology* 2006; 66(10): 1485–9.
5. Frohman EM, Wingerchuk DM. Clinical practice. Transverse myelitis. *N Engl J Med* 2010; 363(6): 564–72.

CASE

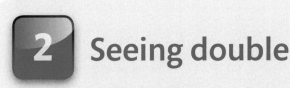

2 Seeing double

Anish N. Shah

Expert commentary Paul Riordan-Eva

Case history

A 27-year-old woman presented to her optician having woken that morning with horizontal double vision. Visual acuity was normal at 6/5 in each eye. There was reduced abduction of the right eye. The optic discs were thought to be swollen and immediate attendance at the local hospital's emergency department was recommended.

At the hospital the patient also gave a history of a few weeks of noticing her vision 'greying out' for a few seconds whenever she bent forwards. She admitted to a three-month history of frontal headaches, worsened by coughing, for which she had been taking increasing quantities of over-the-counter analgesia. She was sometimes nauseated, but denied any vomiting or pulsatile tinnitus. She reported no previous ocular history. Two weeks previously, she had developed a right external ear infection (otitis externa) that was resolving following microsuction in the ENT clinic and treatment with antibiotic drops. She had not experienced any hearing impairment or balance problems and she no longer had any discharge from the ear.

Learning point Neuroimaging in suspected raised intracranial pressure

In the emergency department, the finding of optic disc swelling (papilloedema) usually leads to an urgent unenhanced CT head scan, but this cannot exclude many causes of raised intracranial pressure (ICP), including cerebral venous sinus thrombosis (CVST), meningeal disease, and some neoplasms.

Both CT venography (CTV) and MR venography (MRV) can detect CVST, but CTV provides better assessment of the bony canal in which the transverse sinuses lie thus making it easier to identify congenital anomalies [1].

Contrast-enhanced CT can identify meningeal disease and many neoplasms, but contrast-enhanced MRI is the definitive investigation.

MRI or CT even with contrast enhancement cannot exclude raised ICP. (Dilatation of the cerebral ventricles is a feature of hydrocephalus but its absence does not mean that intracranial pressure is normal.)

Imaging features indicative of raised ICP are an empty sella, dilatation of the optic nerve sheaths, and prominence of the optic nerve heads. Hence the traditional concept that imaging is normal in idiopathic intracranial hypertension (IIH) is incorrect.

Prior to lumbar puncture cerebellar tonsillar ectopia needs to be excluded.

Clinical tip Ear infections and raised ICP

Otitis externa is not associated with intracranial complications, except for the rare necrotizing or malignant form.

Otitis media rarely leads to intracranial complications such as cerebral abscess or transverse sinus thrombosis, which results in the syndrome of **otitic hydrocephalus** (headache, papilloedema, sixth nerve paresis, and otorrhoea) originally described in 1931 in children with acute suppurative otitis media by the British neurologist Sir Charles Symonds. The availability of antibiotics made it a rare entity, but in recent years several cases have been reported in both older patients and those with chronic otitis media and/or mastoiditis without obvious suppuration.

In **Gradenigo syndrome**, direct spread of middle ear infection to the petrous apex causes deep facial pain and an ipsilateral sixth nerve paresis in the setting of a discharging ear.

Any ear symptom in the context of possible raised ICP mandates thorough otologic examination.

Six months earlier the patient had started the combined oral contraceptive pill with subsequent weight gain. She was not taking any other medications. She drank alcohol occasionally and was a non-smoker.

Vital signs, including temperature, were within normal limits. Body mass index was elevated (32kg/m^2). The admitting doctor and a neurologist identified a right sixth cranial nerve palsy and confirmed bilateral optic disc swelling. No other neurological abnormalities were identified. An urgent unenhanced computed tomography (CT) head scan was normal.

The patient was admitted for further investigation of presumed raised intracranial pressure. Lumbar puncture (LP) on the ward was unsuccessful and thus was repeated under fluoroscopic (X-ray) guidance. The CSF opening pressure was elevated (36cmH_2O in the relaxed lateral decubitus position) and a total of 15ml of CSF was removed. CSF constituents were normal. Magnetic resonance imaging (MRI) of the head was normal and a CT venogram (CTV) showed no cerebral venous sinus thrombosis (CVST). A diagnosis of idiopathic intracranial hypertension (IIH) was made. Oral acetazolamide 250mg bd was started and weight loss was recommended.

The patient was referred for ophthalmological assessment. Visual acuity was normal (6/5) in each eye. Colour vision was normal, with all Ishihara colour plates rapidly and correctly identified with each eye. There was no relative afferent pupillary defect (RAPD). Visual field examination by Goldmann kinetic perimetry revealed bilateral enlarged blind spots and generalized constriction of the visual fields, which was worse in the left eye (Figure 2.1).

Expert comment Visual parameters in IIH

In IIH visual acuity and colour vision are regularly measured, but are usually normal until there is severe optic nerve dysfunction (assuming that there are no other causes of reduced visual acuity). A clinically detectable RAPD is only present if there is markedly asymmetric optic nerve dysfunction, which is unusual in IIH. Visual field testing is a much better measure of optic nerve dysfunction in IIH.

Clinical tip Colour vision testing

Acquired colour vision deficit is a characteristic sign of optic neuropathy but it manifests at different stages, being an early sign in compressive or inflammatory optic neuropathy but a late sign in optic nerve dysfunction due to papilloedema or glaucoma.

1. Red desaturation/comparison
   - A sensitive easily performed test for reduced colour vision is assessment and comparison of the intensity of colour of a red object viewed with each eye in turn.
2. Pseudo-isochromatic plates
   - **Ishihara colour plates** were designed to identify congenital colour vision deficit, particularly in the red–green axis. Nevertheless, they are commonly used to detect acquired deficit. The first plate (number 12) is a test plate, which even colour-blind individuals are

(Continued)

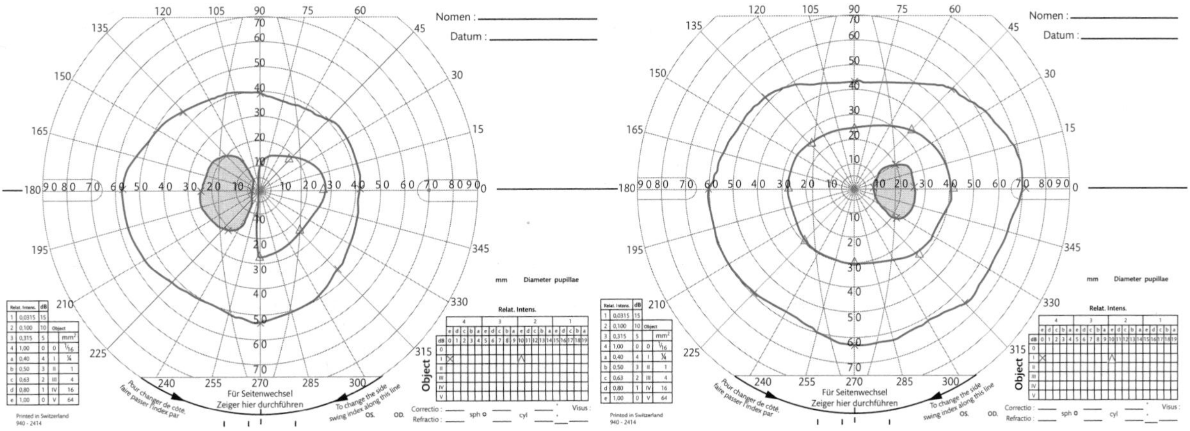

Figure 2.1 Goldmann kinetic perimetry (visual field testing) plots showing enlarged blind spots and generalized constriction worse in the left eye. The solid and dotted lines are the isoptres (lines connecting points of equal sensitivity) for the I4e and less bright I2e stimuli, respectively.

able to identify correctly. It may not be identified correctly in severe visual loss (visual acuity less than 6/60), simultanagnosia, or functional visual loss, in which case the rest of the test is invalidated.

- **Hardy-Rand-Rittler plates** are probably more sensitive than Ishihara plates but are infrequently used in the UK.

3. Colour arrangement tests
   - **Farnsworth-Munsell 100 hue test**—a thorough but very time-consuming arrangement of 85 coloured caps in order.
   - **Farnsworth D-15 test**—a reduced version with 15 coloured caps.
   - **Lanthony desaturated D-15 test**—a more sensitive reduced version with less saturated colours.

A cover test revealed a right esotropia (manifest convergent squint) with reduced abduction of the right eye, and to aid monitoring this was quantified by plotting a Hess chart (Figure 2.2).

Learning point Strabismus in IIH

There are three reasons why a patient with IIH might develop ocular motility deficits.

1. **Sixth nerve palsy**
   - A common false localizing sign of intracranial hypertension (very rarely fourth and seventh nerve palsies occur, but investigation to exclude other causes is required)
   - Following LP
2. **Sensory strabismus**—most normal individuals have a latent ocular misalignment (**heterophoria**) that is not manifest because the brain maintains ocular alignment to avoid diplopia and the superimposition of dissimilar visual images (visual confusion). If one eye becomes poorly-sighted the latent squint can become manifest (**heterotropia**), usually as a divergence of that eye.
3. **After optic nerve sheath fenestration**, temporarily or permanently, which usually requires detachment of the medial rectus muscle from the globe to provide access to the optic nerve sheath.

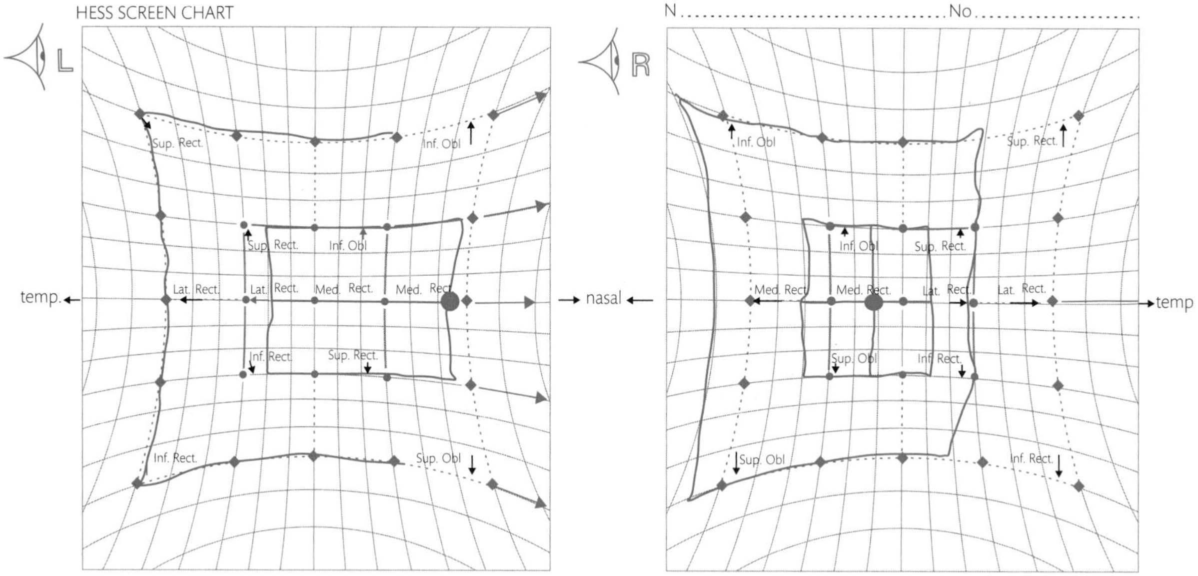

Figure 2.2 Hess chart plots showed that the left and right central spots (filled black circles) are closer together than normal, which indicates convergent ocular deviation. In the right eye, there is also an abnormally short distance from the central spot to the lateral side of the outer square (the black line shows the patient's response; the dotted line is the normal response). This suggests under-action of the right lateral rectus muscle. There is also compensatory over-action of the medial rectus of the left eye (shown by the arrows).

Hess charts are plotted by orthoptists and require the equipment of an eye clinic. They allow quantification and monitoring of ocular motility deficits and thus are useful in monitoring patients with third, fourth, or sixth cranial nerve palsies. They also aid differentiation between neurological and restrictive (orbital) abnormalities. They only show movements of one eye compared with the other and are not an indicator of actual range of movement. Hess chart and Lees screen examinations provide the same information.

Anterior segment ocular examination was normal. Fundal examination following pupil dilation revealed bilateral swollen optic discs (Figure 2.3) with normal retinas and retinal vasculature.

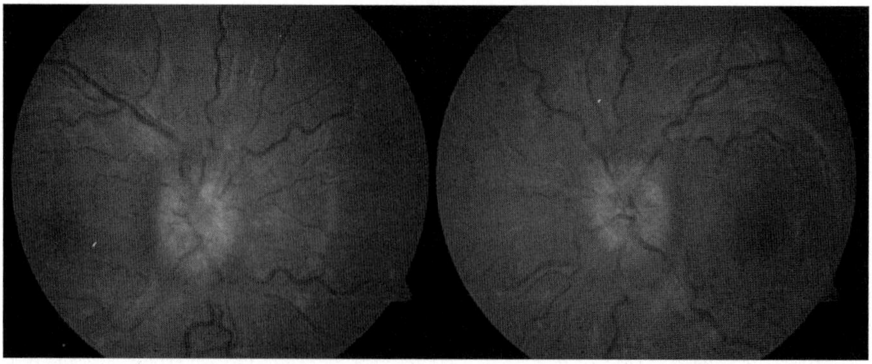

Figure 2.3 Fundus photographs showing bilateral optic disc swelling. Please see colour plate section.

Learning point Optic disc oedema

As the axons of the 1.2 million retinal ganglion cells course into the optic disc they form the **neuroretinal rim (NRR)** around the central physiological 'cup'. Oedema of the NRR ('optic disc swelling') causes elevation of the surface of the disc. This may be apparent only on stereoscopic examination using a slit lamp, but on direct ophthalmoscopy in marked cases there is a clear difference in the lens settings required to focus on the optic disc and retina. 'Greying out' of vision for several seconds, often in association with postural changes (transient visual obscuration), is a characteristic symptom of optic disc oedema.

With a direct ophthalmoscope, also look for:

- blurred ('indistinct') disc margin
- absence of or preferably, because it is absent in 10–20 per cent of normal patients, disappearance of previously documented spontaneous venous pulsation (SVP)
- peripapillary haemorrhages or cotton-wool spots (signs of acute change)
- obscuration (by the swelling of the NRR) of the retinal vessels as they leave the disc
- dilatation (hyperaemia) of capillaries on the surface of the disc (best seen with the green (red-free) light)
- whitish sheathing of the retinal vessels as they leave the disc (sign of previous swelling).

The first two are classic 'textbook' features, but the next three are more reliable, and the last is uncommon.

Papilloedema

There are many causes of optic disc oedema. The term 'papilloedema' should be reserved for optic disc oedema due to raised ICP.

Optic disc elevation

The main causes of elevated discs with blurred margins which may be mistaken for optic disc oedema are as follows.

- Congenitally 'full' or 'crowded' discs, characterized by small size with no physiological cup and often associated with hypermetropia (long-sightedness)—sometimes referred to as 'pseudo-papilloedema'.
- Optic disc drusen are calcified accretions that are not visible initially ('buried') but cause an elevation of the optic disc surface and then gradually become visible with time ('exposed') to produce a 'lumpy' appearance of the surface of the optic disc. (They should not be confused with the much more common retinal drusen that occur in age-related macular disease.)
- Myelinated retinal nerve fibres.

Investigations relevant to assessment of optic disc swelling

- **Fundus fluorescein angiography (FFA)** involves serial fundus photography after intravenous injection of sodium fluorescein (a fluorescent dye). In optic disc oedema the dye initially accentuates the capillary dilatation on the surface of the disc and then leaks out of the disc to produce marked hyperfluorescence in later images.
- **Fundus autofluorescence (FAF)** is similar to FFA but without injection of fluorescein. Exposed optic disc drusen exhibit autofluorescence.
- **Optical coherence tomography (OCT)** measures retinal nerve fibre layer (RNFL) thickness and thus can be used to monitor the severity of optic disc oedema. However, reduction of RNFL thickness can be due to atrophy as well as resolution of oedema, so clinical correlation is essential.
- **B-mode ultrasound ('B-scan')** of an eye with optic disc drusen usually shows them as highly reflective bodies at the optic nerve head.
- **CT scan** of the orbits may also demonstrate disc drusen as highly attenuating lesions at the optic nerve head but it is rarely performed solely for this purpose.

In the few weeks following LP the patient reported resolution of headaches and diplopia, and repeat visual fields demonstrated improvement (Figure 2.4).

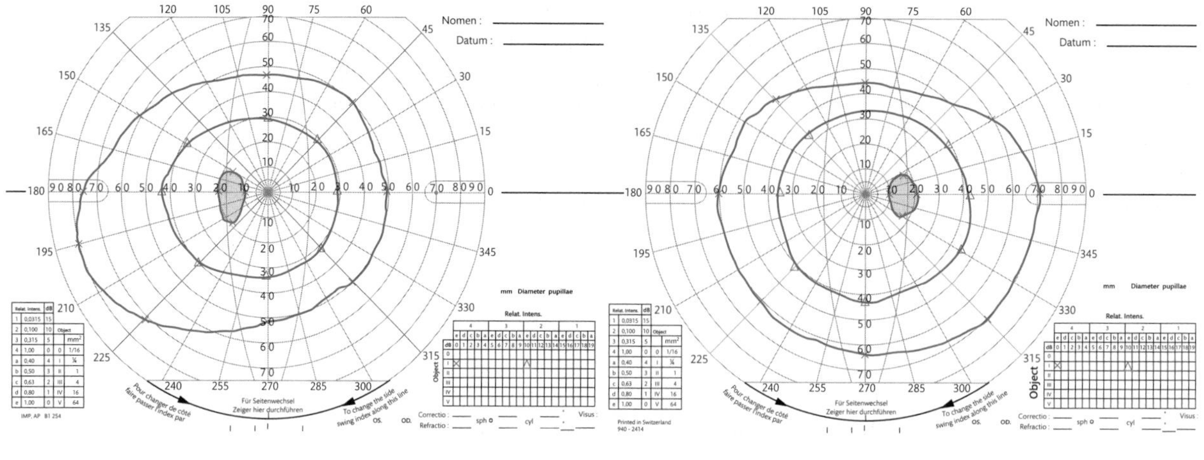

Figure 2.4 Repeat Goldmann perimetry shows a reduction in the size of the blind spots and expansion of the same isoptres as shown in Figure 2.3.

Clinical tip Visual field testing

Visual fields are displayed from the patient's point of view.

In **kinetic perimetry** a stimulus is moved, generally centripetally, along multiple meridians with the subject responding when it is seen such that the boundary of equal sensitivity in the visual field (**isoptre**) is determined. Confrontation visual field testing is an example of kinetic perimetry. The most commonly used kinetic perimeter is the Goldmann, which provides white light stimuli of standardized size and brightness. It is operated manually, usually by an orthoptist. It can be used as a static perimeter by turning the stimulus on momentarily at different points in the visual field. Automated kinetic perimeters are available but are not yet commonly used.

In **automated static perimetry** light stimuli of the same size but varying brightness are presented in the visual field to determine the threshold brightness (at which the stimulus is seen by the subject 50 per cent of the time) at multiple set points. The automation also allows the reliability of the subject's responses to be tested. Common automated perimeters are the Humphrey and Octopus machines. The commonly used Humphrey programme is the 24-2 which tests the central 24° of the visual field.

Automated static perimetry is less labour-intensive and often more sensitive than Goldmann perimetry, but it is difficult to perform well and thus may give spurious results, especially in subjects who are unwell. Both are used in the management of IIH.

Learning point Diagnosing idiopathic intracranial hypertension

1. If symptoms present, they may only reflect those of generalized intracranial hypertension or papilloedema.
2. If signs present, they may only reflect those of generalized intracranial hypertension or papilloedema.
3. Elevated intracranial pressure measured in the lateral decubitus position with the patient relaxed.
4. Normal CSF composition.
5. No evidence of hydrocephalus, mass, structural, or vascular lesion on MRI or contrast-enhanced CT for typical patients, and on MRI and MR venography for all others.
6. No other cause of intracranial hypertension identified.

Over the next few months her headaches and visual obscurations recurred and did not respond to either higher-dose acetazolamide (500mg bd) or oral topiramate (up to 50mg bd). The patient had not been able to lose weight. Acetazolamide 1g bd was restarted in place of topiramate. Upon repeat LP, the CSF opening pressure was elevated at 32cmH_2O and CSF was again drained with improvement in the patient's symptoms. She mentioned that she was planning to stop the oral contraceptive pill as she wished to have a baby. It was explained that stopping the pill might assist with weight loss. Several issues relating to the management of IIH during pregnancy were discussed.

During further follow-up, visual function was stable but the headaches became more troublesome. CSF shunting was discussed but declined.

Discussion

This case illustrates the importance of eliciting specific features in the history of patients with raised ICP, including the chronology of weight gain and any CVST risk factors (e.g. oral contraception or middle ear infections) in relation to the onset of symptoms. Her medication–refractory disease and refusal to consider CSF shunting in the context of possible imminent pregnancy raise several issues regarding her management.

Learning point Considerations in IIH

1. **Medication-induced intracranial hypertension** Several medications are known to cause intracranial hypertension particularly tetracyclines, such as for acne rosacea or malaria prophylaxis, and vitamin A or related agents, such as retinoids for acne, retinoic acid for leukaemia, and over-the-counter vitamin supplements. It may be unclear whether the medication is fully or only partly responsible, but its withdrawal is an important part of treatment.
2. **Fulminant IIH** IIH may cause rapidly progressive severe bilateral visual loss for which urgent surgery is likely to be required
3. **Acephalgic IIH** IIH can be associated with little or no headache [3] leading to late presentation with severe bilateral visual loss.
4. **Chiari malformation** There is an increased prevalence of cerebellar tonsillar ectopia in IIH [4–8]. It is unclear whether it is causative, secondary, or coincidental (Chiari 1 malformation), but it is a relative contraindication to LP and to lumboperitoneal shunt.
5. **Jugular vein obstruction** Intracranial hypertension, with clinical and imaging features mimicking IIH, can be caused by internal jugular vein obstruction due to thrombosis (e.g. from central venous catheterization) or skull base, neck, or mediastinal tumours or surgery.
6. **Diffuse glioma** Diffuse cerebral glioma may present as pseudotumour cerebri but should be identified by MRI.

Although many hypotheses have been proposed, there is no accepted aetiological theory for IIH, including the preponderance of obese women of child-bearing age, who account for up to 90 per cent of patients [15]. In one series of over 400 patients with IIH, 80 per cent of patients had a BMI above 30kg/m^2, and patients with a BMI above 40kg/m^2 were more likely to have severe papilloedema than those with lower BMI [16].

The choice of terminology for patients being investigated for raised ICP is important. In particular, premature labelling of the condition as IIH should be avoided. Intracranial hypertension can be labelled idiopathic (IIH) if no specific cause is identified, but when investigations cannot be completed (e.g. if LP is contraindicated), it may be better to diagnose 'unexplained intracranial hypertension' or to use the older term pseudotumour cerebri (PTC) which carries no aetiological implication.

Expert comment

IIH patients frequently also suffer from other types of headache which are not necessarily related to raised ICP, including tension headache and migraine [2]. Careful history-taking may help to distinguish a relapse of IIH symptoms from the onset of a new and different headache disorder.

It has been suggested that PTC is retained for intracranial hypertension not due to hydrocephalus or mass lesion and for which a cause has been established or BMI is not elevated, so that IIH is reserved for unexplained intracranial hypertension associated with elevated BMI but without obstructive sleep apnoea (OSA) [15]. This emphasizes the need for a continuing search for an underlying cause in atypical cases, such as non-obese men, but fails to encompass IIH in non-obese patients [17]. Conversely, the labelling of intracranial hypertension due to CVST or medications as IIH has been reiterated [18]. Given these conflicting viewpoints, any identified underlying cause (whether wholly or partly responsible) such as CVST, medications, or OSA should be clearly stated, and PTC or 'unexplained intracranial hypertension' should be used except when IIH can be diagnosed confidently, i.e. after suitably extensive investigations have excluded an underlying cause.

Final word from the expert

Although IIH seems to be a specific disease entity, diagnosis largely depends on the absence and not presence of features. It needs to be kept in mind constantly that, although there is a strong association with obese adult females, IIH is a diagnosis of exclusion and must be preceded by a careful search for other causes of raised ICP.

Several attempts have been made to establish diagnostic criteria for IIH [19–22]. The emphasis is on ensuring that no other cause for raised ICP is identifiable; that CSF constituents are normal; and that symptoms, signs, and imaging abnormalities are fully explained by raised ICP. A difficulty is that the required extent of investigations is determined by the clinical circumstances. For instance, more extensive investigation is required in a non-obese young adult male than in an obese young adult female [21]. It is now generally accepted that either CT or MR venography is required in all cases (even if the presentation is typical) to exclude CVST [23–27].

Cerebral venous sinus stenosis rather than thrombosis, usually transverse sinus stenosis (TSS), has been implicated as a causative factor in IIH but may be a secondary phenomenon, coincidental, or in a few cases a consequence of thrombosis [1, 28–32]. At present cerebral venous sinus stenosis is not considered to be a reason to refute a diagnosis of IIH unless it is thought to be due to CVST.

Significant weight loss can markedly improve symptoms and signs, but subsequent weight gain can cause relapse. A prospective study showed that a three-month low-energy diet can reduce weight, ICP, headache, and papilloedema—benefits which remained three months after cessation of the low-energy diet [33].

Medical management of IIH usually begins with acetazolamide, a carbonic anhydrase inhibitor which reduces CSF production [34]. The usual dose is 250–500mg bd, but up to 1g bd may be necessary. Second-line agents include other diuretics such as bendrofluazide and furosemide. Topiramate (usually 25–50mg bd but up to 100mg bd) is a weak carbonic anhydrase inhibitor. It is effective for chronic headache, especially migraine, and has the additional benefit of suppressing appetite. In one randomized study of IIH it was as effective as acetazolamide and associated with significant weight loss [35]. Corticosteroids promote weight gain and are generally avoided, although in high doses they may have a temporizing role in managing patients with rapidly progressive visual loss ('fulminant IIH') [36].

Traditionally IIH has been treated by repeated LP but the reduction in ICP after LP usually lasts only a few days. Rarely, symptomatic relief after LP can last much longer, possibly by breaking the cycle of raised ICP causing TSS which in turn increases ICP [37]. Thus repeated LPs are usually only useful when CSF shunt surgery is indicated but has to be delayed for some reason, or when the options for medical and surgical treatment are limited, such as during pregnancy.

The main indications for surgery are progressive visual loss or headache which are uncontrolled by medical treatment, or intolerance of medical treatment. The choice of surgery is guided by symptoms. CSF diversion procedures have a role when there is rapidly progressive bilateral visual loss, when ICP is markedly elevated, or when headache is a predominant problem. Optic nerve sheath fenestration (ONSF) is favoured when the predominant problem is visual loss with little or no headache, particularly if the visual loss is unilateral. ONSF is not thought to have more than a temporary effect on ICP. However, some investigators have found unilateral ONSF to ameliorate papilloedema and visual field defects in both eyes, often obviating the need for surgery on the second optic nerve [38]. There are no prospective randomized studies comparing the outcome of CSF diversion surgery and ONSF.

CSF diversion procedures include lumbo-peritoneal shunt (LPS) and ventriculo-peritoneal shunt (VPS). There are no prospective randomized trials comparing them. Several retrospective series have demonstrated their ability to reduce papilloedema, preserve vision, and improve headaches. However, the principal complications of low-pressure headache, shunt obstruction, migration, or infection, and acquired cerebellar tonsillar ectopia after LPS remain relatively prevalent, with over half of patients requiring shunt revision and a third needing multiple revisions [39]. There is some evidence that fewer revisions are required for VPS than for LPS [40], but in-hospital mortality is over four times more likely with VPS [41]. Recent developments in shunt surgery include antibiotic-impregnated shunts to reduce infection rates [42], programmable valves to control CSF egress [43], and stereotactic guidance to improve VPS placement [44].

For ONSF, a medial or lateral approach with manoeuvres to aid exposure of the optic nerve (eg. temporary detachment of medial rectus, or removal of bone from the lateral orbital rim) or a supero-medial approach can be used. An initial incision in the nerve sheath should be accompanied by egress of CSF, and a window of dura and arachnoid is then excised [45]. An endoscopic ONSF method using free electron lasers has been developed [46–49] but has not found its way into routine practice. Complications of ONSF include visual loss from iatrogenic optic nerve damage [50], progressive optic neuropathy despite surgery [51], retinal vascular occlusions [52] or choroidal infarction [53], and damage to orbital structures causing pupil dysfunction [52] and ocular motor nerve paresis [54]. There have been no prospective randomized trials of the efficacy of ONSF, but many retrospective reviews have found the procedure to be effective in improving or stabilizing papilloedema, visual acuity, and visual field in IIH [38, 55–58]. Some surgeons have attempted to prevent late scarring of the incised dural window by applying mitomycin C to the nerve sheath prior to incision, which it is claimed may also reduce orbital scarring and adhesions [59].

Unilateral or bilateral TSS, but not thrombosis, is a common imaging finding in IIH, some groups finding it in the majority of IIH patients [60] and a number of studies identifying an associated pressure gradient along the transverse sinus. Resolution of the TSS and the pressure gradient after reduction of ICP by drainage of CSF [61–64] or LPS insertion [65] has been reported. Several studies have reported resolution of symptoms and signs in IIH after endovascular stenting of the stenotic transverse sinus [30]. A recent review of 143 patients undergoing venous sinus stenting found that most patients experienced improvement in headache, visual symptoms, papilloedema, and tinnitus [32]. As yet, this treatment is not being performed routinely in the UK.

The efficacy of weight loss in symptom resolution, coupled with its other medical benefits, has led to bariatric surgery being performed for IIH. Although a review only found weak evidence for benefit [66], over 90 per cent of operated patients experienced resolution of papilloedema and improvement of visual field deficits. It is unknown how long these benefits last post-operatively and whether they are dependent on weight maintenance.

Since most IIH patients are young females of child-bearing age, the need to manage IIH in pregnancy is common and requires special considerations.

Learning point IIH and pregnancy

Pregnancy occurs in IIH patients at a similar rate to the general population. IIH can first present during pregnancy or in any trimester. Since IIH can be exacerbated by pregnancy, close monitoring is required.

1. **Contraception** Oral contraceptive pill (OCP) users are at higher risk of CVST and this must be excluded before IIH is diagnosed. Topiramate accelerates oestrogen and progestogen metabolism, thereby reducing the efficacy of contraceptives. Oestrogens reduce the diuretic effect of diuretics.
2. **Medication** Some IIH medications pose a risk to the fetus, so all IIH patients should be asked whether they are planning to have a child and counselled on the potential teratogenicity of their medications. Topiramate is associated with a higher risk of cleft palate if taken in the first trimester. Acetazolamide has shown some teratogenicity in animal studies, but has been found to be safe in human pregnancy (even in the first trimester) and can be used after appropriate discussion of the risks and benefits [9, 10].
3. **Surgery** LPS surgery to prevent visual loss during pregnancy has been described [11].
4. **Anaesthesia and labour** Spinal anaesthesia for Caesarean section is safe in IIH patients without prior LPS and allows therapeutic drainage of CSF prior to delivery. Epidural and spinal anaesthesia can also be performed with pre-existing LPS, although with the latter technique there are theoretical risks of shunt damage and inadequate anaesthesia due to anaesthetic escape into the peritoneal cavity [12]. There is no clear evidence on the superiority of vaginal delivery or Caesarean section in IIH patients, so this is normally guided by obstetric indication. Straining during the second stage of vaginal delivery will raise ICP, especially in those with a CSF shunt. In the presence of severe papilloedema or marked visual field loss, assistance during the second stage, or Caesarean section, may be indicated.
5. **Abortion and termination** The rate of spontaneous abortion is no higher in IIH patients than in the general population [13]. Some women experience severe relapses of IIH in successive pregnancies [14], and severe sight-threatening disease refractory to treatment may require consideration of termination of pregnancy.

References

1. Connor SE, Siddiqui MA, Stewart VR, O'Flynn EA. The relationship of transverse sinus stenosis to bony groove dimensions provides an insight into the aetiology of idiopathic intracranial hypertension. *Neuroradiology* 2008; 50(12): 999–1004.
2. Friedman DI, Rausch EA. Headache diagnoses in patients with treated idiopathic intracranial hypertension. *Neurology* 2002; 58(10): 1551–3.
3. De Simone R, Marano E, Bilo L, et al. Idiopathic intracranial hypertension without headache. *Cephalalgia* 2006; 26(8): 1020–1.

4. Aiken AH, Hoots JA, Saindane AM, Hudgins PA. Incidence of cerebellar tonsillar ectopia in idiopathic intracranial hypertension: a mimic of the Chiari I malformation. *Am J Neuroradiol* 2012; 33(10): 1901–6.
5. Banik R, Lin D, Miller NR. Prevalence of Chiari I malformation and cerebellar ectopia in patients with pseudotumor cerebri. *J Neurol Sci* 2006; 247(1): 71–5.
6. Bejjani GK. Association of the adult Chiari malformation and idiopathic intracranial hypertension: more than a coincidence. *Med Hypotheses* 2003; 60(6): 859–63.
7. Kumpe DA, Bennett JL, Seinfeld J, et al. Dural sinus stent placement for idiopathic intracranial hypertension. *J Neurosurg* 2012; 116(3): 538–48.
8. Milhorat TH, Chou MW, Trinidad EM, et al. Chiari I malformation redefined: clinical and radiographic findings for 364 symptomatic patients. *Neurosurgery* 1999; 44(5): 1005–17.
9. Lee AG, Pless M, Falardeau J, et al. The use of acetazolamide in idiopathic intracranial hypertension during pregnancy. *Am J Ophthalmol* 2005; 139(5): 855–9.
10. Falardeau J, Lobb BM, Golden S, et al., The use of acetazolamide during pregnancy in intracranial hypertension patients. *J Neuroophthalmol* 2013; 33(1): 9–12.
11. Shapiro S, Yee R, Brown H. Surgical management of pseudotumor cerebri in pregnancy: case report. *Neurosurgery* 1995; 37(4): 829–31.
12. Abouleish E, Ali V, Tang RA. Benign intracranial hypertension and anesthesia for cesarean section. *Anesthesiology* 1985; 63(6): 705–7.
13. Tang RA, Dorotheo EU, Schiffman JS, Bahrani HM. Medical and surgical management of idiopathic intracranial hypertension in pregnancy. *Curr Neurol Neurosci Rep* 2004; 4(5): 398–409.
14. Gumma AD. Recurrent benign intracranial hypertension in pregnancy. *Eur J Obstet Gynecol Reprod Biol* 2004; 115(2): 244.
15. Fraser C, Plant GT. The syndrome of pseudotumour cerebri and idiopathic intracranial hypertension. *Curr Opin Neurol* 2011; 24(1): 12–17.
16. Szewka AJ, Bruce BB, Newman NJ, Biousse V. Idiopathic intracranial hypertension: relation between obesity and visual outcomes. *J Neuroophthalmol* 2013; 33(1): 4–8.
17. Bruce BB, Kedar S, van Stavern GP, et al., Atypical idiopathic intracranial hypertension: normal BMI and older patients. *Neurology* 2010; 74(22): 1827–32.
18. Bruce BB, Biousse V, Newman NJ. Update on idiopathic intracranial hypertension. *Am J Ophthalmol* 2011; 152(2): 163–9.
19. Dandy WE. Intracranial pressure without brain tumor: diagnosis and treatment. *Ann Surg* 1937; 106(4): 492–513.
20. Friedman DI, Jacobson DM. Diagnostic criteria for idiopathic intracranial hypertension. *Neurology* 2002; 59(10): 1492–5.
21. Shaw GY, Million SK. Benign intracranial hypertension: a diagnostic dilemma. *Case Report Otolaryngol* 2012; 2012: 814696.
22. Smith JL. Whence pseudotumor cerebri? *J Clin Neuroophthalmol* 1985; 5(1): 55–6.
23. Agarwal P, Kumar M, Arora V. Clinical profile of cerebral venous sinus thrombosis and the role of imaging in its diagnosis in patients with presumed idiopathic intracranial hypertension. *Indian J Ophthalmol*; 2010: 58(2): 153–5.
24. Biousse V, Ameri A, Bousser MG. Isolated intracranial hypertension as the only sign of cerebral venous thrombosis. *Neurology* 1999; 53(7): 1537–42.
25. Lin A, Foroozan R, Danesh-Meyer HV, et al. Occurrence of cerebral venous sinus thrombosis in patients with presumed idiopathic intracranial hypertension. *Ophthalmology* 2006; 113(12): 2281–4.
26. Mrfka M, Pistracher K, Schökler B, et al. An uncommon case of idiopathic intracranial hypertension with diagnostic pitfalls. *Acta Neurochir Suppl* 2012; 114: 235–7.
27. Sylaja PN, Asan Moosa NV, Radhakrishnan K, et al. Differential diagnosis of patients with intracranial sinus venous thrombosis related isolated intracranial hypertension from those with idiopathic intracranial hypertension. *J Neurol Sci* 2003; 215(1–2): 9–12.

28. Ahmed RM, Wilkinson M, Parker GD, et al., Transverse sinus stenting for idiopathic intracranial hypertension: a review of 52 patients and of model predictions. *Am J Neuroradiol* 2011; 32(8): 1408–14.
29. Burger BM, Chavis PS, Purvin V. A weed by any other name. *Surv Ophthalmol* 2013; 58(2): 176–83.
30. Bussière M, Falero R, Nicole D, et al. Unilateral transverse sinus stenting of patients with idiopathic intracranial hypertension. *Am J Neuroradiol* 2010; 31(4): 645–50.
31. Fargen KM, Siddiqui AH, Veznedaroglu E, et al. Concomitant intracranial pressure monitoring during venous sinus stenting for intracranial hypertension secondary to venous sinus stenosis. *J Neurointerv Surg* 2012; 4(6); 438–41.
32. Puffer RC, Mustafa W, Lanzino G. Venous sinus stenting for idiopathic intracranial hypertension: a review of the literature. *J Neurointerv Surg*, 2013; 5(5): 483–6.
33. Sinclair AJ, Burdon MA, Nightingale PG, et al. Low energy diet and intracranial pressure in women with idiopathic intracranial hypertension: prospective cohort study. *BMJ* 2010; 341: c2701.
34. Rubin RC, Henderson ES, Ommaya AK, et al., The production of cerebrospinal fluid in man and its modification by acetazolamide. *J Neurosurg* 1966; 25(4): 430–6.
35. Celebisoy N, Gökçay F, Sirin H, Akyürekli O. Treatment of idiopathic intracranial hypertension: topiramate vs acetazolamide, an open-label study. *Acta Neurol Scand* 2007; 116(5): 322–7.
36. Thambisetty M, Lavin PJ, Newman NJ, Biousse V. Fulminant idiopathic intracranial hypertension. *Neurology* 2007; 68(3): 229–32.
37. Pickard JD, Czosnyka Z, Czosnyka M, et al. Coupling of sagittal sinus pressure and cerebrospinal fluid pressure in idiopathic intracranial hypertension—a preliminary report. *Acta Neurochir Suppl* 2008; 102: 283–5.
38. Alsuhaibani AH, Carter KD, Nerad JA, Lee AG. Effect of optic nerve sheath fenestration on papilledema of the operated and the contralateral nonoperated eyes in idiopathic intracranial hypertension. *Ophthalmology* 2011; 118(2): 412–14.
39. Sinclair AJ, Kuruvath S, Sen D, et al. Is cerebrospinal fluid shunting in idiopathic intracranial hypertension worthwhile? A 10-year review. *Cephalalgia* 2011; 31(16): 1627–33.
40. Tarnaris A, Toma AK, Watkins LD, Kitchen ND. Is there a difference in outcomes of patients with idiopathic intracranial hypertension with the choice of cerebrospinal fluid diversion site: a single centre experience. *Clin Neurol Neurosurg* 2011; 113(6): 477–9.
41. Curry WT, Jr, Butler WE, Barker FG, 2nd. Rapidly rising incidence of cerebrospinal fluid shunting procedures for idiopathic intracranial hypertension in the United States, 1988–2002. *Neurosurgery* 2005; 57(1): 97–108.
42. Farber SH, Parker SL, Adogwa O, et al. Effect of antibiotic-impregnated shunts on infection rate in adult hydrocephalus: a single institution's experience. *Neurosurgery* 2011; 69(3): 625–9.
43. Nadkarni TD, Rekate HL, Wallace D. Concurrent use of a lumboperitoneal shunt with programmable valve and ventricular access device in the treatment of pseudotumor cerebri: review of 40 cases. *J Neurosurg Pediatr* 2008; 2(1): 19–24.
44. Kandasamy J, Hayhurst C, Clark S, et al. Electromagnetic stereotactic ventriculoperitoneal csf shunting for idiopathic intracranial hypertension: a successful step forward? *World Neurosurg* 2011; 75(1): 155–60; discussion 32–3.
45. Tse DT, Nerad JA, Anderson RL, Corbett JJ. Optic nerve sheath fenestration in pseudotumor cerebri. A lateral orbitotomy approach. *Arch Ophthalmol* 1988; 106(10): 1458–62.
46. Shah RJ, Shen JH, Joos KM. Endoscopic free electron laser technique development for minimally invasive optic nerve sheath fenestration. *Lasers Surg Med* 2007; 39(7): 589–96.
47. Joos KM, Shah RJ, Robinson RD, Shen JH. Optic nerve sheath fenestration with endoscopic accessory instruments versus the free electron laser (FEL). *Lasers Surg Med* 2006; 38(9): 846–51.

48. Joos KM, Mawn LA, Shen JH, Casagrande VA. Chronic and acute analysis of optic nerve sheath fenestration with the free electron laser in monkeys. *Lasers Surg Med* 2003; 32(1): 32–41.
49. Joos KM, Shen JH, Shetlar DJ, Casagrande VA. Optic nerve sheath fenestration with a novel wavelength produced by the free electron laser (FEL). *Lasers Surg Med* 2000; 27(3): 191–205.
50. Brodsky MC, Rettele GA. Protracted postsurgical blindness with visual recovery following optic nerve sheath fenestration. *Arch Ophthalmol* 1998; 116(1): 107–9.
51. Wilkes BN, Siatkowski RM. Progressive optic neuropathy in idiopathic intracranial hypertension after optic nerve sheath fenestration. *J Neuroophthalmol* 2009; 29(4): 281–3.
52. Plotnik JL, Kosmorsky GS. Operative complications of optic nerve sheath decompression. *Ophthalmology* 1993; 100(5): 683–90.
53. Rizzo, J.F., 3rd and S. Lessell, Choroidal infarction after optic nerve sheath fenestration. Ophthalmology, 1994. 101(9): 1622-6.
54. Smith KH, Wilkinson JT, Brindley GO. Combined third and sixth nerve paresis following optic nerve sheath fenestration. *J Clin Neuroophthalmol* 1992; 12(2): 85–8.
55. Spoor TC, McHenry JG. Long-term effectiveness of optic nerve sheath decompression for pseudotumor cerebri. *Arch Ophthalmol* 1993; 111(5): 632–5.
56. Agarwal MR, Yoo JH. Optic nerve sheath fenestration for vision preservation in idiopathic intracranial hypertension. *Neurosurg Focus* 2007; 23(5): E7.
57. Chandrasekaran S, McCluskey P, Minassian D, Assaad N. Visual outcomes for optic nerve sheath fenestration in pseudotumour cerebri and related conditions. *Clin Experiment Ophthalmol* 2006; 34(7): 661–5.
58. Corbett JJ, Nerad JA, Tse DT, Anderson RL. Results of optic nerve sheath fenestration for pseudotumor cerebri. The lateral orbitotomy approach. *Arch Ophthalmol* 1988; 106(10): 1391–7.
59. Spoor TC, McHenry JG, Shin DH. Long-term results using adjunctive mitomycin C in optic nerve sheath decompression for pseudotumor cerebri. *Ophthalmology* 1995; 102(12): 2024–8.
60. De Simone R, Ranieri A, Bonavita V. Advancement in idiopathic intracranial hypertension pathogenesis: focus on sinus venous stenosis. *Neurol Sci* 2010; 31(Suppl 1): S33–9.
61. Dykhuizen MJ, Hall J. Cerebral venous sinus system and stenting in pseudotumor cerebri. *Curr Opin Ophthalmol* 2011; 22(6): 458–62.
62. King JO, Mitchell PJ, Thomson KR, Tress BM. Manometry combined with cervical puncture in idiopathic intracranial hypertension. *Neurology* 2002; 58(1): 26–30.
63. Rohr A, Dörner L, Stingele R, et al. Reversibility of venous sinus obstruction in idiopathic intracranial hypertension. *Am J Neuroradiol* 2007; 28(4): 656–9.
64. Scoffings DJ, Pickard JD, Higgins JN. Resolution of transverse sinus stenoses immediately after CSF withdrawal in idiopathic intracranial hypertension. *J Neurol Neurosurg Psychiatry* 2007; 78(8): 911–12.
65. McGonigal A, Bone I, Teasdale E. Resolution of transverse sinus stenosis in idiopathic intracranial hypertension after L-P shunt. *Neurology* 2004; 62(3): 514–15.
66. Fridley J, Foroozan R, Sherman V, et al. Bariatric surgery for the treatment of idiopathic intracranial hypertension. *J Neurosurg* 2011; 114(1): 34–9.

CASE

3 Recipes no longer a piece of cake

Natalie S. Ryan

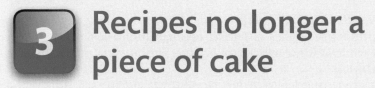

Expert commentary Martin N. Rossor

Case history

A 57-year-old housewife was referred to the neurology clinic with a two-year history of gradually progressive visual symptoms. She complained of frequently misjudging where objects were and of being unable to see things that were right in front of her, such as a cup that she had just put down on a table. Reading had become difficult, and she now needed to use a bookmark to isolate a line of text. She struggled to tell the time on a conventional clock, although she could still manage with a digital clock. She found it hard to iron patterned shirts as the pattern seemed to disappear into the background so that she could no longer tell which part of the shirt she was ironing. On one occasion, this led to her ironing her own hand. She had always enjoyed baking cakes but found it harder to follow recipes and, in particular, judge volumes of ingredients. Her husband noticed that her cakes were no longer accurately square and often had patches left undecorated. She found it difficult now to sew, knit, or even fold a shirt accurately. On driving, she found it hard to stay in lane and on one occasion had attempted to overtake a car turning in her direction ahead. She complained of difficulty recognizing different herbs in her garden and had experienced some unusual colour effects; one day she looked at her tortoiseshell cat and found that he appeared purple. Her calculation and spelling skills also appeared to have deteriorated, and she had occasional word-finding difficulties although these were not pronounced. Her memory for day-to-day events had initially been good, although she felt that this had deteriorated a little in recent months. Her husband did not feel that there had been any change in her behaviour, personality, or mood.

She had no past medical history other than mild hypothyroidism, no vascular risk factors, and no family history of dementia. Her only medication was levothyroxine. She lived with her husband, had never smoked, and did not drink alcohol.

She had initially consulted her optician about her symptoms. The optician detected abnormal visual fields, told her that she may have had a stroke, and referred her to an ophthalmologist. The ophthalmologist found that she had an unusual visual field defect and diagnosed her with a psychosomatic illness. However, he also recommended that she see a neurologist for a second opinion.

On examination, she was engaged and appropriate and cooperated well with cognitive testing. She scored 23 out of 30 on the Mini-Mental State Examination (MMSE). She lost two points on orientation and one on recall, made errors with both serial sevens and reverse spelling, and was completely unable to copy intersecting pentagons. Further bedside cognitive assessment revealed bilateral limb dyspraxia, dyscalculia, and visual disorientation. Visuospatial and visuoperceptual deficits were further indicated by her inability to complete a dot-counting task or perceive fragmented letters (see Figure 3.1). She had jerky pursuit on examination of her eye movements and mild finger myoclonus, but neurological examination was otherwise unremarkable.

Routine blood tests including thyroid function, vitamin B12, and folate were all normal. An MRI brain scan showed mild parietal atrophy bilaterally but well-preserved hippocampal volumes. An EEG demonstrated loss of the alpha rhythm and excess generalized slowing, but no focal or epileptiform features. She underwent formal neuropsychometry. Assessment with the WAIS-R (Wechsler Adult Intelligence Scale—Revised) revealed mild to moderate decline on verbal tasks (verbal IQ 94) and a severe decline on non-verbal tasks (performance IQ 59) compared with premorbid estimates. Visual memory, visuoperceptual and visuospatial skills were gravely impaired, and there was evidence of dyscalculia, limb dyspraxia, and executive dysfunction. There was also some evidence of weak verbal memory, reading, and spelling abilities, although nominal skills were preserved.

She was diagnosed with posterior cortical atrophy (PCA). As the majority of cases of PCA are due to underlying Alzheimer's disease, treatment with the acetylcholinesterase inhibitor donepezil was commenced. She felt that donepezil significantly improved her general cognitive state, and this was reflected in a three-point improvement in her score on the MMSE at her next assessment. She chose to stop driving voluntarily as she no longer felt safe, and she arranged for her husband to have Lasting Power of Attorney. With the help of an occupational therapist, a number of home modifications were made to help her to cope with her visual processing deficits in her day-to-day life, for example using colour contrasts (e.g. red/green) to mark out important areas such as handrails and light switches. Over the subsequent years, she underwent a gradual deterioration, particularly in her visuospatial skills. In view of this, a further ophthalmology referral was made four years after diagnosis in order for her to be registered as severely visually impaired. There has been some gradual deterioration in her episodic memory, but her personality remains unchanged. Her husband has continued to care for her at home with minimal formal help, and their blue badge has allowed them to continue making regular excursions and maintain a good quality of life.

Discussion

This case illustrates some of the symptoms that PCA patients may present with and the initial diagnostic uncertainty that these may provoke. However, it also shows how the syndrome can be readily recognized with careful clinical assessment and appropriate investigation, allowing important management and compensatory strategies to be implemented.

As the name suggests, PCA is a neurodegenerative syndrome that preferentially affects parietal, occipital, and occipito-temporal brain regions. Clinically, it is characterized by progressive deterioration of higher visual processing skills and other posterior cortical functions including literacy, numeracy, and praxis. Alzheimer's disease (AD) is by far the most common underlying cause of PCA [1]. For this reason, the terms 'biparietal AD' and 'visual variant of AD' are sometimes used synonymously with PCA. However, a number of different pathologies can also give rise to PCA, including corticobasal degeneration (CBD), dementia with Lewy bodies (DLB), prion disease, and subcortical gliosis [1–3]. Therefore PCA tends to be the preferred label for this distinct clinical syndrome. Some studies comparing the distribution of pathology in AD cases with PCA and typical amnestic presentations have demonstrated higher amyloid plaque and neurofibrillary tangle burden in primary visual and visual association areas in PCA [4]. Others found increased neurofibrillary tangle but similar amyloid plaque density in visual areas, with fewer tangles or plaques in the hippocampus in PCA compared with typical AD [3].

Estimates of the overall prevalence of PCA are difficult, partly because it tends to be under-diagnosed and because different ways of describing the syndrome are used inconsistently. Criteria for a diagnosis of PCA have been proposed by a number of single centres based on their own experience [3, 5] but no formal consensus criteria yet exist [6]. Only once these have been established and applied to the study of different cohorts of dementia patients will it become clear how common the syndrome is. However, in a study of all AD patients presenting to one specialist centre, 5 per cent were found to have had a visual presentation and 3 per cent an apraxic presentation [7]. Some groups have reported increased prevalence of PCA in women, whilst others have found no difference in sex distribution. One consistent observation is that symptom onset in PCA tends to occur at a much earlier age than in AD in general, typically in the mid-fifties to early sixties [5], although a wider age spread (40–86 years) has been reported [3]. Despite the young age of onset, the available case series indicate that PCA patients do not tend to have any stronger family history of dementia than patients with typical AD. There have only been single case reports of patients with autosomal dominant familial AD due to a Presenilin 1 mutation [8] and familial prion disease due to a 5-octapeptide repeat insertion [9] presenting with PCA. *APOE4* is the strongest genetic risk factor for sporadic AD, and PCA is associated with the same or slightly lower *APOE4* allele frequency as typical AD [3, 5, 7, 10–12]. In a recent large study of patients with a clinical diagnosis of PCA and a separate group of patients lacking clinical information who had posterior AD neuropathologically, *APOE4* did appear to be a risk factor for PCA, and *CLU, BIN1*, and *ABCA7* were identified as additional potential risk loci [13]. Further investigation of genetic risk factors for PCA is likely to require multicentre collaboration to increase sample sizes and will be most informative if the cohorts have both consistent clinical definitions of PCA and known neuropathological diagnoses.

Clinical presentation

Patients with PCA often experience considerable delays in getting a diagnosis. The young age at onset, the unusual nature of their symptoms, and the relative rarity and lack of awareness of the syndrome may all contribute. As the initial symptoms are usually visual, patients tend to present to opticians or ophthalmologists where they may receive reassurance that examination of the eyes is normal. When symptoms persist, it is not uncommon for them to then be attributed to anxiety, depression, or even functional illness. Anxiety does, at least anecdotally; frequently appear to accompany the initial cognitive symptoms. This may relate to the fact that insight is often preserved, at least in the early stages of the illness, making patients painfully aware of their difficulties. The presence of symptoms suggesting impaired higher visual processing skills should prompt the clinician to enquire about other posterior cognitive functions, such as calculation, spelling, and praxis. The impact on other cognitive domains, including memory and language, should also be explored. The impairments in PCA may remain strikingly selective for some time. However, prominent word retrieval deficits may also be evident [14] and, as the disease progresses, memory and global cognitive functions also tend to become affected. Nevertheless, the pattern of deterioration in cognitive skills can vary considerably between individuals, and large prospective group studies of disease progression are lacking.

General neurological examination in PCA is often unremarkable and visual acuity tends to be normal. However, the presence of high order visual attentional deficits can affect performance on visual field testing so that unusual and inconsistent field defects may be apparent, as was the case with this individual.

Clinical tip Examples of symptoms reported by patients with PCA

- Difficulty reading—for example, getting lost on the page, finding that words appear to move around or that small print is easier to read than large print (reverse size phenomena
- Problems judging distance, depth, and speed—for example, tripping over curbs, struggling to negotiate stairs and, in particular, escalators
- Difficulties with driving—for example, clipping wing-mirrors, veering out of traffic lanes
- Perceiving patterns on the floor as three-dimensional
- Experiencing excessive glare from shiny surfaces and particular difficulties with vision in low light conditions
- Problems recognizing household items, familiar faces, or objects from pictures
- Difficulty seeing the whole of a visual scene; instead perceiving only the separate constituent parts of it (simultanagnosia)
- Seeing positive visual phenomena—for example, washes of colour, patterns, or prolonged colour after-images
- Perceiving objects as having an abnormal colour
- Visual misperceptions—for example, shadows on the floor as animals, or hallucinations
- Getting lost on familiar routes and even within their own home (topographical disorientation)
- Difficulty with writing and spelling words
- Difficulty with calculations and with recognizing and writing numbers—for example, handling change, issuing cheques, managing household finances.
- Problems with dextrous tasks—for example, sewing, DIY, tying shoelaces

Finger myoclonus is relatively common in PCA and extrapyramidal signs, which are often asymmetric, may occur. Studies investigating clinicopathological correlations in PCA have so far been relatively small, so it remains unclear how well the phenotype may predict the underlying pathology. Some PCA patients with asymmetric Parkinsonism and apraxia have been found to have underlying CBD [15], although others have had AD [16]. The presence of Parkinsonism and visual hallucinations has been associated with coexisting AD and Lewy body pathology [3] in some cases, although it should be noted that concomitant Lewy body pathology is observed in up to 60 per cent of AD patients at post-mortem according to some series [17].

Expert comment

Patients with PCA may have great difficulty locating objects in their visual field because of their visual disorientation (see below). This often results in profound mis-reaching, which can be demonstrated by asking the patient to take your hand, which you hold out in their peripheral visual space whilst they sit opposite you looking at your face. Gently moving your fingers may help them to locate your hand, as they often find it easier to detect motion than static stimuli.

Cognitive assessment is central to making a clinical diagnosis of PCA. Visuospatial and visuoperceptual impairments are usually the most striking deficits, and these often first become apparent during the MMSE when the patient struggles to copy intersecting pentagons accurately and may have difficulty reading and writing a sentence. Visuospatial deficits are often best demonstrated by asking the patient to copy patterns or count dots in an array—they will typically count more dots than are present. Visuoperceptual deficits can be demonstrated by asking the patient to identify pictures of objects or letters that have been fragmented or distorted (see Figure 3.1). They may have particular difficulty recognizing silhouettes or unusual views of familiar objects. This inability to identify objects from their distinctive structural

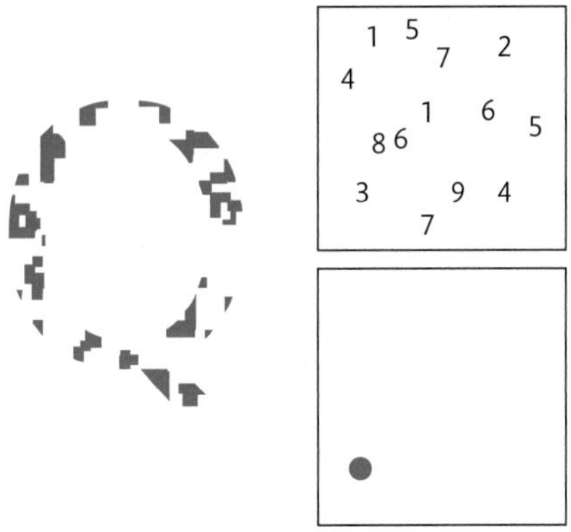

Figure 3.1 Example of neuropsychological test stimuli for assessing patients with PCA. On the left is a fragmented letter, which is used to test visuoperceptual ability. On the right is a number location stimulus, used to test visuospatial ability. The patient is asked which number lies in the same place as the dot.

Reproduced from *Optometry in Practice*, 13(4), Shakespeare TJ, Ryan NS, Petrushkin H, Crutch SJ, Identifying cortical visual in posterior cortical atrophy, pp. 159–62, © 2012, with permission from The College of Optometrists.

features, despite changing viewpoints, is described as apperceptive visual agnosia. In addition to higher-order visual processing deficits such as impaired space and object perception, basic visual impairments including abnormal perception of colour, form, and motion may also be evident.

Other features that may be present on examination include simultanagnosis, oculomotor apraxia (difficulty directing the eyes towards objects), and optic ataxia (difficulty performing visually guided movements)—a triad of signs that is sometimes collectively described as Balint's syndrome. There may also be features indicating dominant parietal involvement: agraphia, acalculia, left–right disorientation, finger agnosia (difficulty naming each finger or moving a finger when its name is given), impaired working memory, and difficulties with limb praxis. Digit span, where the patient is asked to repeat back progressively lengthening strings of numbers, is commonly used to assess working memory. Apraxia may be demonstrated by assessing the patient's ability to perform meaningless hand gestures or meaningful actions such as waving or pantomiming the use of an object such as a toothbrush or screwdriver. So-called constructional apraxia (impaired ability to copy drawings) and dressing apraxia are in fact probably largely attributable to visuospatial impairment and are commonly observed in PCA.

Investigations

Investigations in patients with PCA, as in other dementia syndromes, aim first to exclude a reversible underlying cause and, secondly, to ascertain the likely neurodegenerative pathology. The approach taken will depend upon the individual case, with more intensive investigation appropriate if the presentation is particularly rapid, atypical, or early onset.

Learning point Investigations in PCA

Brain imaging

All patients with dementia should have structural brain imaging with CT or MRI to exclude a reversible cause (e.g. tumour, subdural haematoma). MRI provides particularly useful information in PCA, especially if a range of sequences is acquired.

- The volumetric T1 sequence typically demonstrates a posterior pattern of atrophy with preserved hippocampal volumes. This supports the clinical diagnosis of PCA and indicates the presence of neurodegenerative pathology (see Figure 3.2).

(Continued)

- T2-weighted/FLAIR sequences indicate whether there is significant cerebrovascular disease, which may coexist with degenerative pathology and highlights the need to optimize management of vascular risk factors. If there are prominent white matter hyperintensities, susceptibility-weighted imaging (SWI)/T2* may be useful to look for microbleeds, which may indicate the presence of cerebral amyloid angiopathy if they have a predominantly cortical distribution.
- Diffusion-weighted imaging (DWI) excludes an infarct on the rare occasion that a PCA patient presents acutely and lacks the insight to provide a history of insidious onset of symptoms. DWI and FLAIR should be acquired in any patient with rapid onset of symptoms to look for abnormally high signal in the striatum, thalamus, or cortex, which may be seen in prion disease.

Functional imaging may sometimes be indicated if MRI is normal, CSF examination is unhelpful (see below), and the presence of a neurodegenerative disease is unclear. Single photon emission computed tomography (SPECT) and fluorodeoxyglucose (FDG)-Positron emission tomography (PET) scanning in PCA has demonstrated parieto-occipital hypometabolism. Hypometabolism in the frontal eye fields has also been found using FDG-PET.

Neuropsychometry

Formal neuropsychometry should be acquired in all patients with suspected PCA to characterize the cognitive profile and compare the individual's performance with estimates of premorbid ability and normative data from the age-matched population. In cases where the diagnosis is unclear, for example when there is significant anxiety which may also be impacting upon performance, a repeat assessment after an interval may be particularly informative.

EEG

EEG should be performed if there is any suspicion of Creutzfeldt–Jakob disease (CJD) (to look for periodic sharp wave complexes) or seizures. It may also be useful if there is uncertainty as to the presence of a neurodegenerative disease. In AD, the EEG typically shows generalized slowing and loss or degeneration of the alpha rhythm, although it can be normal early in the illness.

Lumbar puncture

CSF examination may be appropriate and should certainly be performed in younger patients and those with rapid onset cognitive decline. Assessment of basic constituents may identify an inflammatory or infective process, whilst assay for disease-specific proteins may suggest the underlying degenerative pathology. Raised 14-3-3 protein is associated with CJD (in which CSF tau also tends to be very high). Reduced amyloid $\beta_{1\text{-}42}$ and raised tau concentrations support a diagnosis of AD.

Genetic testing

If there is a strong family history of early onset dementia with a pattern suggesting autosomal dominant inheritance, testing for mutations in presenilin 1 and the prion protein gene should be discussed, although this is very rarely the case in PCA.

Clinical tip Interpretation of neuropsychological tests in PCA

Predictably, PCA patients perform poorly on neuropsychological tests with any visual component. Thus there tends to be a marked discrepancy between verbal and performance IQ, with performance IQ often 30–40 points lower. Some neuropsychological tests, including tests of visual recall memory, object naming, and executive function such as the trail-making and Stroop tests, are not designed to assess visual function but require intact visual processing skills to be performed. These assessments should be interpreted with caution in PCA, and alternatives without a verbal component, such as auditory-verbal memory tasks and naming from verbal description, should be used in preference

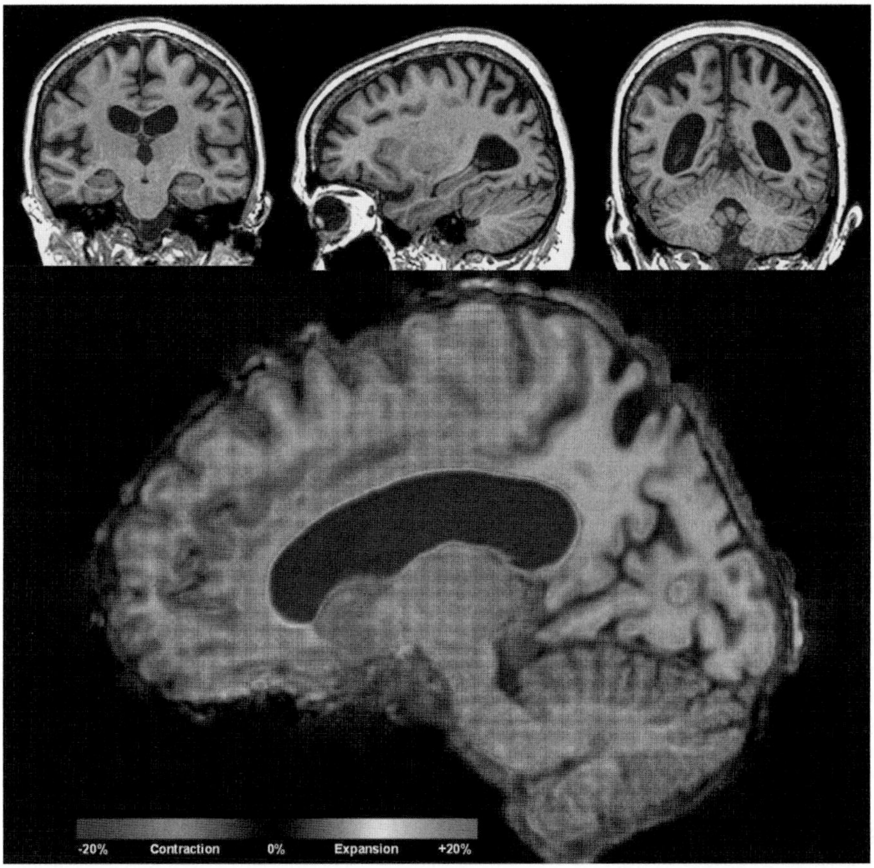

Figure 3.2 MRI of the PCA patient in this case study. The top images show coronal, sagittal, and axial views of a volumetric MRI brain scan acquired four years after symptom onset as part of a research study. There is parieto-occipital atrophy with relatively well-preserved hippocampal volumes, which is typical of PCA. A repeat scan two years later has been fluid registered to the baseline scan to produce the voxel compression map shown in the bottom image. The scale shows the percentage volume change per voxel (−20–20%) with green and blue representing contraction and yellow and red representing expansion. Atrophy over this interval is greatest in the parietal and occipital regions. Please see colour plate section.

Image courtesy of Tim Shakespeare and Shona Clegg.

Management

The approach to management in PCA should be holistic and multidisciplinary. No studies specifically assessing medications in PCA have yet been published. However, as the majority of patients with PCA have AD as the underlying pathology, it is appropriate to offer symptomatic treatment with a cholinesterase inhibitor (donepezil, galantamine, or rivastigmine). Several large randomized controlled trials have shown statistically significant, although clinically modest, symptomatic benefits of cholinesterase inhibitors on cognitive function in AD. However, on an individual basis even small effects can significantly improve quality of life for patients and their carers.

Expert comment

When prescribing a cholinesterase inhibitor for PCA, it is important not to rely too heavily on the results of cognitive testing when making judgements about disease severity and response to treatment. Commonly used assessments like the MMSE are heavily weighted on memory and orientation and place much less emphasis on the deficits that are relevant in PCA.

Although a minority of patients with PCA will have non-AD pathology, such as CBD, it remains uncertain how such patients may be identified from their phenotype. Pragmatically, it therefore seems appropriate to offer cholinesterase inhibitor treatment to all PCA patients (unless there is clear biomarker evidence of a non-AD cause such as CJD), including those with prominent motor features. As diagnostic criteria for PCA are refined and our understanding of predictors of the underlying pathology increases, hopefully there will come a time when PCA patients have the opportunity to enter clinical trials designed specifically for them, assessing therapies with the potential for disease modification.

Learning point Management in PCA

- Discuss starting treatment with a cholinesterase inhibitor and consider memantine (an NMDA receptor antagonist) for patients in whom cholinesterase inhibitors are contraindicated (e.g. heart block), cause side effects, or are thought to have lost efficacy.
- Look for and have a low threshold for treating coexistent depression or anxiety. Avoid anticholinergic medications.
- Optimize management of vascular risk factors to minimize the impact of mixed disease on cognition.
- Discuss driving. Many patients with PCA stop driving voluntarily, but they may need to be advised to stop if they lack insight and they must be made aware of their legal obligation to inform the DVLA of their diagnosis.
- Consider referral to an ophthalmologist so that they can be registered as partially sighted.
- Ensure that they have information about the financial and social assistance they may benefit from and access to post-diagnosis counselling if required.
- Give practical advice on aids for the visually impaired (e.g. talking clocks, audiobooks) and home modifications (e.g. keeping rooms well lit, minimizing patterns on floors and walls that could be misperceived as obstacles). Involve an occupational therapist.
- Support the carer and provide information on patient support groups (e.g. <http://www.pcasupport.ucl.ac.uk>
- Provide opportunities to discuss future planning (e.g. establishing Lasting Power of Attorney) at a stage where the patient is able to express their wishes.

A final word from the expert

This case history illustrates the diagnostic challenge of patients with posterior cortical atrophy. The features are dominated by visual impairments, and so understandably patients will often start with opticians and then move on to ophthalmologists. The clinical features can be very confusing, and patients may see many different specialists before the diagnosis is arrived at. Moreover, many of the symptoms that patients describe are easily dismissed or misunderstood. Another key message from this case history is that not all Alzheimer's disease presents with an impairment of memory, and indeed many patients will have well-preserved episodic memory until late into the illness.

References

1. Renner JA, Burns JM, Hou CE, et al. Progressive posterior cortical dysfunction: a clinicopathologic series. *Neurology* 2004; 63(7): 1175–80.
2. Victoroff J, Ross GW, Benson DF, et al. Posterior cortical atrophy. Neuropathologic correlations. *Arch Neurol* 1994; 51(3): 269–74.
3. Tang-Wai DF, Graff-Radford NR, Boeve BF, et al. Clinical, genetic, and neuropathologic characteristics of posterior cortical atrophy. *Neurology* 2004; 63(7): 1168–74.
4. Hof PR, Vogt BA, Bouras C, Morrison JH. Atypical form of Alzheimer's disease with prominent posterior cortical atrophy: a review of lesion distribution and circuit disconnection in cortical visual pathways. *Vision Res* 1997; 37(24): 3609–25.
5. Mendez MF, Ghajarania M, Perryman KM. Posterior cortical atrophy: clinical characteristics and differences compared to Alzheimer's disease. *Dement Geriatr Cogn Disord* 2002; 14(1): 33–40.
6. Crutch SJ, Lehmann M, Schott JM, et al. Posterior cortical atrophy. *Lancet Neurol* 2012; 11(2): 170–8.
7. Snowden JS, Stopford CL, Julien CL, et al. Cognitive phenotypes in Alzheimer's disease and genetic risk. *Cortex* 2007; 43(7): 835–45.
8. Sitek EJ, Narozanska E, Peplonska B, et al. A patient with posterior cortical atrophy possesses a novel mutation in the presenilin 1 gene. *PLoS One* 2013; 8(4): e61074.
9. Depaz R, Haik S, Peoc'h K, et al. Long-standing prion dementia manifesting as posterior cortical atrophy. *Alzheimer Dis Assoc Disord* 2012; 26(3): 289–92.
10. Balasa M, Gelpi E, Antonell A, et al. Clinical features and APOE genotype of pathologically proven early-onset Alzheimer disease. *Neurology* 2011; 76(20): 1720–5.
11. Schott JM, Ridha BH, Crutch SJ, et al. Apolipoprotein e genotype modifies the phenotype of Alzheimer disease. *Arch Neurol* 2006; 63(1): 155–6.
12. van der Flier WM, Schoonenboom SN, Pijnenburg YA, et al. The effect of APOE genotype on clinical phenotype in Alzheimer disease. *Neurology* 2006; 67(3): 526–7.
13. Carrasquillo MM, Khan Q, Murray ME, et al. Late-onset Alzheimer disease: genetic variants in posterior cortical atrophy and posterior AD. *Neurology* 2014; 82(16): 1455–62.
14. Crutch SJ, Lehmann M, Warren JD, Rohrer JD. The language profile of posterior cortical atrophy. *J Neurol Neurosurg Psychiatry* 2013; 84(4): 460–6.
15. Tang-Wai DF, Josephs KA, Boeve BF, et al. Pathologically confirmed corticobasal degeneration presenting with visuospatial dysfunction. *Neurology* 2003; 61(8): 1134–5.
16. Ryan NS, Shakespeare TJ, Lehmann M, et al. Motor features in posterior cortical atrophy and their imaging correlates. *Neurobiol Aging* 2014; 35(12): 2845–57.
17. Hamilton RL. Lewy bodies in Alzheimer's disease: a neuropathological review of 145 cases using alpha-synuclein immunohistochemistry. *Brain Pathol* 2000; 10(3): 378–84.

CASE

4 Getting your head out of a spin

Diego Kaski

Expert commentary Adolfo M. Bronstein

Case history

A 62-year-old woman was admitted to the emergency department with a rapid onset of rotational vertigo, which she described as 'seeing the world spin in front of me', over a few minutes. The symptoms were continuous and she had felt nauseated and vomited a number of times prior to the arrival of the ambulance. She was unsteady on her feet, needing to hold on to furniture to make her way to the bathroom. She described a constant sensation of movement of both the world around her and as if she herself were spinning. Head movements worsened her symptoms, but these were present even when her head was held completely still. There were no flu-like symptoms preceding this event. There was no significant travel history. She did not describe any additional symptoms. In particular, there was no hearing loss, no altered sensation or weakness in the face or limbs, and no speech disturbance.

There was a past medical history of hypertension, hypercholesterolaemia, and psoriasis. There was a strong family history of malignancy, with breast cancer in her mother, sister, and an aunt. The patient was taking amlodipine 10mg and there were no known drug allergies. She was a retired legal secretary. She drank alcohol socially, and had never smoked cigarettes.

On general examination, the patient was sweaty and clammy. Her temperature was 36.8°C, pulse rate was 96bpm, blood pressure was 162/80mmHg, and respiratory rate was normal. She appeared anxious and lay on the couch with her eyes closed and head held still. Neurological examination revealed normal tone, power, reflexes, and sensation in the upper and lower limbs. Plantar responses were flexor bilaterally. Coordination was normal in the upper and lower limbs. The patient was able to stand unaided, although this worsened her nausea. Romberg's test was negative, but the patient was unable to tandem walk, with a tendency to veer to the sides. Gait was unsteady and broad-based.

Neuro-otological examination revealed spontaneous right-beating unidirectional horizontal nystagmus when looking straight ahead. The intensity of the nystagmus increased on right gaze. Although present, and still right-beating, the intensity decreased with the eyes looking left. Otherwise, the range of eye movements was full. Pursuit movements were difficult to assess because of the presence of nystagmus, but appeared normal. Saccades were of normal latency, accuracy, and velocity. The head impulse test (a clinical bedside test of the vestibulo-ocular reflex (VOR) (Figure 4.1)) was abnormal to the left. The Hallpike positional manoeuvre increased the magnitude of the nystagmus but did not induce a change in her symptoms, or additional nystagmus. The remainder of

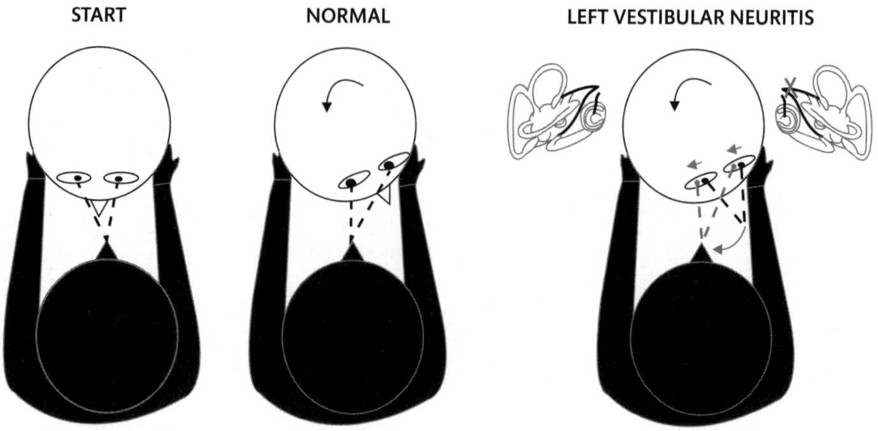

Figure 4.1 Head impulse test. This bedside manoeuvre tests the integrity of the VOR which is designed to keep images stable on the retina during head movements. The patient starts facing the examiner, and is asked to fixate on the examiner's nose throughout (left panel). The examiner then performs a high-acceleration but low-amplitude head movement to the side. The normal response (middle panel) is a movement of the eyes in the opposite direction, but at the same velocity to the head, and thus the eyes remain fixed on the examiner's nose. In vestibular neuritis (right panel) the VOR is absent on one side (left ear in this example), and the eyes move with the head, away from the examiner's nose, and a re-fixation saccade is required to bring them back. This is the abnormality detected.

the cranial nerve examination (fifth, seventh, ninth, tenth, eleventh, and twelfth) was normal.

The patient was started on intravenous (IV) fluids, and was given IV cyclizine for the nausea. Symptoms improved over the subsequent 48 hours, and the drip was discontinued. A bithermal caloric was arranged and a pure tone audiogram was normal. The patient was encouraged to mobilize, and discharged home on day three of admission.

Two months later she arranged to see her GP following a sudden-onset attack of rotational vertigo when brushing her teeth. She felt nauseated and off balance following this episode. In the GP surgery she suffered a further attack of brief vertigo when looking up to read a sign on the wall. She was diagnosed with a recurrence of labyrinthitis, prescribed cinnarizine, and advised complete bed rest for a week.

A month later, the patient continued to experience attacks of vertigo when turning over in bed. She finally admitted herself to the emergency department, with worsening vertigo and nausea. She was markedly unsteady and complained of neck stiffness. She was reviewed by the neuro-otology team. Examination revealed no evidence of spontaneous nystagmus. Cranial nerve and general neurological examination were normal. The sideways Hallpike manoeuvre (Figure 4.2) revealed right-beating torsional nystagmus on right ear down, with a 3sec latency and 7sec duration. The Hallpike manoeuvre with the left ear down was normal. The diagnosis was consistent with right posterior canal BPPV, perhaps related to a previous episode of vestibular neuritis (VN). The patient was treated with a Semont repositioning manoeuvre (Figure 4.2c), which is similar to the Epley manoeuvre and just as effective.

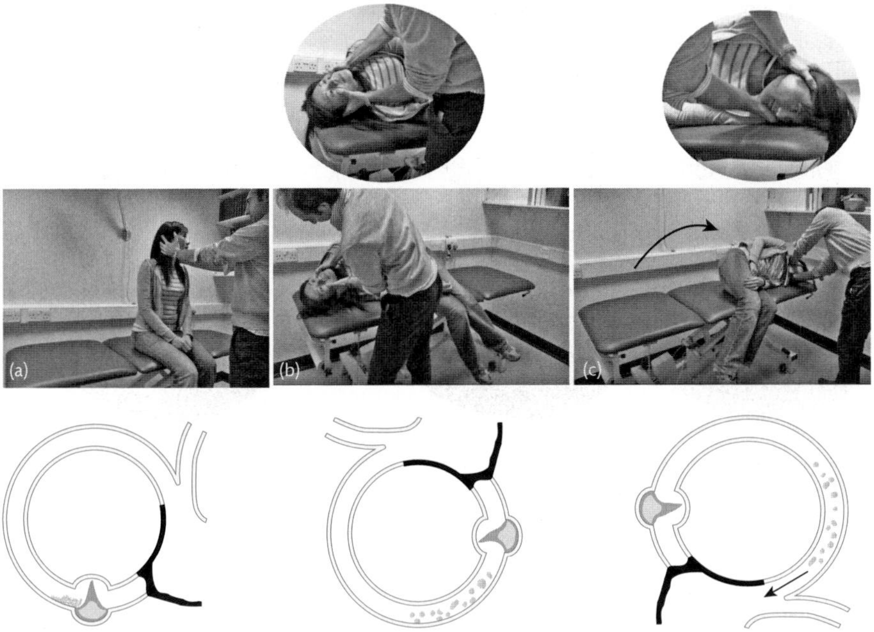

Figure 4.2 Sideways Dix–Hallpike manoeuvre (above) and trajectory of otolith crystals during the manoeuvre (below). (a) The patient begins seated in the centre of the couch, with the legs hanging down the side. The patient's head is then turned **away** from the ear being explored (the right ear in this case). (b) The patient is then rapidly tipped sideways, making sure that the head does not change position. Note that the nose should be pointing upwards, in which case it will be easy to see the eyes (inset). In the presence of BPPV there will be upbeat and torsional nystagmus beating towards the ground. The patient is held in that position for 30sec. (c) To treat the BPPV (in this case right-sided), the patient is then rapidly 'swung' from this position, by 180° to the opposite side, ensuring that the head is not moved. Note that in the starting position the nose is facing upwards, but then faces downwards at the end of the manoeuvre. The manoeuvre is reversed for treatment of left-sided BPPV.

Discussion

Vertigo is the illusion of movement, and thus is a **sensation**. It is important to recall that many patients will use the word 'dizziness' to describe a variety of complaints, ranging from imbalance, to vertigo, light-headedness, and even headache. Therefore it is imperative to understand what the patient means by the word 'dizziness'. Patients may find this difficult, so one may need to offer some words to try to characterize their sensation—for example, spinning like a merry-go-round, rocking like on a boat, off-balance, etc.

One approach to dealing with a patient with acute vertigo, such as the case presented here, is to first consider the common diagnoses, which are benign paroxysmal positional vertigo (BPPV), vestibular neuritis, brainstem or cerebellar stroke, vestibular migraine, and Menière's disease.

The most common cause of vertigo is BPPV. This is characterized by brief attacks of rotational vertigo ('spinning') triggered by changes in head position. Attacks last only a few seconds but, given their severity, patients may often subjectively feel that they last for several minutes. Typical triggers for BPPV include

Expert comment

The patient in this case described two separate phases of vertigo. The first phase is an acute episode of vertigo and oscillopsia (nystagmus), even when the head is held completely still, without other central neurological features. Although there has been no viral prodrome, the clinical picture is most compatible with acute vestibular neuritis (VN), sometimes termed viral labyrinthitis. The second phase of vertigo relates to recurrent (or episodic) vertigo typical of BPPV, triggered by head movement, and occurring when turning over in bed.

turning over in bed, lying down, bending forwards, or looking up (e.g. to reach a high shelf or hang the washing up). Attacks are typically associated with nausea (although not usually vomiting given the brevity of the attack) and marked imbalance. In some patients, the sensation of imbalance may outlast the vertiginous sensation.

There is a murky puddle of ambiguity regarding vestibular neuritis that relates to the terminology used. For many non-specialists, the term 'vertigo' has become synonymous with labyrinthitis. Thus, labyrinthitis has become a common label attached to acute and chronic dizziness that is considered to be benign. For specialists, however, labyrinthitis refers to an inflammation of the whole labyrinth (i.e. vestibular (balance) **and** cochlear (hearing) regions), which is actually very rare in clinical practice. VN refers to inflammation of the vestibular nerve with sparing of hearing, which is much more common, but confusingly is often also referred to as 'labyrinthitis'. VN has an incidence of ~3.5 per 100,000 per year, and so is less common than emergency department or GP referral letters might suggest.

Whatever term is used, this syndrome presents as a single acute attack of rotational vertigo, nausea, and often vomiting, as well as imbalance. The vertigo and nausea typically last hours to days, during which the vertigo is constant, even when the head is held completely still (which contrasts with BPPV). The imbalance in VN consists of the 'furniture-walking' type in contrast with cerebellar stroke where patients are unable to stand.

Patients with acute VN will have **spontaneous nystagmus**, i.e. with the eyes looking forward. The presence of nystagmus is why patients report that the world is spinning. The nystagmus of VN is mostly horizontal with some rotatory (torsional) component and is **unidirectional**—for example, right-beating whether looking to the left, right, or centre. If there are no other CNS symptoms or signs **spontaneous** and **unidirectional** nystagmus is usually peripheral. In VN it is useful to confirm the unilateral loss of the vestibulo-ocular reflex (VOR) (see Figure 4.1), the key function of the vestibular system. Hearing and otoscopy are normal in VN and most other harmless causes of dizziness. The diagnosis of acute VN can be made on clinical grounds based on these features, and therefore is a diagnosis of inclusion, not exclusion.

A patient such as the one described in this case will not need further specialist investigations. The treatment of VN is conservative, with bedrest and anti-emetics recommended for a maximum of three days, but thereafter they are not beneficial and may actually delay the recovery. The recovery from VN occurs as a result of a process of central compensation as the brain re-learns to interpret head motion signals. Therefore patients should be encouraged to move as much as possible once the acute vertigo has subsided. In some countries, steroids are given acutely. However, the advice regarding steroid treatment in VN is inconsistent. Whilst early intervention with corticosteroids may improve vestibular function test results in the long term [1], a Cochrane review [2] concluded that the utility of steroids in relation to long-term outcome in VN remains unclear. Of note, it is exceptionally rare for VN to recur in the same patient; if it does, a diagnosis of BPPV or vestibular migraine should be considered. Given the rich interplay between dizziness and psychological factors, an incomplete and false understanding of the symptoms can lead to long-term dizziness and handicap [3].

Red flags in cases of acute dizziness include unilateral hearing loss, abnormal neurological symptoms or signs, new headache, and a **normal** VOR as assessed by the head impulse test (as this would imply that the vertigo is not originating in the peripheral vestibular system). In such cases, the clinician should think of potentially more serious causes such as posterior circulation stroke, which is an important differential diagnosis here. Posterior circulation strokes present with headache (usually occipital), and typically with vertigo, vomiting, and imbalance. Acute deafness may result from occlusion of the internal auditory artery, which is a branch of the anterior inferior cerebellar artery [4] which supplies both the vestibular and cochlear organs in 90 per cent of the population. Occasionally, hearing loss can result from a pontine lesion affecting the crossing of auditory pathways (lateral lemniscus) [5]. Oculomotor disturbances may also aid diagnosis and allow a topographical diagnosis to be made. When present, the nystagmus may be gaze-evoked (beating in the direction of gaze), spontaneous (with the patient looking straight ahead), or positional. In fact, positional downbeat nystagmus is a strong pointer to a central cause of vertigo (usually of the cerebellar nodulus or uvula), particularly if the nystagmus has no latency, fatiguability, or habituation. These features help distinguish central from peripheral types of positional nystagmus (e.g. BPPV). Therefore performing a positional manoeuvre by tipping the patient backwards (as for a Hallpike test but without turning the head to the side) is an important clinical test in patients with a suspected posterior fossa stroke. From a practical perspective, whilst isolated vertigo is unlikely to be the only manifestation of a brainstem stroke, there may be a paucity of clinical signs and a degree of suspicion may be required to make the diagnosis.

A further common cause of vertigo to consider in this patient is vestibular migraine. The typical patient is one with a previous history of migrainous headaches or motion sickness in whom the symptoms change to include episodes of dizziness. Although typically of the 'rocking' type, the dizziness may take any form, including true rotational vertigo. Attacks usually last minutes to hours, but it is not uncommon to see patients in whom symptoms last several days or weeks. Attacks of vertigo are often associated with other migrainous features, such as nausea, photophobia, phonophobia, osmophobia, and increased motion sensitivity—an aversion to self-movement and external motion. Clinical examination during an attack may reveal a number of different oculomotor abnormalities, including nystagmus of a central type, or may be normal. As such, the diagnosis relies on a previous history of similar symptoms, or a strong personal or family history of migraine. Clinicians must be careful not to over-diagnose vestibular migraine: BPPV, Menière's disease, anxiety disorders, and orthostatic hypotension are more common in migraine patients than in controls [6].

Finally, Menière's disease should be considered in a patient presenting with an acute attack of vertigo, vomiting, and imbalance. However, such attacks are often accompanied by aural symptoms, such as hearing loss, a feeling of fullness or pressure in the ear, tinnitus, or otalgia. Although Menière's disease is the most common cause of acute vertigo with deafness [7], remember that acute unilateral hearing loss with vertigo is a red flag, so all patients presenting with a suspected first attack of Menière's disease should have neuroimaging performed to exclude a stroke. Clinical examination during an attack reveals peripheral vestibular nystagmus with a positive head impulse test to the affecting side. Progressive unilateral audiovestibular loss typically ensues, with lessening of the severity of acute attacks. Sudden drop attacks (Tumarkin attacks) related to otolithic disturbances may occur in the absence of other audiovestibular symptoms.

Acoustic neuromas typically present with gradually progressive unilateral hearing loss and tinnitus. Although reported [8], vertigo is rare in uncomplicated acoustic neuroma because the slow growth of the tumour allows brainstem mechanisms to compensate well for the vestibular deficit. Labyrinthine haemorrhage is a rare cause of vertigo presenting with severe and permanent hearing and vestibular loss. It is diagnosed with imaging which shows a hyperintense signal in the membranous labyrinth and cochlea, and has been associated with bleeding diatheses of varying aetiologies.

Clinical tip Vertigo versus oscillopsia

Vertigo is the sensation (i.e. a feeling) or illusion of motion, and may or may not be associated with nystagmus. Oscillopsia refers to a movement of the external world and implies the presence of nystagmus or an impaired vestibulo-ocular reflex. The patient with oscillopsia may describe that the world moves, shakes, or bounces, or may report blurring of vision. One must consider the possibility of oscillopsia in a patient with blurred vision or difficulty focusing, and probe the history further. It can be categorized into (i) continuous, (ii) paroxysmal, (iii) associated with head movements, and (iv) positional.

Learning point Types of vertigo

Vertigo can be divided into single episode, recurrent, and chronic. A single episode of vertigo may be related to acute vestibular neuritis or 'labyrinthitis', cerebellar stroke, migrainous vertigo, 'missed' BPPV, or bilateral vestibular failure. Recurrent attacks of vertigo are usually caused by BPPV. Other causes include migrainous vertigo, Menière's disease, vertebrobasilar TIAs, and perilymph fistula, or, more rarely, syphilis of the inner ear, acoustic neuroma, vestibular epilepsy, episodic ataxia type 2, and familial hemiplegic migraine. Chronic vertigo may have started with one or more attacks of vertigo. There may be a history of progressive disequilibrium, or there may be neither, in which case investigating other general medical conditions such as postural hypotension, anaemia, hypothyroidism, or a functional disorder will be warranted.

Clinical tip Vestibulo-ocular reflex (VOR)

The VOR is the fastest human reflex, occurring with a latency of < 16msec. Its role is to keep images steady on the fovea during rapid head movements (e.g. when walking or running). It works rather like a 'steadycam' by generating eye movements in the opposite direction to the head movement, but at the same velocity. This is shown in Figure 4.1.

Learning point Oscillopsia

Oscillopsia refers to an oscillation of the visual environment. Oscillopsia that is present only during head movements relates to bilateral vestibular failure as a result of an absent VOR. Patients typically describe difficulty recognizing people's faces or reading road signs while walking, running, or riding in a car, with 'bouncing' or 'blurring' of images. The oscillopsia disappears when the head is held completely still. Bilateral vestibular failure can be identified by the bedside with a bilaterally-impaired head impulse test (see Figure 4.1) or with dynamic visual acuity tests. Here, visual acuity is compared with and without head oscillation. Common causes are meningitis, ototoxicity (usually gentamicin), idiopathic, and miscellaneous (cranial neuropathies, severe head trauma). This condition is often overlooked by clinicians because the imbalance is not severe and there are no significant abnormalities on general neurological examination. Bilateral vestibular failure should be considered in patients with gait unsteadiness, particularly in the dark, or unusual visual symptoms during movement.

When oscillopsia is continuous and unrelated to movement, the most likely diagnosis is an acquired nystagmus of central origin—acquired pendular nystagmus or downbeat nystagmus (DBN). The most common causes of DBN are cerebellar disorders, including multiple system atrophy (MSA), vascular demyelination, or other miscellaneous disorders [9]. Paraneoplastic disease may also cause DBN, particularly if associated with anti-GAD antibodies.

Oscillopsia may also be paroxysmal, in which case it may be spontaneous or triggered. The latter usually relates to the Tullio phenomenon, or sound-induced vertigo, which typically results from a dehiscence of the superior semicircular canal and the direct stimulation of the labyrinth with sound. Patients with the Tullio phenomenon report oscillopsia and imbalance in response to loud sounds, in addition to diplacusis (an echoing of sounds) and autophony (an amplification of internally-generated sounds). Paroxysmal oscillopsia in just one eye is usually related to superior oblique myokymia, whereas transient, brief, and very frequent attacks with shaking of visual images with an electric-shock quality may represent vestibular paroxysmia [10].

Expert comment

The treatment of oscillopsia depends on the cause and is often unsuccessful. In a subset of patients downbeat nystagmus may respond to gabapentin, memantine, baclofen, clonazepam, or the aminopyridines [11]. Superior oblique myokymia is a spasm of the superior oblique muscle causing paroxysmal oscillopsia, and responds to low doses of carbamazepine. The Tullio phenomenon can be treated either conservatively or surgically by plugging the hole in the superior semicircular canal when a dehiscence is identified and symptoms are very severe.

Learning point Central positional nystagmus

Oscillopsia triggered by lying down or changes in head position signifies the presence of positional central nystagmus. This type of nystagmus has characteristic features that differentiate it from 'benign' peripheral causes such as BPPV. First, the nystagmus will start as soon as the head is put in that position (i.e. it has no latency), which contrasts with the nystagmus of BPPV that has a latency of a few seconds. Secondly, it does not fatigue—the nystagmus continues for as long as the head is held in that position. Thirdly, the nystagmus does not habituate, meaning that it will be present every time the head is put in that position. Again, this contrasts with peripheral causes of positional nystagmus where the intensity of the nystagmus decreases with repeated sequential positional manoeuvres.

Clinical tip Red flags for vertigo

Red flags in cases of acute dizziness include unilateral hearing loss, abnormal neurological symptoms or signs, new headache, and a **normal** VOR as assessed by the head impulse test (as this would imply that the vertigo is not originating in the peripheral vestibular system).

Final word from the expert

This case exemplifies not one but two common clinical problems—the patient with acute vertigo and the patient with recurrent (or episodic) vertigo. For the acute vertigo scenario the doctor's mind has to go into 'Has this patient had a stroke?' mode, regardless of age or vascular risk factors. In this patient's acute situation the lack of symptoms and signs indicating brainstem/cerebellar damage (e.g. no speech or fifth and sixth nerve involvement, no 'weird' nystagmus) suggests a peripheral vestibular cause. Furthermore, the presence of a positive (abnormal) head impulse test strongly suggests that the vertigo arises from an imbalance in vestibular nerve function. This combination of features would make the diagnosis of vestibular neuritis (or 'labyrinthitis'). In contrast, when the patient comes back a few weeks or months later again with vertigo, vestibular neuritis (or 'labyrinthitis') is never the right diagnosis—lightning rarely strikes twice! However, this patient's second phase of vertigo illustrates, first, a common complication of VN and, secondly, that common things are common. BPPV is by far the most common cause of recurrent vertigo—and remember that it is easily cured in five minutes with a repositioning manoeuvre (Figure 4.2c), not with drugs.

References

1. Okinaka Y, Sekitani T, Okazaki H, et al. Progress of caloric response of vestibular neuronitis. *Acta Otolaryngol Suppl* 1993; 503: 18–22.
2. Fishman JM, Burgess C, Waddell A. Corticosteroids for the treatment of idiopathic acute vestibular dysfunction (vestibular neuritis). *Cochrane Database Syst Rev* 2011; (5): CD008607.
3. Yardley L, Beech S, Weinman J. Influence of beliefs about the consequences of dizziness on handicap in people with dizziness, and the effect of therapy on beliefs. *J Psychosom Res* 2001; 50(1): 1–6.
4. Lee H, Sohn SI, Jung DK, et al. Sudden deafness and anterior inferior cerebellar artery infarction. *Stroke* 2002; 33(12): 2807–12.
5. Doyle KJ, Fowler C, Starr A. Audiologic findings in unilateral deafness resulting from contralateral pontine infarct. *Otolaryngol Head Neck Surg* 1996; 114(3): 482–6.
6. Lempert T, Neuhauser H, Daroff RB. Vertigo as a symptom of migraine. *Ann NY Acad Sci* 2009; 1164: 242–51.
7. Minor LB, Schessel DA, Carey J. Menière's disease. *Curr Opinion Neurol* 2004; 17(1): 9–16.
8. Sugimoto T, Tsutsumi T, Noguchi Y, et al. Relationship between cystic change and rotatory vertigo in patients with acoustic neuroma. *Acta Otolaryngol Suppl* 2000; 542: 9–12.
9. Wagner JN, Glaser M, Brandt T, Strupp M. Downbeat nystagmus: aetiology and comorbidity in 117 patients. *J Neurol Neurosurg Psychiatry* 2008; 79(6): 672–7.
10. Brandt T, Dieterich M. Vestibular paroxysmia: vascular compression of the eighth nerve? *Lancet* 1994; 343(8900): 798-9.
11. Kalla R, Glasauer S, Büttner U, et al. 4-Aminopyridine restores vertical and horizontal neural integrator function in downbeat nystagmus. *Brain* 2007; 130(Pt 9): 2441–51.

CASE

5 A delayed diagnosis in delirium

Benedict D. Michael and David J. Stoeter

Expert commentary Hadi Manji

Case history

A 43-year-old right-handed successful deputy director of a London-based company was brought to hospital after marked changes in behaviour and personality.

During the morning of that day, he left his office desk and was finally found by his colleagues around the back of their office building. At this time he was said to have been looking for a fire. The man was adamant that he could intermittently smell smoke, although his colleagues thought that there was no evidence of a fire. They persuaded him to return to his desk where he appeared calmer. In the early afternoon he was again absent from his desk. This time his colleagues were unable to find him anywhere on the premises. Eventually he was found after finally answering his mobile telephone. He was in a service station about 150 miles from the office.

An ambulance was sent to bring him to hospital. On admission to the emergency department, his Glasgow coma scale (GCS) score was 14/15 (eyes 4; motor 6; verbal 4) and he had an Abbreviated Mental Test Score (AMTS) of 8/10. The initial neurological examination did not identify any abnormality. There was no evidence of meningism or rash and no stigmata of alcoholic liver disease or intravenous drug abuse. He was found to have a slightly elevated serum white cell count (13.2×10^9cells/ml) and C-reactive protein (12mg/dl), normal urea, and normal electrolytes. Arterial blood gas showed normal pH, po_2, pCo_2, and bicarbonate levels. Urine dipstick test showed blood (1+) and leucocytes (1+), and was sent for formal microscopy and culture. He was started on oral trimethoprim and transferred under the care of a surgical team to await urology review.

The next day, he was reported to be acting in an increasingly bizarre manner, which was disturbing to both the nursing staff and other patients on the ward. He appeared to have strange ideas about the nursing staff, claiming that they were refusing to give him painkillers for his headache, although he had been given both oral paracetamol and tramadol. The security service and doctor on-call were contacted and he was given an intramuscular injection of haloperidol. The junior doctor noticed that he had been recorded as having an intermittent low-grade pyrexia for the previous six hours, although he was not febrile on admission or that morning. His GCS at this time was recorded as 13/15 (eyes 4; motor 5; verbal 4). Intravenous cefotaxime was started after blood cultures were sent.

A CT scan without intravenous contrast was performed the next day and was reported as normal. Once a formal radiology report of the CT scan was available, 24 hours after the patient was first given intravenous antibiotics, a lumbar puncture

(LP) was performed. Cerebrospinal fluid (CSF) analysis showed 4 RBCs, 45 WBCs (85% lymphocytes, 15% neutrophils), protein 0.65mg/dl, and CSF glucose 52mg/dl; microscopy did not identify any organisms and a bacterial culture was awaited. Opening pressure was not measured, a serum glucose sample was not sent, and no CSF sample was sent for virological analysis.

On the basis of the lymphocyte predominance, intravenous aciclovir 10mg/kg eight-hourly was started alongside cefotaxime. However, as there was a mixed lymphocyte and neutrophil picture and there were delays in performing the LP after starting antibiotics, the team decided to continue the cefotaxime as well.

On the morning of day six of admission, the patient was found to have a GCS of 7/15 (eyes 2; verbal 2; motor 3). His pupils were equal and reactive, and his plantar responses were flexor; he was thought to have bilateral papilloedema. He had a repeat CT scan, again without intravenous contrast, which did not identify any specific focal abnormality, although there was some suggestion of effacement of the sulci, possibly more of the right hemisphere.

The on-call neurology registrar was contacted and found that the GCS had actually been fluctuating between 6/15 and 13/15 over the previous one to two hours and that there had been some subtle twitching movements of the lower part of the right side of his face. An urgent electroencephalogram (EEG) was arranged, a HIV test was requested, and the team were requested to ask the microbiology laboratory to find the CSF sample and send it for viral polymerase chain reaction (PCR) at the virology laboratory. The EEG confirmed complex partial status epilepticus, so intravenous lorazepam and then phenytoin were given. The patient was transferred to the intensive care unit. His GCS improved to 14 over the next two days. The CSF culture and viral PCR were negative for herpes simplex virus (HSV) types 1 and 2, varicella zoster, and enterovirus. Aciclovir was continued but cefotaxime was stopped. A repeat LP on day eight showed an opening pressure of 28cmH_2O, WBCs 32 (90% lymphocytes, 10% neutrophils), RBCs 6, and protein 0.83g/dl; the CSF:serum glucose ratio was 78 per cent. Again, CSF microscopy did not identify any organisms and the bacterial culture was negative. This time a CSF sample was sent to virology directly; this was antibody-positive for HSV type 1 (serum:CSF albumin ratio confirmed intrathecal production) and subsequently PCR was reported as positive for HSV type 1.

His HIV antigen and antibody test were negative, his GCS returned to 15/15, and he was discharged after 12 days of intravenous aciclovir.

At 12-month follow-up he reported impaired short-term memory and frequent headaches, both of which were limiting his ability to work. He was continuing to suffer with simple partial seizures every couple of months, although this was some improvement on the previous frequency. He had no further complex partial seizures on combination anti-epileptic drug therapy.

Discussion

Definition of encephalitis

'Encephalitis' is inflammation of the brain parenchyma [1]. Therefore, fundamentally, this diagnosis can only be established by histopathological examination of brain tissue. However, as this is only possible either post-mortem, or only justified ante-mortem in a minority of patients, proxy markers of brain inflammation are routinely used [1]. Whilst there is some role for neuroimaging, it is the presence of an elevated leucocyte count in the CSF that is most often used clinically to establish the presence of inflammation, and culture and molecular analysis of the CSF that identifies the aetiology [1,2]. Encephalitis can present with an encephalopathic picture, for which there is a broad range of differential diagnoses including systemic, metabolic, toxic, endocrine disturbances, neoplastic or vascular processes, and infection outside of the CNS. However, these are distinguished from encephalitis by the absence of evidence of inflammation in the CSF or on imaging [1]. Nevertheless, there is a broad range of aetiologies even once encephalitis has been established.

Epidemiology

The estimated incidence of encephalitis is reported as 0.7–13.8 per 100,000 per year, equating to approximately 700 cases per year in the UK and approximately 70–140 deaths [2–4]. Although a relatively rare diagnosis, it may be as common a cause of stupor or coma as subarachnoid haemorrhage in patients for whom a neurological opinion is requested [5]. Moreover it is important for two further reasons; first, cases of **suspected** encephalitis are not uncommon and, secondly delays in establishing the diagnosis and starting treatment can result in significant morbidity and mortality for many causes. For example, in encephalitis due to HSV type 1, the most common sporadic cause, mortality can be as high as 70–90 per cent in those who are untreated or treated late and can be reduced to 20–30 per cent if treatment is started early [3].

Aetiology of encephalitis

The most common cause of encephalitis is infection; encephalitis can occur due to direct infection of the CNS or due to para- or post-infectious immune-mediated processes, such as acute disseminated encephalomyelitis (ADEM) or cerebelitis [1]. An immune-mediated encephalitis can also occur as part of a paraneoplastic disease for which specific antibodies directed against CNS antigens may be identified. Additionally, some forms of antibody-associated encephalitis can occur as part of a primary autoimmune process in the absence of neoplasia [5], although this appears to be a relatively less common cause of encephalitis compared with cases related to infection [4].

Herpes simplex virus encephalitis

HSV encephalitis has an estimated annual incidence of 1 in 250,000–500,000 [2, 4]. Approximately 90 per cent of cases of HSV encephalitis are due to HSV type 1 and approximately 10 per cent are due to HSV type 2 which more often causes meningitis [1]. HSV is an alpha herpes DNA virus. Whereas HSV type 2 is transmitted sexually. The majority of the population are exposed to HSV type 1 during childhood, and by adulthood almost all have been infected through transmission by droplet spread [6]. The virus crosses the oral mucous membrane and travels by retrograde axonal transport along the trigeminal nerve to then establish latency in the trigeminal ganglion. Periodically the virus reactivates and travels by antegrade axonal transport to be shed; this usually occurs asymptomatically, but in a small proportion will be manifest as a herpes labialis [6]. Rarely, the virus will replicate in the brain, resulting in encephalitis; it is not clear whether this follows directly from further retrograde axonal transport after reactivation in the trigeminal ganglion or is due to reactivation of virus latent within the brain. Indeed, a proportion of people who die without evidence of any neurological disease will have the nucleic acid of this highly neurotropic virus within the brain parenchyma [7]. HSV type 1 encephalitis occurs in a bimodal distribution with peaks in incidence in young adults and the elderly [4].

The clinical picture is typically an alteration in cognition, consciousness, personality, or behaviour which occurs either during or following a febrile or coryzal illness [1]. Associated clinical features include headache, which may be severe, features of meningism (neck stiffness and photophobia), seizures, or features suggesting raised intracranial pressure, such as papilloedema [3]. Traditionally, seizures reflecting involvement of the frontal lobes, or temporal lobes, as in the case described, were thought to be specific for HSV encephalitis. However, it is now considered that no clinical features, or combination thereof, are sufficiently sensitive or specific to diagnose or exclude encephalitis overall or indeed the specific aetiology of the encephalitis. Therefore examination of the CSF and, to a lesser extent neuroimaging, are vital in establishing the diagnosis of encephalitis and the aetiology [1–3]. Nevertheless, some clinical features can act as pointers for possible diagnoses:

Learning point Pearls and pitfalls in the history and examination

It is increasingly recognised that the GCS is a very crude proxy of cerebral dysfunction; rather, the clinician should look for the, sometimes more subtle, features of alterations in personality, behaviour, or cognition [1,2]. Certainly a comment from a relative or friend stating that the patient is not 'themselves' should not be disregarded.

Moreover, although fever was once considered the ubiquitous feature of CNS infection, it is now realized that as many as 28 per cent of patients with acute encephalitis may not have a fever on admission, and up to 24 per cent of those with proven HSV type 1 encephalitis may not be febrile on admission [4].

Therefore, the clinician must be vigilant in asking about a history of recent fever prior to admission and keep a close eye on the observation chart for episodes of low-grade pyrexia [1].

Because of the non-specific nature of the presentation, in the early stages the differential diagnosis is broad. Nevertheless, as in the case described here, the cause of the acute confusional state should not be attributed to an infection outside the CNS in an otherwise fit and healthy individual when there is limited evidence to support it [3]. The elderly patient with long-term oxygen-dependent chronic obstructive pulmonary disease who has an acute severe multilobar pneumonia and type 2 respiratory failure is clearly quite different from the 43-year-old previously well patient described here, where the only evidence to support an infection outside the CNS was some minor changes on ward test urinalysis. Indeed, 10–50 per cent of patients may have coexistent urinary, respiratory, or gastrointestinal symptoms [4]. However, there are two important caveats to consider. First, HSV encephalitis has a bimodal distribution with peaks in both the young and older adults [3, 4]. Secondly, whilst patients with physiological alcohol dependence often present with an acute confusional state due to toxic, withdrawal, or nutritional causes, infectious encephalitis is also more common in this group [1].

With the emergence of novel pathogens, the spread of previously geographically restricted pathogens, and the expansion of global travel a thorough travel and vaccination history is vital—for example, travel to areas with arboviral encephalitides, such as Japanese encephalitis virus in east Asia or West Nile virus in the Middle East, Southern Europe, and North America. Also liaise closely with your regional infectious disease team when there may be a significant travel history and/or Public Health England for advice on samples required for specific tests and disease notification [1].

(Continued)

Focal neurological signs may be present, such as multiple cranial nerve palsies reflecting brainstem involvement, which is more commonly seen as a rhombencephalitis due to flaviviruses, enterovirus, or listeria [1]. However, cranial nerve palsies may also be a false localizing sign due to brain shift or may be due to infiltration of the basal meninges in mycoplasma tuberculosis infection, although this history is typically longer [3].

Recent years have seen improved understanding of the role of antibody-mediated encephalitides. Clinical clues to these disorders include features such as a sub-acute presentation (weeks to months), movement disorders (such as orofacial dyskinesia, choreoathetosis or faciobrachial dystonia) or seizures, particularly if intractable [1,8]. Additionally, hyponatraemia may be present, but this is not specific to antibody-mediated encephalitis [3,4].

Learning point When to do a LP, when to get a CT first

As interpretation of the CSF is vital to directing treatment (Table 5.1). A LP is a crucial investigation in the work-up of a patient with suspected encephalitis and therefore should be considered in all patients as soon as possible [1]. Although concerns have been raised about LP and the risk of herniation of the cerebellar tonsils and uncus, national guidelines from the National Institute for Health and Care Excellence (NICE), the British Infection Association, and the Association of British Neurologists have all confirmed that neuroimaging cannot accurately predict the risk of herniation, and therefore a LP should be performed without the need to wait for neuroimaging in patients with suspected meningoencephalitis unless clear **clinical** contraindications are present (Table 5.2) [1, 9, 10]. If these clinical contraindications are present, neuroimaging should be performed to identify a possible alternative diagnosis or significant brain shift caused by, or causing, obstructive raised intracranial pressure. If they are excluded, then a LP should be performed as soon as possible after neuroimaging [1, 9, 10]. In the case presented here, the on-call doctor was unable to perform the LP without the assistance of the medical registrar. Several studies have identified delayed LPs as a major component of the sub-optimal care that many patients receive [2]. To help to address such issues we have published an educational video tutorial [11]. Moreover, interpretation of the CSF glucose is significantly impaired if the concomitant serum glucose is not known, as in the first LP of the case described here [1]. In addition, measurement of the opening pressure and, to a greater extent, virology PCR analysis are important in determining the aetiology [1,3]. PCR is a highly specific and sensitive test, but may be negative in the first few days or later on in the disease, particularly after aciclovir has been started [1]. Therefore in such cases CSF viral antibodies, which are typically present from days seven to ten of the disease, can be useful. Rieber's formula comparing the CSF with the serum albumin ratio is required to confirm intrathecal antibody production [12]:

$$\text{antibody index} = \frac{(\text{CSF antibody concentration/serum antibody concentration})}{(\text{CSF albumin concentration/serum albumin concentration})}.$$

In the case described here none of these investigations were performed on the first LP. We have published a lumbar puncture pack to try to encourage doctors to perform the necessary investigations (Figure 5.1) [13].

In the case described here the clinicians were unclear as to whether the lymphocyte predominance in the CSF reflected viral infection or partially treated bacterial infection, because the patient had been on antibiotics prior to the LP. In addition, starting antibiotics prior to performing the LP can reduce the chance of culturing a bacterial pathogen [14]. Nevertheless, polymerase chain reaction for bacteria and viruses is likely to remain positive in the early period following treatment [12].

Table 5.1 Interpretation of investigations performed at the time of lumbar puncture

Investigation	Normal	Bacterial	Viral	Tuberculous	Fungal	Antibody-associated
Opening pressure	10–20cm*	High	Normal-high	High	High-very high	Normal-high
Colour	Clear	Cloudy	Clear (so-called 'gin clear')	Cloudy/yellow	Clear/cloudy	Clear
Cells/mm^3	<5†	High-very high (100–50,000)	Slightly increased (5–100)	Slightly increased (25–500)	Normal-high (0–1000)	Normal-slightly increased (<5–500)
Predominant differential	Lymphocytes	Neutrophils	Lymphocytes	Lymphocytes	Lymphocytes	Lymphocytes
CSF:plasma glucose ratio	66%‡	Low	Normal-slightly low	Low-very low (<30%)	Normal-low	Normal
Protein (g/L)	<0.45	High >1	Normal-high (0.5–1)	High-very high (1.0–5.0)	Normal-very high (0.2–5.0)	Normal-high (0.5–1)

*Normal opening pressure is less than ~20cm in adults.

†A 'bloody tap' will falsely elevate both CSF white cell count and protein. To approximately correct for this subtract one white cell/mm^3 for every 700 red blood cells/mm^3 and 0.1g/dL of protein for every 1000 red blood cells/mm^3.

‡'Normal' CSF glucose ratio is typically quoted as 66%, although in practice only values below 50% are likely to be significant.

Some important exceptions:

- in viral CNS infections, an early or late LP may not demonstrate a pleocytosis or an early LP may show neutrophil predominance
- in partially treated bacterial meningitis the CSF pleocytosis may be low and/or may show a lymphocytic predominance
- early CSF in *Mycobacterium tuberculosis* may have predominant polymorphs
- listeria can give a similar CSF picture to tuberculous meningitis
- CSF findings in cases of a bacterial abscess range from near normal to purulent depending on the location and whether there is associated meningitis or rupture
- a cryptococcal antigen test and India ink stain should be performed on all CSF samples of immunocompromised patients.

Adapted from *J Infect* 64(4), Solomon T, Michael BD, Smith PE, et al., On behalf of the National Encephalitis Guidelines Development Group, Management of suspected viral encephalitis in adults: Association of British Neurologists and British Infection Association National Guideline, pp. 347–73, © 2012, with permission from Elsevier.

Table 5.2 Clinical contraindications to lumbar puncture without neuroimaging

Signs of raised ICP	Cushing's reflex, papilloedema, abnormal respiratory pattern, decorticate/decerebrate posturing, altered pupillary response, absent doll's eye reflex
Seizure	If convulsive and within 30min or lasting >30min or if focal or tonic
Focal neurological signs	Hemi/monoparesis, extensor plantars, ocular palsies
Glasgow coma score	<13 or deterioration by >2 points
Strong suspicion of meningococcal sepsis	Typical purpuric rash in an ill child
Systemic shock	
Local superficial infection	At potential LP site
Coagulation disorder	
Immunocompromised	

Some have also suggested that those aged > 60 years should undergo a CT scan first as there is a higher proportion with other diagnoses such as strokes and neoplasia

Data from *N Engl J Med* 345(24), Hasbun R, Abrahams J, Jekel J, et al., Computed tomography of the head before lumbar puncture in adults with suspected meningitis, pp. 1727–33, © 2001, with permission from Massachusetts Medical Society.

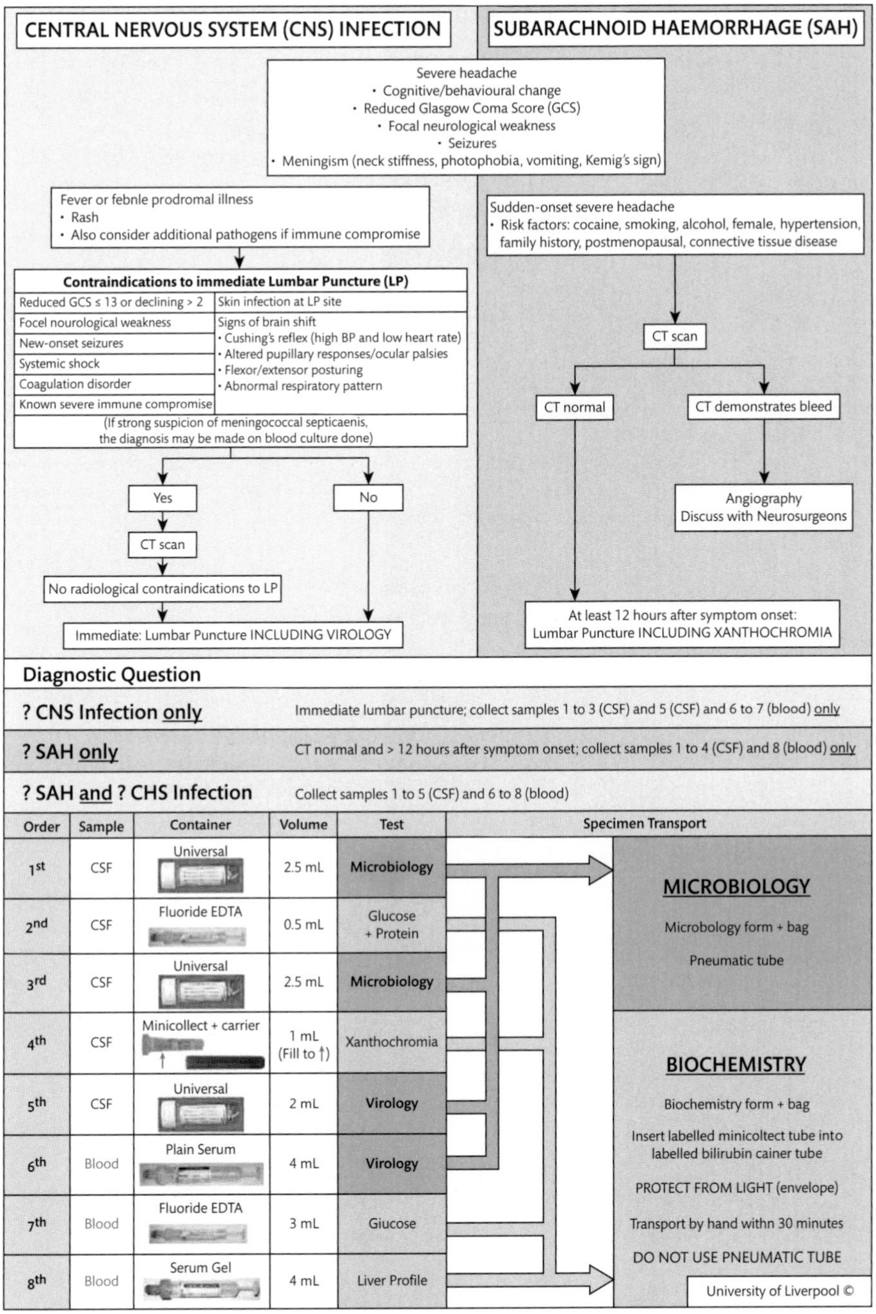

Figure 5.1 Lumbar puncture pack, (with thanks to Dr Sarah Curtis).

> **Clinical tip** When can one have safely excluded viral encephalitis?
>
> Recent UK guidelines have recommended that aciclovir can be stopped in immunocompetent patients if an alternative diagnosis has been made, or if HSV PCR in the CSF is negative on two occasions 24–48 hours apart and MRI is not characteristic for HSV encephalitis (Figure 5.2), or if HSV PCR in the CSF is negative once >72 hours after neurological symptom onset, with unaltered consciousness, normal MRI (performed >72 hours after symptom onset), and a CSF white cell count <5/mm^3 [1].

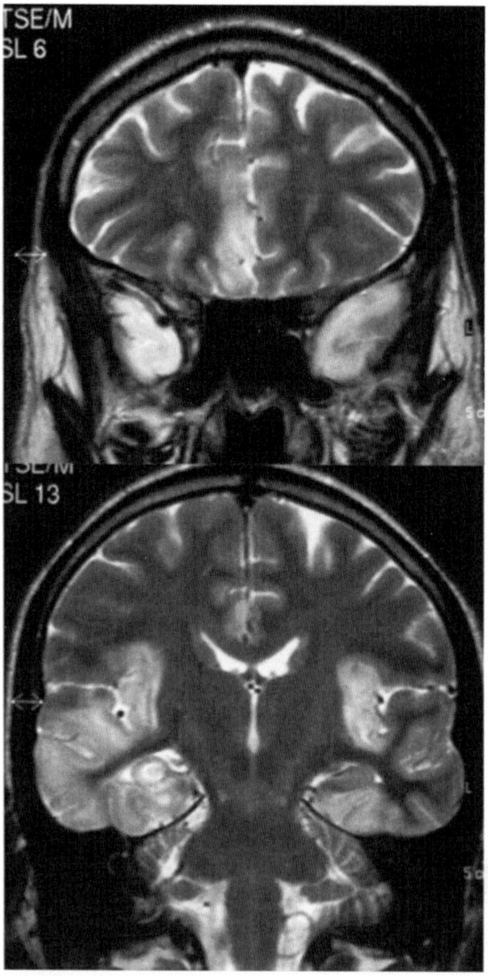

Figure 5.2 T2-weighted MRI in a patient with encephalitis due to HSV type 1: upper panel demonstrates right frontal hyperintensity, predominantly in the orbitofrontal cortex; lower panel demonstrates bilateral, but asymmetrical, hyperintensity of the temporal lobes and hippocampi.

Courtesy of Dr Ian Turnbull.

Clinical tip When can aciclovir be safely stopped in HSV encephalitis?

Recent UK guidelines recommend that in immunocompetent patients with proven HSV encephalitis intravenous aciclovir be continued for at least 14 days, and a repeat LP performed at this time to confirm that the CSF is negative for HSV by PCR. If the CSF is still positive, aciclovir should be continued intravenously, with weekly CSF PCR until it is negative [1].

If the patient is imunocompromised or aged between three months and 12 years the minimum course of treatment, before repeating the LP, should be 21 days as these groups are at higher risk of relapse [15].

Learning point Use and misuse of electroencephalography (EEG)

An EEG is not required for every patient with suspected or proven encephalitis, and periodic lateralizing epileptiform discharges (PLEDs), although once considered pathognomonic for HSV encephalitis, are now known to be non-specific features of many pathologies [16]. However, EEG does have two important roles. In a patient with clinical features that raise uncertainty as to whether there is an underlying organic or psychiatric cause, an EEG can be useful to assess encephalopathic changes [1]. Also, in patients with suspected non-convulsive status epilepticus (Figure 5.3), as in the case described here, an EEG should be performed for diagnosis. EEG monitoring can also be valuable in assessing response to treatment [1].

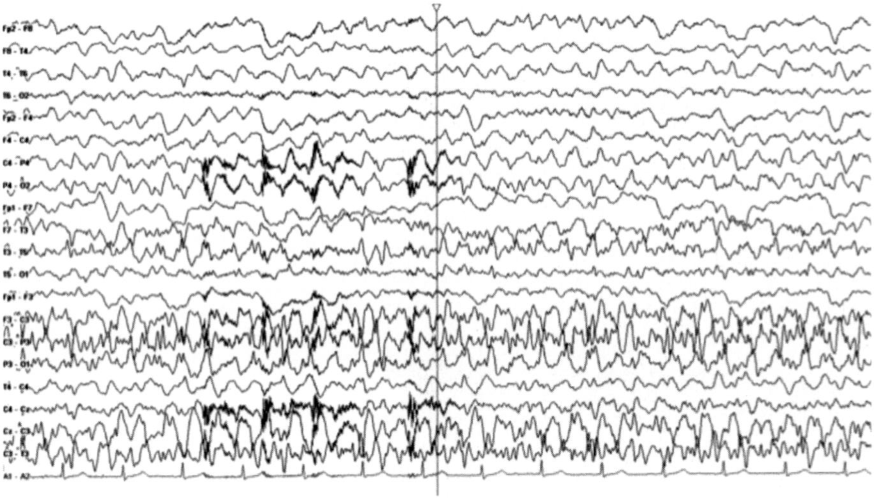

Figure 5.3 EEG demonstrating non-convulsive motor status epilepticus.

Courtesy of Dr Radhika Manohar.

Learning point Acute complications of CNS infections

If the conscious level of a patient who is being investigated or treated for encephalitis deteriorates, non-convulsive status epilepticus should be considered as specific anti-epileptic drug treatment will be required, particularly in patients who are experiencing fluctuations in their conscious level or who are demonstrating subtle motor features, such as twitching of the fingertips [1].

If a patient with an acute CNS infection develops seizures or their conscious level deteriorates, whilst this might be due to the underlying pathophysiology, it is necessary to consider para-infectious processes, including hyponatraemia and venous sinus thrombosis, which may be important [1, 3, 17]

Evidence base

In 1986 Whitley et al. [18] published a randomized controlled trial of 69 patients with biopsy-proven HSV encephalitis in which they report that 28 per cent of the 32 who received aciclovir 30mg/kg/day and 54 per cent of the 37 who received vidarabine 15mg/kg/day ($p = 0.008$) died. In addition, six-month morbidity, using the adapted scoring system, identified that 12 (38 per cent) of those who received aciclovir were functioning normally, as opposed to five (14 per cent) of those who received vidarabine ($p = 0.02$). This study also identified, that, in those treated with aciclovir, a GCS >10, 7–10, or <7 at the time of commencing treatment was associated with a six-month mortalities of 0 per cent, 25 per cent, and 25 per cent respectively.

This landmark study dramatically changed the way in which we treat patients with suspected HSV encephalitis in terms of both the drug of choice and the emphasis on early treatment before there is a significant decline in the GCS, and therefore often before the diagnosis has been confirmed. However, in 2015, it is disappointing to think that the most recent trial that improved practice for a condition that continues to have high rates of morbidity and mortality was performed nearly three decades ago. It is hoped that the growing field of neuroimmunological modulation may provide adjunctive therapies to improve practice, and therefore patient outcomes, in the future.

Expert comment

Features that suggest a systemic cause, such as toxic, metabolic, or endocrine disturbance or a locus of infection outside the CNS include a history of previous such episodes, symmetrical neurological findings, such as positive or negative myoclonus, a profound acid-base disturbance, or a clear and severe locus of infection, particularly in patients with prior cognitive impairment [1]. The features of a bimodal age distribution, or possibly degrees of immunosuppression such as chronic alcohol dependence, may be more common in those with HSV encephalitis. However, HSV encephalitis can present at any age and typically without any history to suggest an impaired immune response. Therefore, when a patient presents with acute changes in cognition, consciousness, personality, or behaviour, particularly in the context of current or antecedent febrile illness, even if low-grade, we would argue that the CNS requires urgent investigation, especially with a LP where possible, before attributing CNS symptoms and signs to a problem outside the CNS.

Final word from the expert

Many patients present to general clinicians and neurologists with alterations in consciousness every day, up and down the country, and, whilst around 80 per cent will not have a CNS infection and maybe only six per cent will have encephalitis, the consequences of delayed or missed diagnoses, which include death in 70-90 per cent of patients with HSV encephalitis are such that a low threshold for investigation and treatment is demanded [2,18]. It is hoped that recent National Encephalitis Guidelines will go some way to addressing this as, unfortunately, cases such as that described here are all too common currently [1,15].

The authors acknowledge the work of Andy Roberts in the development of the Liverpool Lumbar Puncture Pack video [11].

References

1. Solomon T, Michael BD, Smith PE, et al. Management of suspected viral encephalitis in adults: Association of British Neurologists and British Infection Association National Guideline. *J Infect* 2012; 64(4): 347–73.
2. Michael BD, Sidhu M, Stoeter D, et al. The epidemiology and management of adult suspected central nervous system infections—a retrospective cohort study in the NHS Northwest Region. *Q J Med* 2010; 103(10): 749–5.
3. Solomon T, Hart IJ, Beeching NJ. Viral encephalitis: a clinician's guide. *Pract Neurol* 2007; 7: 288–305.
4. Granerod J, Ambrose HE, Davies NW, et al. Causes of encephalitis and differences in their clinical presentations in England: a multicentre, population-based prospective study. *Lancet Infect Dis* 2010; 10: 835–44.
5. Posner JB, Saper CB, Schiff ND, et al. *Plum and Posner's Diagnosis of Stupor and Coma* (4th edn) (Oxford: Oxford University Press); 2007: 4–5.
6. Whitley RJ (2006) Herpes simplex encephalitis: adolescents and adults. *Antiviral Res.* 71: 141–8.
7. Wozniak MA, Shipley SJ, Combrinck M, et al. Productive herpes simplex virus in brain of elderly normal subjects and Alzheimer's disease patients. *J Med Virol* 2005; 75(2): 300–6.
8. Jarius S, Hoffmann L, Clover L, et al. CSF findings in patients with voltage gated potassium channel antibody associated limbic encephalitis. *J Neurol Sci* 2008; 268(1–2): 74–7.

9. Heyderman RS, British Infection Society. Early management of suspected bacterial meningitis and meningococcal septicaemia in immunocompetent adults–second edition. *J Infect* 2005; 50: 373–4.
10. Visintin C, Mugglestone MA, Fields EJ, et al. Management of bacterial meningitis and meningococcal septicaemia in children and young people: summary of NICE guidance. *BMJ* 2010; 340: c3209.
11. Michael BD, Roberts A. Liverpool lumbar puncture pack—How to video: <http://www.youtube.com/watch?v=TYB7kyiic0Y> accessed 23 July 2012).
12. Ambrose HE, Granerod J, Clewley JP, et al. Diagnostic strategy used to establish etiologies of encephalitis in a prospective cohort of patients in England. *J Clin Microbiol* 2011; 49(10): 3576–83.
13. Michael BD, Powell GA, Curtis S, et al. Improving the diagnosis of central nervous system infections in adults through introduction of a simple lumbar puncture pack: a quality improvement project. *Emerg Med J* 2013; 30(5): 402–5.
14. Michael BD, Menezes BF, Cunniffe J, et al. The effect of delayed lumbar punctures on the diagnosis of acute bacterial meningitis in adults. *Emergency Med J* 2010; 27(6): 433–8.
15. Kneen R, Michael BD, Menson E, et al. Management of suspected viral encephalitis in children: Association of British Neurologists and British Paediatric Allergy, Immunology and Infection Group National Guideline. *J Infect* 2012; 64(5): 449–77.
16. Kate MP, Dash GK, Radhakrishnan A. Long-term outcome and prognosis of patients with emergent periodic lateralized epileptiform discharges (ePLEDs). *Seizure* 2012; 21(6): 450–6.
17. Irani SR, Alexander S, Waters P, et al. Antibodies to Kv1 potassium channel-complex proteins leucine-rich, glioma inactivated 1 protein and contactin-associated protein-2 in limbic encephalitis, Morvan's syndrome and acquired neuromyotonia. *Brain* 2010; 133: 2734–48.
18. Whitley RJ, Alford CA, Hirsch MS, et al. Vidarabine versus acyclovir therapy in herpes simplex encephalitis. *N Engl J Med* 1986; 314: 144–9.

CASE

6 Writer's cramp

Anna Sadnicka

Expert commentary: Mark J. Edwards and Kailash P. Bhatia

Case history

A right-handed 35-year-old woman working as a legal secretary was referred to clinic. For approximately six months she had been having increasing difficulty writing. After writing a few words the middle, ring, and little fingers of her right hand started to curl uncontrollably and she found that she needed to grip the pen tightly. She previously had excellent handwriting, but when seen in clinic she complained that it was barely legible, slow, and laborious. There were no problems with other manual tasks such as putting on make-up or using cutlery. She did not associate the onset of symptoms with any local injury or precipitating factor. She was otherwise well and there was no family history of a similar disorder.

An examination of the patient demonstrated flexion of the three lateral fingers of her right hand during writing and an abnormal (probably compensatory) flexion and elevation of the wrist. There was no evidence of dystonia at rest or on posture, or evidence of tremor. The neurological examination was otherwise normal.

The patient was referred for electromyography-guided botulinum toxin injections. There was good response to this therapy, and it was continued for the next ten years until she felt that the injections were having no effect. Over the next four years there was a clear progression of her symptoms. She developed a prominent jerky tremor of the right arm and abnormal postures of the left arm. Her head turned involuntarily to the left, which was relieved to some extent by touching the side of her face. Her voice because strangulated and irregular in pitch. She experienced involuntary clenching of the jaw, particularly during speech (Figure 6.1). Her left foot started turning in when she was walking, and noticed that she was scuffing her foot when she walked. There was a deterioration in her symptoms throughout the day and she thought that there was a benefit from sleep. A detailed neurological examination at this time did not reveal any other neurological signs. An MRI scan of the brain was normal.

Expert comment

Initially the patient fitted well into the diagnostic category of action-specific focal hand dystonia (Table 6.1). Over the previous two years this has clearly changed. Although there is no family history, she should be tested for mutations in the *TOR1A* (*DYT1*) and, if negative, *THAP1* (*DYT6*) genes (Table 6.2). These are the most common inherited causes of generalized dystonia. Dopa-responsive dystonia is important to consider, as response to treatment is usually dramatic. The disease classically presents at a younger age, but adult cases have been described and the diurnal fluctuation described by the patient is suggestive of this disorder. The history is against an acquired dystonia due to a known specific cause; for example, she has not previously been exposed to dopamine-receptor-blocking drugs which can cause tardive dystonia. One should always exclude Wilson's disease, which is treatable, and also investigate other causes of dystonia in which there is prominent bulbar involvement such as neuroacanthocytosis and neuronal brain iron accumulation.

Learning point Definition of dystonia

The history is suggestive of writing dystonia/writer's cramp—a focal form of dystonia. The dystonias are a heterogenous group of hyperkinetic movement disorders. A recently revised formal definition of dystonia is [1]:

Dystonia is a movement disorder characterized by sustained or intermittent muscle contractions causing abnormal, often repetitive movements, postures or both. Dystonic movement are typically patterned, twisting and may be tremulous. Dystonia is often initiated or worsened by voluntary action and associated with overflow muscle activation.

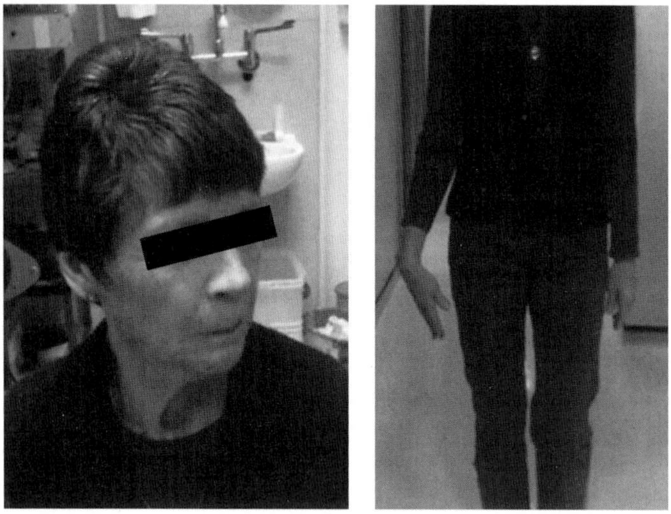

Figure 6.1 Clinical involvement of oromandibular, cervical, and upper limb muscles is demonstrated.

Table 6.1 The classification of dystonia

Axis I. Clinical characteristics	
Clinical characteristics of dystonia	
(i) Age at onset	Infancy (birth to 2 years) Childhood (3–12 years) Adolescence (13–20 years) Early adulthood (21–40 years) Late adulthood (>40 years)
(ii) Body distribution	Focal Segmental Multifocal Generalized Hemidystonia
(iii) Temporal pattern	Disease course Static Progressive Variability Persistent Action-specific Diurnal Paroxysmal
Associated features	
(iv) Isolated dystonia or combined with another movement disorder	
(v) Occurrence of other neurological or systemic manifestations	
Axis II. Aetiology	
(i) Nervous system pathology	Evidence of degeneration Evidence of structural (often static) lesions No evidence of degeneration or structural lesion
(ii) Inherited or acquired	Inherited Acquired (e.g. infection, drug, psychogenic) Idiopathic (sporadic or familial)

Reproduced from *Movement Disorders* 28(7), Albanese A, Bhatia K, Bressman SB, et al., Phenomenology and classification of dystonia: a consensus update, pp. 863–873, © 2013, with permission from John Wiley and Sons.

Table 6.2 Investigations to consider in the work-up of dystonia

Bloods	Copper, ceruloplasmin (Wilson's disease) Acanthocytes (neuroacanthocytosis, NBIA) Creatine kinase (neuroacanthocytosis) Plasma amino acids (amino acidaemias) White cell enzymes (GM1/2 gangliosidosis) Alphafetoprotein (ataxia telangieactasia) Immunoglobulins (ataxia telangiectasia)
Urine	24hour urinary copper (Wilson's disease) Urinary organic acids (amino-acidaemias)
Genetic tests	*TOR1A*, *THAP1* (*DYT1*, *DYT6*) Huntingtin (Huntington's disease) *PANK2* (NBIA) Ferritin light chain (NBIA) *SCA1, 2, 3, 5, 7, 17* (spinocerebellar ataxia) *DRPLA* gene (dentatorubral-pallidoluysian atrophy) *NPC1/2* (Niemann pick C) *ATM* (ataxia telangiectasia) *TIMM8A* (Mohr-Tranebjaerg syndrome) *PLA2G6* (*PLA2G6*-associated neurodegeneration) *ATP13A2* (Kufor-Rakeb syndrome)
Imaging	
MRI brain	Iron deposition (NBIA) Caudate atrophy (Huntington's disease) White matter high signal (amino-acidaemias)
CT brain	Calcium deposition can be missed on MRI (mitochondrial disorders)
Functional imaging	DaT scan (abnormal in Parkinson's disease, progressive supranuclear palsy, multiple system atrophy, corticobasal degeneration)
Other	Slit-lamp examination (Wilson's disease) Nerve conduction studies Electro-retinography (e.g. retinitis pigmentosa seen in NBIA)

Further investigations were sent and no evidence of a metabolic or neurodegenerative disorder were found (blood tests for Wilson's disease, neuroacanthocytosis, and neuronal brain accumulation syndromes were negative). Genetic tests for *DYT1* and *DYT6* dystonia were also negative, and a trial of levodopa (given the possibility of dopa-responsive dystonia) was ineffective. Trihexyphenidyl was started with limited response (Table 6.3). Because of the severity of her symptoms and the limitation of speech the patient was keen to discuss the possibility of deep brain stimulation. She was reviewed by the deep brain stimulation multidisciplinary team and was offered bilateral internal globus pallidum stimulation.

Discussion

This case illustrates some of the clinical spectrum of dystonia and treatment strategies. It is unusual because the patient initially appeared to have a focal dystonia which later became more generalized. It also emphasizes the need for a clinician to be alert to changes in phenotype that do no fit with the original diagnosis so that appropriate investigations can be initiated.

Table 6.3 Treatment of dystonia

Therapy	Individualized retraining programmes can be effective in relieving the symptoms of both generalized and focal dystonia. These use a variety of techniques which aim to increase control and range of movement and retrain the brain towards healthy non-dystonic movements.
Medication	A trial of levodopa is appropriate in any patients in which dopa-responsive dystonia is a possibility. Trihexiphenidyl, an anticholinergic medication, is often used as first-line therapy. Trihexiphenidyl is usually gradually titrated to a dose of 2-4mg tds. Second-line medications that may be of benefit include clonazepam, tetrabenazine, and baclofen. It is uncommon, but not unknown, for focal dystonias to respond to drug therapy.
Botulinum toxin	Botulinum toxin treatment continues to be the mainstay of treatment for most types of focal dystonia. The injection pattern depends on the distribution of dystonia and severity. Injections usually take 2-3 days to start working, have their peak effect by 2 weeks, and wear off in approximately 2-4 months Repeat injections are necessary to maintain effect. The toxin works primarily by reducing neurotransmitter release in the presynaptic terminal and thus weakening the target muscle. It may also desensitize sensory receptors in the muscle (muscle spindles). Use in generalized dystonia is usually limited to focal disability which is resistant to treatment (medication or deep brain stimulation).
Deep brain stimulation	Long-term bilateral electrical stimulation of the internal globus pallidum is now established as an effective treatment for various types of dystonia.

Adapted from *European Journal of Neurology* 13(5), Albanese A, Barnes MP, Bhatia KP, et al., A systematic review on the diagnosis and treatment of primary (idiopathic) dystonia and dystonia plus syndromes: report of an EFNS/MDS-ES Task Force, pp. 433–44, © 2006, with permission from John Wiley and Sons; *Current Treatment Options in Neurology*, 14(3), Batla A, Stamelou M, Bhatia KP, Treatment of focal dystonia, pp. 213–29, © 2012, with permission from Springer.

The diagnosis of dystonia is clinical. It is characterized by abnormal posture (with or without tremor) due to excessive flexion, extension, or torsion of body regions [2]. Another feature suggestive of dystonia is the presence of *gestes antagonistes* [3]. These are sensory tricks, typically described in cervical dystonia, in which a light touch to the face or chin can relieve both dystonic postures and dystonic movements. The examination of patients with dystonia should include an assessment of body posture for each major body region during rest, during particular postures and during movement in order to delineate the extent of clinical involvement. Associated signs such as pyramidal disturbance, parkinsonism, and cerebellar features suggest an alternate diagnosis. Electromyography is rarely used in diagnosis, but if performed frequently reveals coactivation of agonist and antagonist muscles and overflow into adjacent muscle groups that are not usually activated by a given task. An MRI scan is often not required in adult-onset dystonia with no other neurological features.

Clinical tip Dystonia syndromes

Commonly encountered patterns of dystonia are described below.

Generalized isolated dystonia

Onset is usually in late childhood or adolescence with dystonia of the lower limbs which spreads over months to years to become generalized (in a minority of patients the dystonia remains focal). There is an equal sex ratio. Symptoms typically plateau, although they may fluctuate throughout the years. Specific gene mutations of *TOR1A* (*DYT1*) and *THAP1* (*DYT6*) cause dystonia and both are inherited in an autosomal dominant manner with reduced penetrance (approximately 30 per cent for *DYT1* and 60 per cent for *DYT6*). These two mutations account for over half the cases of generalized dystonia.

Focal or segmental isolated dystonia

Onset is usually in adulthood. Limb dystonia typically occurs in the third and fourth decades and is more common in men, whereas craniocervical dystonia usually has its onset in the fifth decade and is more common in women.

Writer's cramp/writing dystonia usually starts as an action-specific dystonia but can progress so that dystonia is present when performing other manual tasks. If patients learn to write with the other hand, about a third will develop dystonia bilaterally. Pain is not usually prominent; however, tremor on writing can coexist or be the dominant feature. There are many other types of task-specific or occupational focal dystonias. For example, in musicians' dystonia the abnormal movement can be very subtle, but because of the exceptional spatiotemporal control that their occupation demands the dystonia can be devastating for careers. Similarly, the fast footwork required for flamenco dance predisposes to dystonia of the foot [4].

Cervical dystonia (or spasmodic torticollis) usually starts with gradual discomfort in the neck followed by involuntary pulling of the head in a particular direction. A jerky tremor is common and can be the predominant clinical feature. Symptoms usually progress over 6–12 months and then plateau.

Oromandibular dystonia affects the muscles of mastication with additional involvement of the platysma. Initially, dystonia may be triggered by speaking or chewing, but later will occur spontaneously. This can look very similar to the abnormal movements caused by long-term use of dopamine-receptor-blocking drugs, so a careful drug history should always be elicited.

Laryngeal dystonia affects the vocal cords. The most common is adductor dystonia in which the vocal cords are held together; this classically causes a strangled voice with frequent variations in pitch. Less commonly, abductor dystonia holds the vocal cords apart, resulting in a whispering breathy voice.

Blepharospasm affects the muscles around the eyes and tends to have an older age of onset than the other craniocervical dystonias (mean age of onset is 63 years). There is often a gritty or uncomfortable feeling in the eyes before the onset of the spasm in the orbicularis oculi.

Learning point Phenomena suggestive of dystonia

A hallmark of dystonia which emphasizes the important role of the sensory system in its pathophysiology is the sensory trick. It was first described by the French school of neurology in the late nineteenth century (*geste antagoniste*) [3]. Some patients with cervical dystonia have reported useful control of their dystonia using sensory tricks for more than 20 years. The mechanisms of *geste antagoniste* are poorly understood; it seems that by changing the sensory information sent to the brain improved control over dystonic contractions can be achieved.

Additionally, there can be a paradoxical improvement in dystonia symptoms with motor activity. With dystonia of the lower extremity running or walking backwards frequently fails to trigger the abnormal posture [5]. Patients with torticollis describe improvement in their symptoms while playing tennis or can watch TV better while knitting. One amateur musician demonstrated a dramatic improvement in his generalized dystonia while playing the piano [6].

The current classification of dystonia incorporates recent research findings and defines patients along two axes (details shown in Table 6.1). The first axis uses five descriptors of the clinical characteristics of the dystonia. The structure aims to provide a useful framework for prognostic purposes and for identifying management strategies [1]. The second axis addresses aetiology, and the two descriptors (identifiable pathology and pattern of inheritance) are considered to be complementary. The term 'primary dystonia' is now discouraged as it is currently used as an aetiological descriptor which includes both genetic and idiopathic cases, and as such this dual meaning does not aid clarity [7].

The pathophysiology of dystonia remains poorly understood. There has been a rapid increase in the speed of genetic discoveries over recent years because of advances in sequencing technologies. Monogenic forms of dystonia currently include *TOR1A* mutations (*DYT1*, usually generalized), *THAP1* mutations (*DYT6*, usually generalized), *ANO3* (*DYT23*, craniocervical dystonia), *GNAL* (usually cervical), *CIZ1* (cervical), and *TUBB4A* (*DYT4*, laryngeal progressing to generalized dystonia) [8]. Furthermore, mutations that confer risk for dystonia are also beginning to be identified[9, 10]. How these mutations translate functionally into dystonia remains to be established, but early data suggest that dystonia can result from dysfunction of a wide variety of cellular pathways [8]. Neurophysiologically, dystonia is characterized by a loss of inhibitory mechanisms [11] and abnormal regulation of synaptic plasticity (within the sensorimotor system) [12]. In addition, the importance of the sensory system in the pathophysiology of dystonia is evident from the occurrence of sensory tricks, and abnormalities in temporal discrimination and vibratory processing have been demonstrated [13]. Finally, the concept that dystonia represents a network disorder has emerged, challenging the traditional view that dystonia is a disorder of basal ganglia dysfunction. In particular, the role of the cerebellum in the pathophysiology of dystonia is receiving much interest [14].

The treatment of dystonia is tailored to the individual's phenotype and aetiology. In some cases the choices are clear. For example, in a child presenting with generalized dystonia due to a *TOR1A* mutation (DYT1), deep brain stimulation will usually be offered in late adolescence. In patients with cervical or laryngeal dystonia, botulinum toxin injections will be offered as the first-line treatment with long-term efficacy in the majority of patients. Some patients with writing dystonia have a good response to therapy, whereas others find botulinum toxin injections more helpful. Combinations of the different types of treatments may be required for optimal symptom control in more severely affected patients. There are many good sources of information for patients, and the Dystonia Society in the UK (http://www.dystonia.org.uk) and similar societies in other countries provide additional forums for patients to obtain more information and to take part in educational events.

Final word from the expert

This patient has a diagnosis of idiopathic generalized dystonia with no identifiable brain pathology or inherited cause. The majority of patients previously labelled as having primary dystonia fall into this category, identifying the major need to understand this disabling condition further. This patient's symptoms were resistant to conservative methods of treatment, and therefore it was appropriate that she was considered and subsequently accepted for deep brain stimulation. There is now good evidence that deep brain stimulation for generalized, segmental, and cervical dystonia is safe and has long-term efficacy [15]. It remains to be seen whether the prominent oromandibular involvement in this patient will be improved by deep brain stimulation, as unfortunately effects on speech are often only marginal [15].

Clinical tip Pointers that suggest a structural, degenerative, or acquired aetiology

- Exposure to dopamine-receptor-blocking drugs (e.g. anti-psychotics, metoclopramide, prochlorperazine)
- Exogenous brain injury (e.g. abnormal birth or perinatal history, head injury or encephalitis)
- An unusual phenotype given the age of presentation (e.g. foot dystonia in young adults can be a presentation of young-onset Parkinson's disease).
- Hemidystonia should always prompt investigation for a lesion of the contralateral hemisphere
- Additional neurological signs or involvement of other systems (e.g. pyramidal signs, cerebellar signs, parkinsonism, cognitive decline, organomegaly)
- Fixed (non-mobile) dystonia is more typical than psychogenic/functional dystonia

References

1. Albanese A, Bhatia K, Bressman SB, et al. Phenomenology and classification of dystonia: a consensus update. *Mov Disord* 2013; 28(7): 863–73.
2. Phukan J, Albanese A, Gasser T, Warner T. Primary dystonia and dystonia-plus syndromes: clinical characteristics, diagnosis, and pathogenesis. *Lancet Neurol* 2011; 10(12): 1074–85.
3. Poisson A, Krack P, Thobois S, et al. History of the 'geste antagoniste' sign in cervical dystonia. *J Neurol* 2012; 259(8): 1580–4.
4. Garcia-Ruiz PJ, del Val J, Losada M, Campos JM. Task-specific dystonia of the lower limb in a flamenco dancer. *Parkinsonism Relat Disord* 2011; 17(3): 221–2.
5. Pont-Sunyer C, Marti MJ, Tolosa E. Focal limb dystonia. *Eur J Neurol* 2010; 17(Suppl 1): 22–7.
6. Kojovic M, Parees I, Sadnicka A, et al. The brighter side of music in dystonia. *Arch Neurol* 2012; 69(7): 917–19.
7. Albanese A, Barnes MP, Bhatia KP, et al. A systematic review on the diagnosis and treatment of primary (idiopathic) dystonia and dystonia plus syndromes: report of an EFNS/MDS-ES Task Force. *Eur J Neurol* 2006; 13(5): 433–44.
8. Charlesworth G, Bhatia KP, Wood NW. The genetics of dystonia: new twists in an old tale. *Brain* 2013; 136(7): 2017–37.
9. Lohmann K, Schmidt A, Schillert A, et al. Genome-wide association study in musician's dystonia: a risk variant at the arylsulfatase G locus? *Mov Disord* 2014; 29(7); 921–7.
10. Lohmann K, Klein C. Genetics of dystonia: what's known? What's new? What's next? *Mov Disord* 2013; 28(7): 899–905.
11. Hallett M. Neurophysiology of dystonia: the role of inhibition. *Neurobiol Dis* 2011; 42(2): 177–84.
12. Quartarone A, Hallett M. Emerging concepts in the physiological basis of dystonia. *Mov Disord* 2013; 28(7): 958–67.
13. Tinazzi M, Fiorio M, Fiaschi A, et al. Sensory functions in dystonia: insights from behavioral studies. *Mov Disord* 2009; 24(10): 1427–36.
14. Sadnicka A, Hoffland BS, Bhatia KP, et al. The cerebellum in dystonia—help or hindrance? *Clin Neurophysiol* 2012; 123(1): 65–70.
15. Vidailhet M, Jutras MF, Roze E, Grabli D. Deep brain stimulation for dystonia. *Handb Clin Neurol* 2013; 116: 167–87.

CASE

7 Being moved to tears

Jonathan D. Virgo and Sui Wong

Expert commentary: Gordon T. Plant

Case history

A 30-year-old British South Asian woman attended the neuro-ophthalmology clinic complaining of tinnitus, left-sided ocular symptoms, and an ipsilateral headache. She had first developed pulsatile tinnitus 11 months ago during the third trimester of a pregnancy, which was later complicated by hypertension requiring treatment with oral labetalol. Eight months ago she delivered a healthy term baby. Secondly, six months previously she had noticed the gradual onset of watering, itching, and reddening of the left eye, which had steadily deteriorated despite topical treatments for both infectious and allergic conjunctivitis. Finally, in the few weeks before presentation she had developed a constant left-sided headache that was exacerbated by movement, especially bending forward, with associated nausea and photophobia. Past medical history included gastro-oesophageal reflux disease and allergic rhinitis. Regular medications included paracetamol, ranitidine, and the oral contraceptive pill. She was a lifelong non-smoker and did not drink alcohol. The family history was unremarkable.

A general physical examination revealed no abnormalities of the cardiovascular, respiratory, or abdominal systems. Temperature, pulse rate, and blood pressure were normal. Gross inspection revealed an obviously bloodshot left eye, and further ophthalmic examination revealed periorbital swelling, injected conjunctival vessels showing 'corkscrew' morphological change, mild chemosis and 4mm exophthalmos (Figure 7.1a). The intra-ocular pressures were 17mmHg in the right eye and 27mmHg in the left. There were no abnormalities of the ocular surface, anterior chamber, or posterior segment, and a cephalic bruit was not heard. Her unaided visual acuities were 6/4 bilaterally, and Ishihara plate colour vision testing was unimpaired (right: 20/21; left: 21/21). Pupil reactions were normal and the visual fields were full to confrontation using a small coloured target. As already mentioned, fundus examination was unremarkable; specifically it did not reveal any abnormalities of the optic discs or retinal vasculature. The eye movements were normal (Figure 7.1b), as were the remaining cranial nerves. The remainder of the neurological examination revealed no limb abnormalities and the gait was normal.

In summary, a previously well 30-year-old female complained of pulsatile tinnitus (11 months duration); watering, itching, and reddening of the left eye (6 months duration); and a left-sided headache (<1 month duration). Previously, a pregnancy had been complicated by hypertension requiring treatment with oral labetalol. Examination revealed left-sided ocular hypertension, periorbital swelling, exophthalmos, and 'corkscrew' injected episcleral and conjunctival vessels with normal vision and ocular motor function.

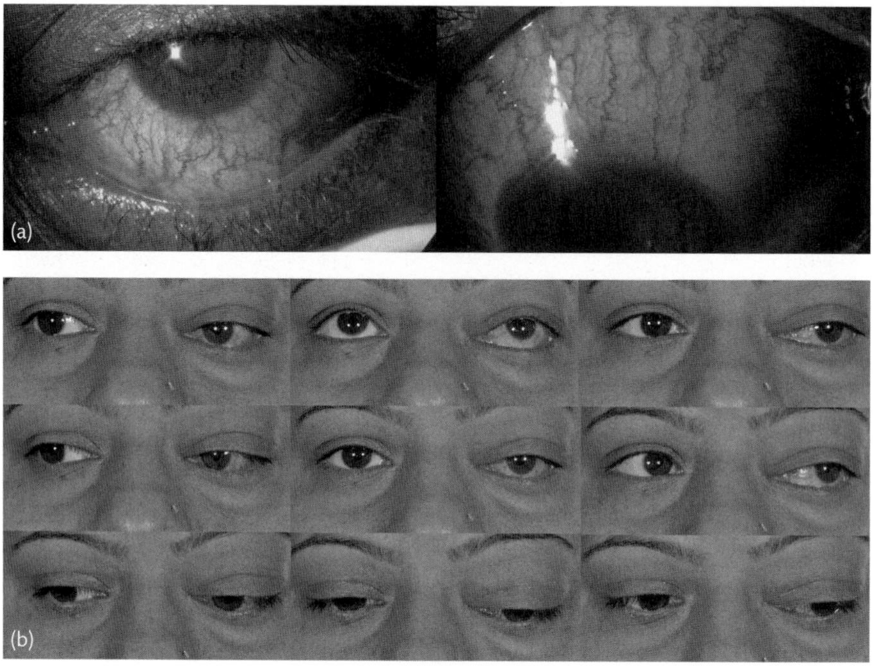

Figure 7.1 Examination findings at the time of presentation. (a) Slit-lamp biomicroscopy images show 'corkscrew' injected episcleral and conjunctival vessels with mild chemosis. Please see colour plate section. (b) The eye movements were normal.

A carotid cavernous fistula (CCF) was suspected at presentation and an orbital Doppler ultrasound that day supported the diagnosis. It showed a grossly dilated (lumen diameter 4.6mm) left superior orbital vein (SOV) with reversed low-velocity high-volume arterialized flow (maximum velocity 7cm/s). Tables 7.1 and 7.2 provide an overview of the subsequent clinical management. The patient was started on timolol (0.25%) drops twice daily, but two weeks later she attended the emergency department complaining of a burning sensation after using timolol. A hypersensitivity reaction was suspected, and she was switched to preservative-free dorzolamide (2%) drops three times daily. She continued to deteriorate despite enhanced treatment with preservative-free dorzolamide/timolol (2.0%/0.5%) drops bd, and latanoprost (0.005%) drops every night. When seen again in the neuro-ophthalmology clinic 23 days after initial presentation her visual acuities were 6/6 in the right eye and 6/9 in the left, with preserved Ishihara plate colour vision (right: 17/17; left: 17/17). However, there was now subtle limitation of left eye movements to 80 per cent of maximum in all directions of gaze. She was admitted to hospital 10 days later electively for investigations, at which point her visual acuities were 6/5 in the right and 6/18 in the left eye and her colour vision was also impaired (right: 17/17; left: 14/17). Periorbital swelling, 'corkscrew' injected conjunctival vessels, chemosis, and exophthalmos were all more pronounced, and there was ongoing left-sided complex ophthalmoplegia (Figure 7.2).

Table 7.1 Overview of the examination findings and clinical management prior to hospital admission

	Intraocular pressure (mmHg)		Visual acuity		Left-sided exophthalmos (mm)	Management
	Right	Left	Right	Left		
Presentation	17	27	6/4	6/4	4	Timolol Orbital ultrasound scan
+14 days	14	33	6/5-3	6/5	4	Switched to preservative-free dorzolamide
+22 days	14	32	6/5+6	6/5+2	5	Switched to preservative free dorzolamide/timolol plus latanoprost
+23 days	14	26	6/6	6/9	6	Neuro-ophthalmology appointment

Table 7.2 Overview of the examination findings and clinical management during hospital admission

	Intraocular pressure (mmHg)		Visual acuity		Left-sided exophthalmos (mm)	Management
	Right	Left	Right	Left		
+33 days	15	24	6/5	6/18	6	ICU admission IV mannitol 1g/kg MRI/MRA
+35 days	14	44	6/5	6/12	6	Diagnostic catheter angiography
+36 days	15	38	6/5	6/12	6	Unsuccessful endovascular intervention
+37 days	14	40	6/5	6/12	6	Successful endovascular intervention (results recorded prior to intervention)
+41 days	11	12	6/4	6/6+2	1	Discharged from hospital

ICU, intensive care unit; IV, intravenous; MRI, magnetic resonance imaging; MRA, magnetic resonance angiography.

Expert comment

This patient's initial complaint was pulsatile tinnitus. As an isolated symptom it may be idiopathic, but it is always important to check if it can be heard on auscultation of the cranium or the orbits. For example, pulsatile tinnitus in raised intracranial pressure does not give rise to an audible bruit because it is caused by transmission of the pulse pressure wave in the cerebrospinal fluid to the cochlea. If there is an audible bruit, a fistula or a vascular malformation is likely. However, it should be noted that a low-flow dural fistula often gives rise to neither tinnitus nor a bruit.

She later developed a red eye. Patients with dural fistula are often treated for conjunctivitis at this stage and may present with a red eye that has failed to respond to treatment. However, the injection in this situation is due to episcleral venous hypertension because the venous compartment is arterialized. This gives rise to 'corkscrewing' of the episcleral and conjunctival vessels which increase in length as well as diameter.

It is the episcleral venous hypertension that leads to the rise in intra-ocular pressure. The development of ocular hypertension is the major cause of visual loss in patients with dural fistula, although damage can occur from ischaemia due to arterialization of the venous compartment. In this situation conventional treatments for glaucoma to lower intra-ocular pressure tend not to be effective, as was the case in this patient, and this is an important indication of the need for closure of the fistula.

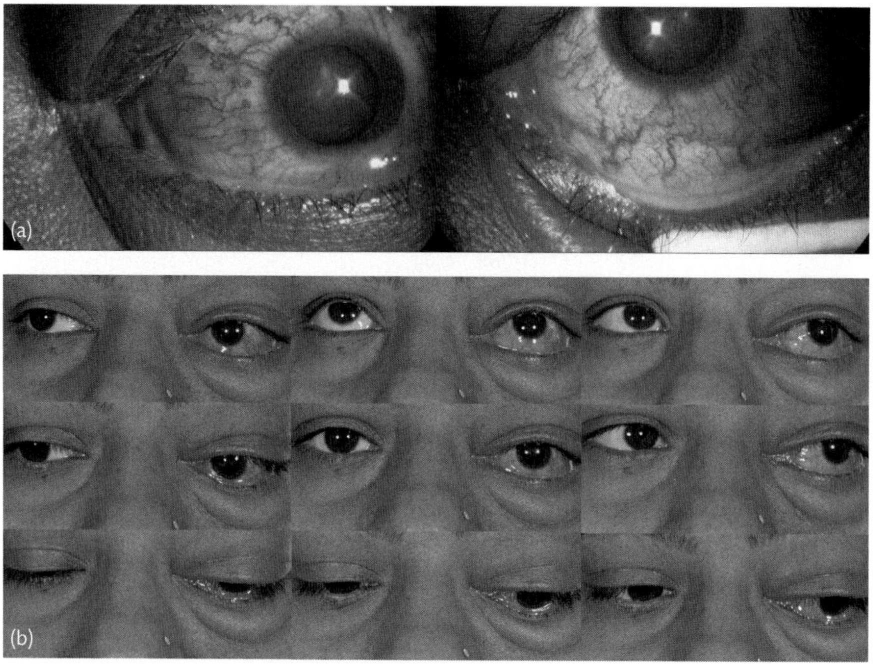

Figure 7.2 Examination findings at the time of admission to hospital 33 days after presentation. (a) Slit-lamp biomicroscopy images show 'corkscrew' injected episcleral and conjunctival vessels with chemosis and lid swelling. Please see colour plate section. (b) Slight limitation of left eye movements in all directions of gaze was observed. Pupil-dilating drops had been instilled into the left eye at the time of photography.

Learning point Pathophysiology and manifestations of carotid-cavernous fistulas

A CCF is an abnormal arteriovenous communication between a component of the carotid arterial tree and the cavernous sinus (CS). A fistula is termed 'direct' if the arterial supply is derived from the internal carotid artery (ICA) itself, and 'indirect' if the supply is via a dural branch (or via multiple dural branches) of the ICA and/or external carotid artery (ECA) (Table 7.3) [1]. If the blood escapes posteriorly through the superior and inferior petrosal sinuses (IPSs), ocular signs may be minimal, although an expanded IPS can cause direct compression of the sixth cranial nerve. When arterial blood is shunted anteriorly into the orbital veins, ocular signs due to raised episcleral venous pressure, reduced arterial perfusion pressure, and venous stasis manifest. Signs are usually ipsilateral to the fistula, but are occasionally contralateral or bilateral because of the variable connections between each CS [2].

Direct fistulas account for 70–90 per cent of cases, and are typically seen in young men secondary to blunt or penetrating head trauma [3–5]. However, about 20 per cent of direct fistulas occur spontaneously, usually in older women, due to the rupture of an aneurysmal, atherosclerotic, or otherwise diseased intracavernous ICA [6]. Risk factors for the development of spontaneous direct CCF include Ehlers–Danlos syndrome, fibromuscular dysplasia, and pseudoxanthoma elasticum [7–9]. As direct fistulas shunt blood at a higher flow rate, they tend to present acutely over days to weeks with a more severe clinical picture. The classic clinical triad is that of pulsatile exophthalmos, a cephalic bruit, and episcleral/conjunctival congestion (corkscrew injection and chemosis). Ophthalmoplegia may develop due to compression of cranial nerves within the CS and/or extraocular muscle hypoxia and oedema. Visual loss can occur due to ischaemic optic neuropathy, retinal ischaemia, retinal vein occlusion, retinal detachment, vitreous haemorrhage, ocular hypertension, or exposure keratopathy.

(Continued)

Bleeding from the mouth, nose, or ears may occur and intracranial haemorrhage is seen in 5 per cent of cases.

Indirect fistulas account for 10–30 per cent of cases and typically occur spontaneously in middle-aged to elderly women [3–5]. A minor, or even asymptomatic, CS thrombosis is thought to be the triggering event [5]. Subsequent venous congestion within the sinusoids of the CS, in combination with thrombus organization and aberrant recanalization, promote fistula formation with adjacent dural branches of the ICA and/or ECA [10, 11]. Risk factors for development of indirect CCF include pregnancy, hypertension, diabetes, sinusitis, and minor trauma [12, 13]. As indirect fistulas shunt blood at a lower flow rate, they tend to present subacutely over weeks to months with a less severe clinical picture. Patients usually develop a chronically red eye, and examination reveals tortuous dilatation of episcleral and conjunctival vessels with ipsilateral ocular hypertension; a cephalic bruit may or may not be heard and chemosis is less likely to be present. All patients with direct CCF will require treatment, whereas 20–50 per cent of patients with indirect CCF will resolve spontaneously, or with medical treatment alone, within days to months of presentation [13, 14]. Venous thrombosis can cause abrupt deterioration in patients with an indirect fistula. In cases where drainage is predominantly orbital, it is likely to be thrombosis of the superior ophthalmic vein giving rise to acute orbital congestion. The risk of cortical vein thrombosis and venous infarction is also significant in cases associated with cortical venous drainage.

Clinical tip Misdiagnosis of carotid cavernous fistulas

Misdiagnosis is common in patients with CCF, especially at an early stage prior to appropriate diagnostic work-up. Fistulas that drain anteriorly causing orbital congestion may be mislabelled as conjunctivitis, dysthyroid orbitopathy, orbital cellulitis, episcleritis, idiopathic orbital inflammatory syndrome, spheno-orbital meningioma, or Tolosa–Hunt syndrome [15]. Posteriorly draining fistulas that cause a sixth nerve lesion with minimal signs of orbital congestion are often mislabelled as a microvascular ischaemic peripheral mononeuropathy.

Table 7.3 Carotidcavernous fistulas

	Anatomical classification	Typical demographics and aetiology
Type A (direct)	Direct communication of ICA and the cavernous sinus	Young males; traumatic
Type B (indirect)	Supplied only by dural branches of the ICA	Middle-aged to elderly women; spontaneous/non-traumatic
Type C (indirect)	Supplied only by dural branches of the ECA	
Type D (indirect)	Supplied by dural branches of the ICA and ECA	

ICA, internal carotid artery; ECA, external carotid artery.

The patient was admitted to the intensive care unit (ICU) for treatment with intravenous mannitol 1g/kg to lower the intra-ocular pressure. MRI and MRA showed a dilated left SOV with adjacent swelling of the extraocular muscles, and a left-sided CCF (Figure 7.3a); however, the exact anatomical location of the fistula could not be determined. Catheter arteriography showed a left-sided Barrow type D indirect fistula. It involved the inferolateral trunk of the ICA and separate dural branches of the internal maxillary artery (IMA), itself a branch of the ECA. Venous drainage from the left CS was via the right and left SOV, and via the right and left IPS. Retrograde flow of contrast into the left SOV was observed (Figure 7.3b). An additional right-sided Barrow type D indirect fistula was detected involving the inferolateral trunk of the ICA and dural branches of the IMA. However, venous drainage from the CS on this side was via the middle cerebral and superficial cortical veins, thus explaining the lack of ocular signs and symptoms on this side. The patient was transferred to the ICU after the procedure and her case was discussed at the neurovascular multidisciplinary team meeting.

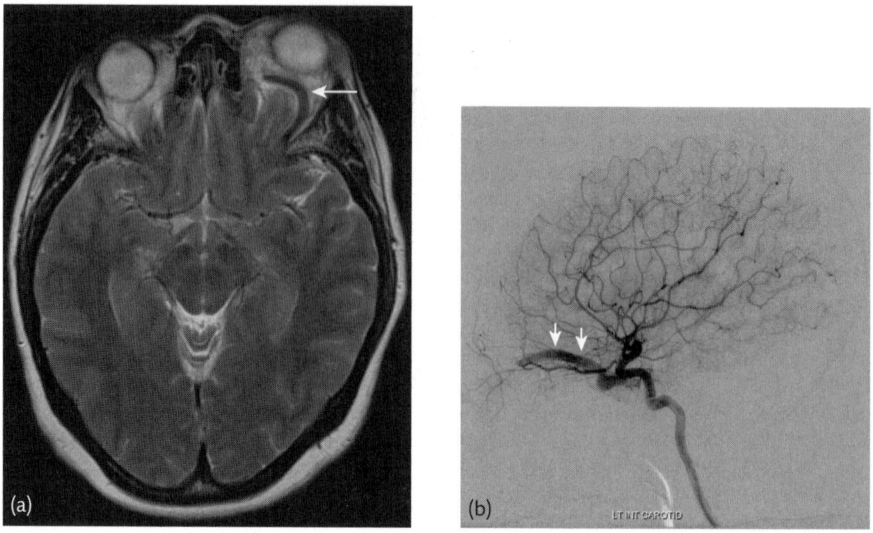

Figure 7.3 Magnetic resonance brain imaging and catheter arteriography. (a) Transverse T2-weighted MRI shows left-sided exophthalmos and dilatation of the left superior ophthalmic vein (white arrow); adjacent cuts showed swelling of the extraocular muscles. (b) Catheter arteriogram (left internal carotid injection) viewed laterally shows early filling of the superior ophthalmic vein (black arrows).

Expert comment

If the diagnosis of a low-flow CCF is suspected, the minimum finding to look for is dilatation of the superior ophthalmic vein. If there are orbital signs, this will invariably be present and can be demonstrated on ultrasound, CT, or MRI of the orbits. The advantage of ultrasound is that it is also possible to demonstrate reverse, often pulsatile, flow. Other imaging signs may be subtle (distension of the CS) or only apparent in more severe cases (swollen extraocular muscles).

Learning point Imaging of carotid cavernous fistulas

Orbital ultrasound, CT, and MRI are frequently used in the initial work-up of patients with CCF [16, 17]. Imaging findings include exophthalmos, swelling of the extraocular muscles, and enlargement of the superior ophthalmic vein and/or ipsilateral CS. Orbital structures are best visualized with fine-cut (≤3mm) CT, or via contrast-enhanced fat-suppressed MRI sequences. Although modern CT and MRA can be used to detect and characterize the fistula tract in the majority of patients with CCF, invasive catheter angiography is considered the gold standard investigation [18, 19]. It provides the highest quality images of the vascular anatomy, and in straightforward cases can be combined with endovascular intervention in one visit to the catheter suite. Bilateral ICA and ECA should be performed in order to detected multiple (Barrow type D) and/or bilateral fistulas. There is considerable normal variation in the route of venous drainage from the CS [20]. Therefore these drainage pathways should be characterized, as this information is used to plan the approach (transarterial or transvenous) of endovascular therapy. Vertebral artery angiography is required in cases where therapeutic ICA sacrifice is considered.

The symptomatic left indirect fistula was targeted first for treatment. On day three of the hospital admission a catheter was passed via a transvenous approach involving the right common femoral vein and left IPS into the posterior portion of the left CS. Injected contrast passed freely into the right and left IPS and also into right SOV. However, very little contrast passed into the left SOV, and the catheter could not be advanced forwards into the anterior portion of the CS. The procedure was abandoned and the patient was returned to the ICU. On the following day a catheter was passed via the left SOV into the anterior portion of the CS adjacent to the point of fistulation with the inferolateral trunk of the left ICA. Metal coils were deployed and simultaneous ICA arteriography demonstrated closure of the fistula. As was anticipated, the reduced rate of blood flow within the left CS led to spontaneous closure of the remaining fistulas (confirmed via ECA arteriography).

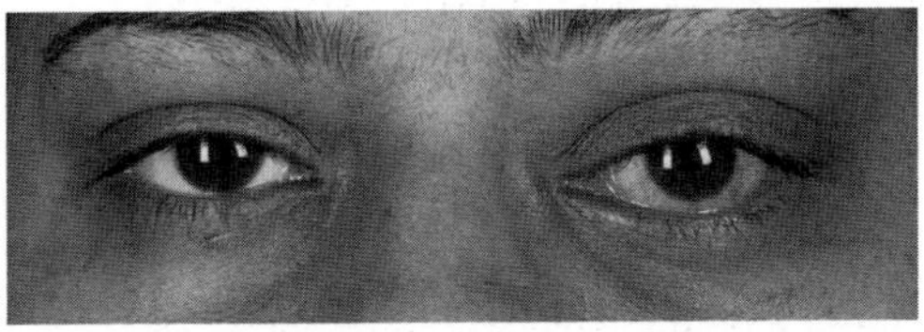

Figure 7.4 The patient's facial appearance six days after successful endovascular treatment. The infra-orbital puncture site through which the superior ophthalmic vein was accessed is just visible.

The patient was discharged three days later with visual acuities of 6/4 in the right eye and 6/6+2 in the left, normal intra-ocular pressures, and almost complete resolution of left exophthalmos. Figure 7.4 shows her facial appearance in clinic six days after successful embolization. The asymptomatic right dural fistula was electively treated six months later. A catheter was passed via a transarterial approach involving the left femoral artery, right ECA, and right IMA with selective catheterization of the offending dural branches. Multiple fistulas were embolized with ethylene vinyl alcohol copolymer injections (confirmed via ECA arteriography). The reduced rate of blood flow within the right CS led to spontaneous closure of the fistula involving the inferolateral trunk of the right ICA (confirmed via ICA arteriography). Left ICA/ECA arteriography showed no recurrence of the previously treated left indirect fistula.

Learning point Treatment for carotid cavernous fistula

All patients with direct CCF should receive urgent endovascular intervention [17]. Monitoring alone may be appropriate for some patients with indirect CCF, but the majority will require medical treatment; endovascular intervention is used in cases with severe or persistent symptoms that do not respond to medical treatment [17]. If cortical venous drainage is demonstrated, this constitutes an indication for endovascular treatment in its own right because of the risk of stroke due to venous infarction. Neurosurgery and stereotactic radiosurgery can be used where endovascular intervention has failed, whilst in selected patients (usually frail or elderly) stereotactic radiosurgery may have a primary role in the treatment of indirect CCF [21, 22].

Medical treatment

Standard topical agents for glaucoma can be used to treat ocular hypertension [13]. Intravenous mannitol can be used for the same indication whilst prepping patients for endovascular intervention [23, 24]. Prism spectacles or patching can be used to treat diplopia, whilst exposure keratopathy can be treated with lubricants and overnight lid-taping [13]. Intermittent manual compression of the carotid artery and jugular vein may encourage closure of the fistula by reducing the rate of blood flow through it [25]. The patient applies pressure with the contralateral arm for 30 seconds frequently each day for 4–6 weeks.

Endovascular treatment

Multiple endovascular therapies have been developed for the treatment of CCF [17]. The technique that is used in individual cases is determined by the subtype of the fistula, by the anatomy of the cavernous sinus, and by the preference of the interventional neuroradiologist, or neuroscience centre.

Direct fistulas are best treated via a transarterial approach. A catheter is passed through the tear in the ICA and directly into the CS. Embolization of the fistula tract is then achieved by inflating a detachable balloon, deploying metallic coils, or injecting a liquid embolic agent (e.g. n-butyl cyanoacrylate glue or ethylene vinyl alcohol copolymer) [26–28]. To reduce the risk of anterior circulation stroke during transarterial embolization, the distal portion of the ICA is temporarily occluded to prevent migration of coils and liquid embolic material. If a transarterial approach is not possible, transvenous embolization can be achieved using metallic coils and liquid embolic agents [29]. In such cases the CS is usually accessed via the IPS or the SOV. Large tears in the ICA that are not amenable to embolization can be treated with ICA stenting [30, 31]. Fistula occlusion is achieved in 55–90 per cent of patients with direct CCF, but 10–40 per cent of patients experience deterioration in ocular symptoms [17].

Indirect fistulas are best treated via a transvenous approach. A catheter is passed into the CS, usually via the IPS or SOV, and embolization is achieved by deploying metallic coils or injecting a liquid embolic agent [29, 32, 33]. Simultaneous ICA/ECA catheter arteriography is used to monitor closure of the fistula tract. Transarterial embolization is less straightforward in cases of indirect CCF, as it usually requires selective catheterization of multiple tiny dural arterioles [13, 34]. Furthermore, it is only safe to perform ICA embolization when super-selective catheterization of the offending dural feeder is achieved, as otherwise the risk of anterior circulation stroke is too high [35]. Multiple techniques may be required in individual cases. Fistula occlusion is achieved in 70–90 per cent of patients with indirect CCF, but 2.3–5 per cent of patients experience complications [17].

Discussion

CCF is a rare, but important, pathology. It is a cause of significant ocular and neurological morbidity and has an overall mortality of about 3 per cent. Patients often present to clinicians who are not familiar with the condition, and this can lead to mismanagement (e.g. misdiagnosis, diagnostic delay, inappropriate treatment, and delay in starting effective treatment). Patients with an indirect CCF who present with less dramatic signs and symptoms are more frequently mismanaged. The diagnosis is most frequently made by ophthalmologists, whilst treatment is best delivered in a tertiary neuroscience centre with on-site neurology, interventional neuroradiology, and neurosurgery teams. Follow-up with a neuro-ophthalmologist is most appropriate. However, when this is not possible, follow-up with both an ophthalmologist and neurologist is required.

A final word from the expert

The take-home message from this case centres on the clinical manifestations of CCF and the appropriate management of patients with the condition. This includes a description of the investigations and treatment options (including medical and endovascular interventions) that are available. In recognition of the fact that cases of direct CCF are far more common than cases of indirect CCF, a discussion of direct CCF has been included in the learning points.

This case was particularly complex because of the presence of multiple bilateral fistulas and the patient's unusual CS and associated venous anatomy. It highlights the need for these patients to be managed in a neuroscience centre under the care of a multidisciplinary team who are experienced in managing patients with CCF.

References

1. Barrow DL, Spector RH, Braun IF, et al. Classification and treatment of spontaneous carotid-cavernous sinus fistulas. *J Neurosurg* 1985; 62: 248–56.
2. Plant G, Acheson J, Clarke C, et al. Carotico-cavernous fistula. In: Clarke C, Howard R, Rossor M, Shorvon SD (eds), *Neurology: A Queen Square Textbook* (Oxford: Blackwell); 2009; 511–12.
3. Locke CE. Intracranial arterio-venous aneurism or pulsating exophthalmos. *Ann Surg* 1924; 80: 1–24.
4. Keltner JL, Satterfield D, Dublin AB, Lee BC. Dural and carotid cavernous sinus fistulas. Diagnosis, management and complications. *Ophthalmology* 1985; 94(12): 1585–1600.
5. Debrun GM, Viñuela F, Fox AJ, et al. Indications for treatment and classification of 132 carotid-cavernous fistulas. *Neurosurgery* 1988; 22(2): 285–9
6. Tomsick TA. Type A (direct) CCF: etiology, prevalence, and natural history. In: Tomsick TA (ed.), *Carotid Cavernous Fistula* (Cincinnati, OH: Digital Educational Publishing); 1997: 35–8.
7. Schievink WI, Piepgras DG, Earnest F 4th, Gordon H. Spontaneous carotid-cavernous fistulae in Ehlers–Danlos syndrome type IV. *J Neurosurg* 1991; 74: 991–8.
8. Hieshman GB, Cahan LD, Mehringer CM, Bentson JR. Spontaneous arteriovenous fistulas of cerebral vessels in association with fibromuscular dysplasia. *Neurosurgery* 1986; 18(4): 454–8.
9. Rios-Montenegro EN, Behrens MM, Hoyt WF. Pseudoxanthoma elasticum. Association with bilateral carotid rete mirabile and unilateral carotid-cavernous sinus fistula. *Arch Neurol* 1972; 26(2): 151–5.
10. Takahashi M, Nakano Y. Magnification angiography of dural carotid-cavernous sinus fistulae with emphasis on clinical and angiographic evolution. *Neuroradiology* 1980; 19: 249–56.
11. Houser OW, Campbell JK, Campbell RJ, Sundt TM Jr. Arteriovenous malformation affecting the transverse dural venous sinus—an acquired lesion. *Mayo Clin Proc* 1979; 54(10): 651–61.
12. Komiyama M, Nakajima H, Nishikawa M, Kan M. Traumatic carotid cavernous sinus fistula: serial angiography studies from the day of trauma. *Am J Neuroradiol* 1998; 19: 1641–4.
13. Miller NR. Diagnosis and management of dural carotid-cavernous sinus fistulas. *Neurosurg Focus* 2007; 23(5): E13.
14. Liu HM, Wang YH, Chen YF, et al. Long-term clinical outcome of spontaneous carotid-cavernous sinus fistulae supplied by dural branches of the internal carotid artery. *Neuroradiology* 2001; 43: 1007–14.
15. Yeh S, Foroozan R. Orbital apex syndrome. *Curr Opin Ophthalmol* 2004; 15: 490–8.
16. Kilic T, Elmaci I, Bayri Y, et al. Value of transcranial Doppler ultrasonography in the diagnosis and follow-up of carotid-cavernous fistulae. *Acta Neurochirurg (Wien)* 2001; 143: 1257–65.
17. Gemmete JJ, Chaudhary N, Pandey A, Ansari S. Treatment of carotid cavernous fistulas. *Curr Treat Options Neurol* 2010; 12: 43–53.
18. Chen CC, Chang PC, Shy CG, et al. CT angiography and MR angiography in the evaluation of carotid cavernous sinus fistula prior to embolization: a comparison of techniques. *Am J Neuroradiol* 2005; 26: 2349–56.
19. Debrun GM. Angiographic workup of a carotid cavernous sinus fistula (CCF) or what information does the interventionalist need for treatment? *Surg Neurol* 1995; 44: 75–9.
20. Yasuda A, Campero A, Martins C, et al. Microsurgical anatomy and approaches to the cavernous sinus. *Neurosurgery* 2008; 62 (6 Suppl 3): 1240–63.
21. Parkinson D, Downs AR, Whytehead LL, Syslak WB. Carotid cavernous fistula: direct repair with preservation of carotid. *Surgery* 1975; 76: 882–9.

22. Hirai T, Korogi Y, Baba Y, et al. Dural carotid cavernous fistulas: role of conventional radiation therapy—long-term results with irradiation, embolization, or both. *Radiology* 1998; 207: 423–30.
23. Quon DK, Worthen DM. Dose response of intravenous mannitol on the human eye. *Ann Ophthalmol* 1981; 13(12): 1392–3.
24. Mauger TF, Nye CN, Boyle KA. Intraocular pressure, anterior chamber depth and axial length following intravenous mannitol. *J Ocul Pharmacol Ther* 2000; 16(6): 591–4.
25. Kai Y, Hamada J, Morioka M, et al. Treatment of cavernous sinus dural arteriovenous fistulae by external manual carotid compression. *Neurosurgery* 2007; 60: 253–8.
26. Goto K, Hieshima GB, Higashida RT, et al. Treatment of direct carotid cavernous sinus fistulae. Various therapeutic approaches and results in 148 cases. *Acta Radiol Suppl* 1986; 369: 576–9.
27. Halbach, VV, Higashida RT, Barnwell SL, et al. Trans-arterial platinum coil embolization of carotid-cavernous fistulas. *Am J Neuroradiol* 1991; 12: 429–33.
28. Luo CB, Teng MM, Chang FC, Chang CY. Transarterial balloon assisted *n*-butyl-2-cyanoacrylate embolisation of direct carotid cavernous fistulas. *Am J Neuroradiol* 2006; 27: 1535–40.
29. Klisch J, Huppertz HJ, Spetzger U, et al. Transvenous treatment of carotid cavernous and dural arteriovenous fistulae: results for 31 patients and review of the literature. *Neurosurgery* 2003; 53: 836–56.
30. Morón FE, Klucznik RP, Mawad ME, Strother CM. Endovascular treatment of high flow carotid cavernous fistula by stent-assisted coil placement. *Am J Neuroradiol* 2005; 26: 1399–1404.
31. Gomez F, Escobar W, Gomez AM, et al. Treatment of carotid cavernous fistulas using covered stents: midterm results in seven patients. *Am J Neuroradiol* 2007; 28: 1762–8.
32. Suzuki S, Lee DW, Jahan R, et al. Transvenous treatment of spontaneous dural carotid-cavernous fistulas using a combination of detachable coils and Onyx. *Am J Neuroradiol* 2006; 27: 1346–9.
33. Wakhloo AK, Perlow A, Linfante I, et al. Transvenous *n*-butyl cyanoacrylate infusion or complex dural carotid cavernous fistulas: technical considerations and clinical outcome. *Am J Neuroradiol* 2005; 26: 1888–97.
34. Cognard C, Januel AC, Silva NA Jr, Tall P. Endovascular treatment of intracranial dural arteriovenous fistulas with cortical venous drainage: new management using Onyx. *Am J Neuroradiol* 2008; 29: 235–41.
35. Borden NM, Liebman K. Endovascular access to the meningohypophyseal trunk. *Am J Neuroradiol* 2001; 22: 725–7.

CASE

8 An urgent and frequent symptom

William M. Stern

Expert commentary Jalesh N. Panicker

Case history

A 43-year-old right-handed woman presented for her annual review in the neurology clinic. She had been diagnosed with relapsing remitting multiple sclerosis (MS) at the age of 30 following an episode of optic neuritis and a subsequent episode of left arm weakness. Imaging at the time showed lesions suggestive of demyelination in the periventricular white matter and cervical spinal cord. A lumbar puncture confirmed the presence of unmatched oligoclonal bands in the CSF. Relapses continued despite disease-modifying therapy, which was subsequently withdrawn when she was diagnosed with secondary progressive MS at the age of 40.

At review, she reported various difficulties including low mood and excessive fatigue. She experienced occasional diplopia. She had difficulty performing fine motor tasks with her left hand, and sometimes dropped objects. She had stiffness affecting her legs and painful muscle cramps in the legs at night. She could walk around 100 metres with a walking aid, and had an Expanded Disability Status Scale (EDSS) score of 6.0. She was taking baclofen for her spasticity and citalopram for her mood.

On specific questioning, she admitted to problems affecting her bladder, including urinary urgency, frequency, and incontinence which was occurring on a daily basis. She also reported urinary hesitancy and double voiding. She had stopped going out socially because incontinence was becoming an embarrassment.

On examination, she had bilateral internuclear ophthalmoplegia, a mild left hemiparesis, bilateral intention tremor, and past pointing on finger–nose testing. Reflexes were brisk and tone was increased in all four limbs, especially the legs. Plantar reflexes were upgoing bilaterally. She had a spastic gait.

Learning point History-taking

Where bladder involvement is suspected in a neurological condition, the following aspects of the history should be ascertained.

- Storage symptoms ('overactive bladder'):
  - urinary frequency
  - nocturia
  - urinary urgency with or without incontinence.
- Voiding symptoms:
  - hesitancy
  - poor or interrupted urinary stream
  - sensation of incomplete bladder emptying
  - double voiding (needing to urinate a second time for relief).
- It is common to have a combination of storage and voiding symptoms.

(Continued)

Clinical tip Ask about urinary symptoms

Many neurological conditions affect bladder function and this may be having a significant impact on quality of life. Patients may be embarrassed to mention such problems, unless specifically asked.

- If a patient reports incontinence, try to ascertain from the history whether this is:
  - urgency incontinence—related to an overactive bladder
  - stress incontinence—due to a weak pelvic floor
  - overflow incontinence—related to incomplete bladder emptying/urinary retention
  - functional incontinence—where the patient is aware of the need to urinate, but is unable to go to a toilet because of physical or mental disabilities, or poorly accessible toilets.
- Medications—drugs that can cause or exacerbate urinary symptoms include the following.
  - Drugs that affect bladder emptying:
    - anticholinergics (e.g. hyoscine)
    - tricyclic antidepressants (e.g. amitriptyline)
    - agents used to treat spasticity (e.g. baclofen)
    - opiates
  - Drugs that exacerbate overactive bladder symptoms:
    - diuretics (e.g. furosemide).
- Medical history:
  - systemic diseases (e.g. diabetes) may cause urinary symptoms
  - urinary tract infections may exacerbate urinary symptoms, and are also a cause of future morbidity if not addressed.
- Urological/gynaecological/obstetric history>.
- Social history.
- Caffeine and fizzy drink intake should be assessed.

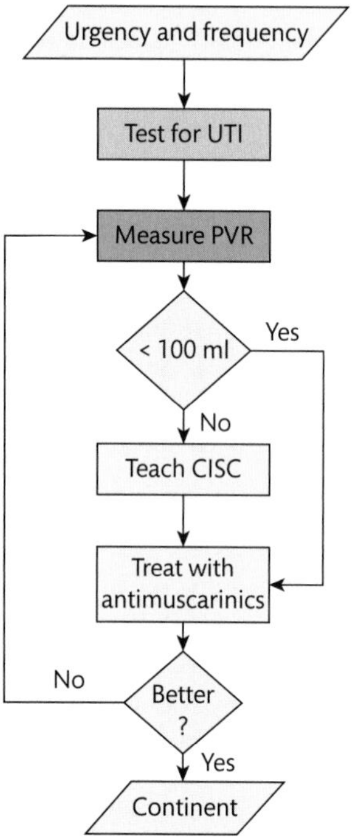

Figure 8.1 An algorithm for the management of neurogenic bladder dysfunction: CISC, clean intermittent self-catheterization; PVR, post-void residual volume; UTI, urinary tract infection.

Reproduced from *J Neurol Neurosurg Psychiatry*, 80(5), Fowler CJ, Panicker JN, Drake M, et al., A UK consensus on the management of the bladder in multiple sclerosis, pp. 470–7, © 2009, with permission from BMJ Publishing Group Ltd.

The patient was further evaluated for her urinary symptoms in the uroneurology clinic. She was assessed based on the algorithm shown in Figure 8.1. Her urine dipstick test did not show presence of nitrites or leucocytes. She had a bladder scan and her post-void residual volume (PVR) was found to be around 150ml on two occasions. She was asked to maintain a bladder diary for three days (Figure 8.2). This showed a daytime urinary frequency of eight visits to the toilet, and she was waking up to pass urine twice at night. She recorded voided volumes which averaged around 125ml. She was incontinent two or three times a day.

Learning point First-line investigations

Bladder diary

- A bladder diary is a useful diagnostic aid, and is essentially an extension of history-taking.
- A frequency–volume chart records the time and volume of urine whenever the patient passes urine. Patients also record the time they go to bed for sleeping and when they wake up in the morning, thus providing information about nocturia.
- A bladder diary provides an opportunity to review fluid intake, as well as the type of fluids, which have an impact on lower urinary tract symptoms.
- If the bladder diary shows multiple small-volume voids, it indicates a reduced functional bladder capacity. This may be due to a number of causes such as reduced bladder capacity, overactivity, or elevated post-void residual volume (see below).

Urine dipstick

Patients with neurological disease reporting urinary symptoms should have a urine dipstick test [1] as part of their initial evaluation, or if there is a recent change in symptoms.

- The presence of nitrites and leucocytes on dipstick is suspicious for infection.
- The urine dipstick has a high negative predictive value and therefore can exclude an infection. However, it has a low positive predictive value and therefore, if positive, should be followed up with a mid-stream urine specimen for microbiology analysis.
- There is a higher false-positive rate in patients who use a urinary catheter.

(Continued)

Measurement of post-void residual volume

- Patients with voiding dysfunction may not report any specific symptoms and therefore the PVR should be measured in all neurological patients with urinary symptoms.
- The PVR can be measured by either a bladder scan or in-out catheterization
- PVR should be measured on more than one occasion.
- Patients with a persistently elevated PVR should be taught catheterization, ideally clean intermittent self catheterization (CISC), before they are started on antimuscarinics for their overactive bladder.
- There is lack of consensus about the PVR volume at which to start catheterization. However, for neurological patients, a PVR persistently greater than 100ml is often used.
- Regular bladder emptying improves the functional bladder capacity and this in itself may improve storage symptoms
- Patients with a persistently raised PVR have a greater likelihood of developing UTIs.

Expert comment

The 'neurogenic bladder' is a common management problem for neurologists. There are a variety of causes. Taking a targeted history and arranging appropriate investigations will help to elucidate these.

Sensation *- What is the reason you went to urinate (pass water)? This can be graded as:*

Grade	*Definition*
0	*Convenience (no urge)*
1	*Mild urge (can hold more than 1 hour)*
2	*Moderate urge (can hold for 10 to 60 minutes)*
3	*Severe urge (can hold less than 10 minutes)*
4	*Desperate urge (must go immediately)*

Time out of bed: 08-30 *Time to bed: 23-15*

Time	*Voided Volume mL*	*Urinary leakage (none, slight, moderate, heavy)*	*Fluid intake*	*Bladder sensation (0 to 4)*
02-00	*100ml*	*slight*	*None*	*3*
06-30	*125ml*	*heavy*	*None*	*4*
08-30	*100ml*	*none*	*400ml*	*1*
11-15	*150ml*	*none*	*300ml*	*3*
13-00	*100ml*	*none*	*500ml*	*1*
15-45	*200ml*	*heavy*	*300ml*	*4*
16-45	*50ml*	*none*	*None*	*2*
18-10	*200ml*	*none*	*500ml*	*3*
20-00	*100ml*	*none*	*None*	*3*
23-15	*125ml*	*none*	*None*	*1*

Figure 8.2 The patient's bladder diary.

The patient was drinking four cups of coffee and fizzy drinks on a daily basis, and was encouraged to replace this, maintaining a daily fluid intake of around 1.5–2 litres. She spent time with a dedicated continence advisor and was taught clean intermittent self catheterization.

She continued to have overactive bladder symptoms and was started on an antimuscarinic drug—solifenacin 5mg daily, which was subsequently increased to 10mg. At subsequent review she was using CISC well, catheterizing twice daily, and reported a marked improvement in urinary urgency and frequency with only minimal incontinence. However she was experiencing troublesome side effects of dry mouth and constipation and was not keen to continue solifenacin.

She was then reviewed by a urologist and was found to be suitable for intradetrusor injections of botulinum toxin type A. The treatment session, performed using a flexible cystoscope under local anaesthesia, lasted 15 minutes and she went home the same day. A total of 200U of onabotulinum toxin A was administered. After the treatment, she was self-catheterizing more often, three or four times a day, but she reported no further episodes of incontinence. Her quality of life improved significantly and she was pleased with the results. The effects lasted for 10 months and she was re-treated when incontinence recurred.

Learning point Clean intermittent self-catheterization

Advantages

- Recommended as first-line method in NICE guidelines [2]
- Lower risk of infection than indwelling catheter
- Allows relative independence
- Better body image than indwelling catheter
- Sexual intercourse possible

Disadvantages

- Requires intact vision, cognition, strength, bimanual dexterity
- Psychologically difficult for some individuals

Expert comment

Bladder dysfunction is dynamic, especially in the context of progressive neurological disease, and the appropriate treatment may change over time. Urological symptoms, if present, should be regularly reviewed.

Evidence base: Efficacy and safety of onabotulinum toxin A in patients with urinary incontinence due to neurogenic detrusor overactivity: a randomised, double-blind, placebo-controlled trial

Cruz et al. [3] studied 275 patients in this trial (91 given placebo), which demonstrated that neurogenic bladder symptoms were effectively treated by onabotulinum toxin A, with a reduction in urinary incontinence and an improvement in quality of life. Patients treated in this way generally require CISC. This study led to the licensing of onabotulinum toxin A for this indication. NICE guidance now recommends this as a second-line treatment in patients who fail a trial of antimuscarinic medication because of either lack of efficacy or side effects [4].

She did well for two years but then developed progressive weakness in her right arm and found it difficult to carry on with CISC. After a short period with a urethral indwelling catheter, she had a suprapubic catheter (SPC) inserted.

Learning point Suprapubic catheter

Advantages

- Eliminates the risk of urethral damage
- More comfortable than urethral catheter
- More conducive to sexual activity than indwelling urethral catheter
- Relatively easy catheter change
- Improved perineal hygiene

Disadvantages

- Insertion requires a surgical procedure, with discomfort and possible complications
- Insertion and catheter changes difficult in obese individuals
- Unwanted urethral voiding may occur

Discussion

Lower urinary tract dysfunction commonly occurs in neurological disease [5] and the pattern of dysfunction varies according to the site of lesion. In health, the bladder is unique amongst visceral organs in that it has a phasic pattern of activity. In the storage phase, the detrusor muscle is relaxed and the urethral sphincters are contracted. In the voiding phase, the detrusor muscle contracts and the sphincters relax, leading to micturition.

Lesions above the level of the pons result predominantly in storage dysfunction due to loss of inhibition of the detrusor muscle, leading to involuntary contractions called detrusor overactivity. Symptoms of storage dysfunction include urinary urgency, frequency, nocturia, and incontinence. Spinal lesions also result in detrusor overactivity, but additionally the activity of the detrusor muscle and urethral sphincters is no longer coordinated, resulting in detrusor–sphincter dyssynergia. Patients may report voiding difficulties as well as incontinence. Lesions of the conus medullaris, the cauda

Table 8.1 The pattern of lower urinary tract dysfunction varies according to the site of neurological lesion

	Suprapontine lesion	Spinal cord lesion	Sacral/infrasacral lesion
Common causes	Stroke Neurodegenerative Tumours Trauma	Multiple sclerosis Trauma Disc prolapse Tumours	Disc prolapse Tumours Pelvic nerve injury Small fibre neuropathy
Symptoms	Storage symptoms	Storage and voiding symptoms	Voiding symptoms
Bladder scan	PVR normal	PVR usually raised	PVR raised
Urodynamics findings	Detrusor overactivity	Detrusor overactivity and detrusor sphincter dyssynergia	Acontractile detrusor

PVR, post-void residual volume.

equina, and the peripheral nerves lead to a paralysed or acontractile detrusor muscle, resulting predominantly in voiding dysfunction. Symptoms of voiding dysfunction include hesitancy, straining to pass urine, and incomplete bladder emptying.

The pattern of symptoms and investigation findings is illustrated in Table 8.1. If the underlying diagnosis is unclear, the type of bladder dysfunction may help to narrow down the site of the lesion.

Even if there is an obvious underlying neurological condition, as in our patient, it is worth taking a careful history, as urinary symptoms can have multiple causes. For example, a multiparous woman with MS may have stress incontinence resulting from obstetric causes. Moreover, a thorough history helps to identify potential barriers to effective bladder management, such as problems with dexterity which might limit the use of CISC.

MS is commonly associated with bladder dysfunction, with around 75 per cent of MS patients believed to be affected [6]. Bladder dysfunction may show temporal fluctuations, reflecting the dynamic course of MS. It may worsen suddenly as a patient experiences a relapse and improve as they recover. Like other symptoms in MS, bladder dysfunction may also be gradually progressive. Spinal cord lesions are particularly associated with urinary difficulties, though the cumulative effect of lesions throughout the central nervous system is likely to contribute. The common symptoms relate to detrusor overactivity and detrusor–sphincter dyssynergia [7].

Regardless of the underlying diagnosis, it is essential to perform a urine dipstick test looking for evidence of a urinary tract infection that can mimic an overactive bladder. A PVR is essential to look for evidence of incomplete bladder emptying. Both these tests are easily available in most centres. Patients with a raised PVR should be taught CISC prior to pharmacological treatment.

Specialist urodynamic testing may be considered if there is diagnostic uncertainty, a poor response to initial treatment, or risk factors for upper urinary tract damage. Urodynamic testing may also provide diagnostic clues if the underlying neurological process is unclear.

Mild storage dysfunction may be amenable to simple non-pharmacological intervention. Regular bladder emptying, regulation of fluid intake, reduction of caffeine and fizzy drinks, and pelvic floor exercises may be effective. If these fail, pharmacological interventions are often useful.

Learning point Pharmacological treatment of storage dysfunction

Antimuscarinic agents

Antimuscarinic agents are included in the first-line management of the neurogenic over-active bladder. Commonly used examples in the UK are oxybutynin, solifenacin, tolterodine, fesoterodine, trospium, and darifenacin [6]. Antimuscarinic agents act through the muscarinic receptors of the detrusor muscle and help with the overactive bladder. Anticholinergic side effects include dry mouth, blurred vision, tachycardia, and constipation. They also exert a central effect and may adversely affect cognition. Some of the newer antimuscarinics are reported to have fewer central side effects. For instance, darifenacin has greater specificity for the M3 muscarinic receptors in the bladder and less affinity for the central muscarinic receptors. Trospium is a quarternary ammonium compound and therefore is less permeable through the blood–brain barrier.

Desmopressin

This drug, which is an analogue of vasopressin, minimizes urine production. It can be used to provide relief from bladder symptoms for 6–8 hours, but can be administered only once over a 24-hour period. For example, it may be taken in the evening to allow uninterrupted sleep. Desmopressin acts at the collecting tubules of the kidneys, minimizing water excretion into urine. The water remains in the circulation and therefore may exacerbate heart failure or leg oedema. Minimizing excretion of water into urine may also cause hyponatraemia, and serum sodium levels must be monitored.

Botulinum toxin type A

This drug blocks neuromuscular transmission, effectively paralysing the targeted muscle. Recent evidence suggests that it also interferes with afferent signalling in the bladder. It is an effective treatment for detrusor overactivity and onabotulinum toxin A has recently been licensed for neurogenic detrusor overactivity. As the detrusor muscle is paralysed following the toxin, patients may retain urine and therefore should be taught intermittent self-catheterization before proceeding with injections.

Neuromodulation has also been used to treat storage dysfunction. Sacral nerve stimulators have been used since the 1990s [8], but require surgical implantation with a risk of complication. Transcutaneous or percutaneous tibial nerve stimulation has recently been shown to be effective, and does not require a surgical procedure [9]. Treatments are given once a week for 12 weeks.

There are few pharmacological solutions for voiding dysfunction. Alpha blockers are sometimes used in men, especially when a concomitant bladder outlet obstruction from an enlarged prostate gland is suspected. Botulinum toxin injections into the external urethral sphincter may also be considered, more often in patients with spinal cord injury. The mainstay of treatment, however, is catheterization. CISC is preferable, in terms of both patient quality of life and infection risk. However, patients with neurological impairments affecting vision, strength, or coordination may be unable to perform this. Our patient's progressive neurological impairment forced her to switch to an indwelling suprapubic catheter after two years.

Untreated incontinence impacts quality of life, with as many as 70 per cent of MS patients reporting a high or moderate impact on their life [10]. Failure to diagnose and treat lower urinary tract dysfunction can also have long-term health sequelae. Urinary tract infections are common in this group of patients, and can lead to systemic infections. Incomplete bladder emptying is associated with renal failure, particularly in patients with neural tube defects or traumatic spinal cord injuries. For unknown reasons, renal failure is rarely seen in MS patients despite the high prevalence of lower urinary tract dysfunction [6].

Final word from the expert

Bladder dysfunction has a major impact on many neurological patients, but may be overlooked by neurologists. Once bladder dysfunction is diagnosed, effective pharmacological and non-pharmacological treatments are available which can significantly improve quality of life and reduce further complications in those affected.

References

1. Lammers RL, Gibson S, Kovacs D, et al. Comparison of test characteristics of urine dipstick and urinalysis at various test cutoff points. *Ann Emerg Med* (2001); 38; 505–12.
2. NICE. *NICE Guideline CG8 Multiple Sclerosis*. Available at: <http://publications.nice.org.uk/multiple-sclerosis-cg8/guidance#treatment>
3. Cruz F, Herschorn S, Aliotta P, *et al*. Efficacy and safety of onabotulinumtoxinA in patients with urinary incontinence due to neurogenic detrusor overactivity: a randomised, double-blind, placebo-controlled trial. *Eur Urol* 2011; 60: 742–70.
4. NICE. *Urinary Incontinence in Neurological Disease. CG 148*. Available at: <guidance.nice.org.uk/cg148>.
5. Panicker JN, Fowler CJ. The bare essentials: uro-neurology. *Pract Neurol* 2010; 10: 178–85 (2010).
6. Fowler CJ, Panicker JN, Drake M, *et al*. A UK consensus on the management of the bladder in multiple sclerosis. *J Neurol Neurosurg Psychiatry* 2009; 80: 470–7
7. Dalton CM, Preziosi G, Khan S, de Seze M. Multiple sclerosis and other non-compressive myelopathies. In: Fowler CJ, Panicker JN, Emmanuel A (eds), *Pelvic Organ Dysfunction in Neurological Disease* (Cambridge: Cambridge University Press); 2010: 220–40.
8. Das AK, White MD, Longhurst PA. Sacral nerve stimulation for the management of voiding dysfunction. *Rev Urol* 2000; 2: 43–60.
9. Peters KM, Carrico DJ, Perez-Marrero RA, *et al*. Randomized trial of percutaneous tibial nerve stimulation versus sham efficacy in the treatment of overactive bladder syndrome: results from the SUmiT trial. *J Urol* 2010; 183: 1438–43.
10. Hemmett L, Holmes J, Barnes M, Russell N. What drives quality of life in multiple sclerosis? *QJM* 2004; 97: 671–6.

CASE

9 Not moving a muscle

Dipa Raja Rayan

Expert commentary Chris Turner

Case history

A 20-year-old man presented to clinic with a history of behavioural problems in childhood, muscle stiffness, and slurred speech. He was the product of a normal pregnancy although he was born two weeks premature by forceps delivery. He had normal motor milestones but had problems with attention, concentration, and behaviour, which were labelled as attention-deficit hyperactivity disorder and Asperger's syndrome. From the age of 14 years, his mother noted that he had speech difficulties and was poor at sport at school. She described him as apathetic with poor motivation. Throughout his childhood he had faecal urgency and constipation. He did not have any cardiac or respiratory symptoms, but did suffer from mild excessive daytime sleepiness (EDS). There was no history of cataracts or diabetes mellitus and there was no known family history of muscle disease. He left school at age 16 years with average qualifications but was unable to maintain employment because of a combination of poor motivation and anxieties related to his jobs.

On examination he had myopathic facies, bilateral ptosis, and bulbar dysarthria. Limb power was normal apart from mild finger flexion weakness (Figure 9.1a). He had myotonia of hand grip but not of eyelid closure.

Learning point Differential diagnosis of myotonia

There are several conditions presenting with myotonia clinically and on EMG which should be considered in the differential diagnosis.

- Myotonic dystrophy type 1 (DM1)—this is the most common cause of myotonia. It is a multisystem disorder. Patients often present with hand-grip weakness and myotonia. They may also have cataracts, frontal balding, cardiac arrhythmias, hypersomnia, IBS-like symptoms, and diabetes mellitus [1].
- Myotonic dystrophy type 2 (DM2)—this is genetically and clinically similar to DM1. Patients often have much milder disease. They may develop proximal rather than distal weakness and often suffer from significant pain. For this reason, it has also been called proximal myotonic myopathy (PROMM). Patients may also develop arrhythmias, cataracts, and EDS [1].
- Non-dystrophic myotonia—this group of diseases classically presents in early childhood with prominent myotonia. Persistent weakness is rare and all symptoms are confined to skeletal muscle with no multisystem effects. The most common form is myotonia congenita in which patients develop muscle hypertrophy and limb myotonia which improves with repeated movement. A less common type is paramyotonia congenita in which patients develop myotonia, mainly in the face and eyes, are extremely sensitive to cold and may have episodic weakness [2].

There are also a number of conditions, such as acid maltase deficiency, which may present with pseudomyotonia on EMG although not clinical myotonia. Very occasionally myopathy or denervation can cause electrical myotonia.

In light of the patient's clinical myotonia and myopathic facies, he underwent neurophysiological studies. Electromyography (EMG) demonstrated both myotonic discharges and myopathic units. His serum creatine kinase (CK), thyroid function tests, and serum glucose were normal. An MRI scan of the brain demonstrated non-specific changes in the cerebellum. Given his behavioural and cognitive problems he had full neuropsychometric testing which did not suggest developmental learning difficulties but demonstrated mild cognitive impairment and reduced reading skills. His verbal IQ was 92 and his performance IQ was 89.

Clinical tip Investigations in DM1

- Routine blood tests: serum CK may be normal, although it can be mildly elevated. Liver function tests may be elevated and IgG levels can be low.
- EMG: often the key investigation that leads to a suspicion of DM1. Patients often have a combination of myotonic discharges and myopathic motor units.
- Genetic testing: looking for the expansion in the *DMPK* gene is the most important test for a definitive diagnosis. All patients with suspected DM1 should have genetic confirmation.
- Muscle biopsy: since the advent of genetic testing, biopsies are rarely performed. They will often demonstrate variation in fibre size, increased internal nuclei, ring fibres, sarcoplasmic masses, and early type 1 fibre atrophy.
- Brain MRI scan: this is not used clinically but white matter changes and cerebral atrophy have been found in studies.

The combination of myotonia and myopathy on EMG suggested a diagnosis of myotonic dystrophy. Subsequent DNA analysis identified an abnormal medium-sized CTG expansion (200–700 repeats) in the myotonin-protein kinase gene *DMPK*, diagnostic for DM1.

Evidence base Prophylactic pacing and survival in adults with DM1 [3]

- A retrospective observational study investigating outcome of intensive cardiac monitoring with an electrophysiological study of survival in DM1 patients with conduction system defects.
- The study compared an invasive strategy (n = 341) with a non-invasive strategy (n = 148) in patients with a PR interval >200ms and/or QRS duration >100ms.
- The invasive strategy group had invasive electrophysiology studies and if they had an HV interval (time from activation of the bundle of His to ventricles) over 70ms or sustained ventricular tachyarrhythmias a pacemaker was inserted.
- The non-invasive strategy group had routine cardiac monitoring without an electrophysiology study.
- Fifty patients in the invasive group died compared with thirty in the non-invasive group, producing a greater nine-year survival rate in the invasive group (hazard ratio, 0.74).
- The improved survival was attributed to a lower incidence of sudden death in those in the invasive strategy group.
- Conclusion: patients have a better outcome with invasive electrophysiology and insertion of a pacemaker if they are demonstrated to have a prolonged HV interval or an implantable cardiac defibrillator (ICD) if they developed ventricular arrhythmia.

The patient was further assessed for systemic complications of DM1. His ECG showed a PR interval of 198ms and mild ST segment elevation in the inferior and lateral leads. An echocardiogram and cardiac MRI scan were normal. He had a sleep study to assess his daytime somnolence which did not show significant oxygen desaturation overnight. At review, his main problems were identified as continuing daytime sleepiness and increased frequency of bowel opening with fluctuating constipation and diarrhoea. Therefore he was prescribed modafinil to treat the daytime sleepiness and cholestyramine for the gastrointestinal symptoms thought to be secondary to poor bile acid absorption in DM1. A 24-hour tape was also scheduled for the patient and the possibility of other cardiac electrophysiology tests was explained to him.

Learning point Multidisciplinary management of DM1

As DM1 is a multisystem disorder it is important that all patients are followed up by a number of different specialists.

- **Cardiology** Cardiac conduction defects are common in DM1 and can lead to cardiac death. Patients should be assessed by a cardiologist after first diagnosis with an ECG, echo, and 24-hour Holter monitoring. Patients with prolonged PR intervals or QRS duration are at higher risk of sudden death and should be followed closely [4]. Those at risk should be further assessed with electrophysiology studies to assess the need for pacemakers or ICDs.
- **Respiratory medicine** Breathing complications account for over 40 per cent of deaths in patients with DM1 [5]. Any patient with EDS should be assessed with a sleep study and offered non-invasive ventilation if appropriate. Central nervous system stimulants such as modafinil, dexamfetamine, or methylphenidate can be used in patients who continue to experience EDS despite treatment of sleep-disordered breathing [1, 6].
- **Gastrointestinal medicine** Patients may develop dysphagia which can lead to aspiration pneumonia. Patients often develop IBS-like symptoms which can have a significant impact on quality of life. Bile acid sequestrants, such as cholestyramine, and antibiotics, such as the quinolones, to treat bacterial overgrowth may help some patients [7, 8].
- **Neurology** Myotonia rarely causes significant problems, but may be associated with marked myalgic pain and symptomatic problems in the early stages of adult-onset disease. A recent trial has demonstrated the benefit of mexiletine, but it should be used with caution because of its pro-arrhythmogenic potential [9]. Other pharmaceutical options include carbamazepine, phenytoin, flecainide and imipramine [10].
- **Ophthalmology** The majority of patients will develop posterior subcapsular cataracts during their lifetime which require removal. Patients should be screened regularly for this, especially if there they note a change in vision.
- **Endocrinology** Patients should be checked for glucose intolerance, hypothyroidism, and gonadal failure.
- **Physiotherapy** can help with management of weakness, especially foot drop and neck flexion, and respiratory failure, with orthotics, exercise regimes, and non-invasive ventilation (IV) support.
- **Speech and language therapy** This is useful in monitoring dysphagia and providing practical advice on swallowing safely.

Evidence base Mexiletine as an effective treatment of myotonia in DM1 [9]

- Mexiletine versus placebo in DM1 patients (n = 20) with grip or percussion myotonia.
- Randomized double-blind placebo-controlled crossover study.
- Two trials were performed, one with mexiletine 150mg three times daily and the other with mexiletine 200mg three times daily given to each group of 20 patients for seven weeks with a four- to eight-week washout.
- Outcome measure: isometric grip relaxation time.
- Significant reduction in grip relaxation time at both doses compared with placebo.
- No serious adverse events reported.

The patient's family was assessed in detail to identify other affected individuals. The patient's mother was unaffected (Figure 9.1a). The patient's father was 50 years old with cataracts diagnosed a year earlier. He had no symptoms of muscle weakness or stiffness and no cardiac or respiratory symptoms. He had noticed mild daytime somnolence and faecal urgency. He was employed in a manual job as a warehouse operative and had never had any problems maintaining employment. His parents and brother were reported to be unaffected (Figure 9.1b). On examination, his head was shaved bald. He had mild weakness of eye closure and percussion myotonia of the thenar muscles. His ECG showed sinus bradycardia at a rate of 51bpm and a prolonged PR interval of 220ms, but was otherwise normal.

The patient's 18-year-old brother had a history of hand and leg cramps beginning in the last few years with no history of weakness. He had no cardiac or respiratory symptoms and no daytime somnolence, with an Epworth Sleepiness score of only 2/24. He had mild dyslexia and had obtained only two qualifications after secondary education. On examination, he had myopathic facies with mild eye closure weakness (Figure 9.1a). He had hand-grip myotonia and mild weakness of the forearm and finger extensors. His ECG was normal apart from a minor QRS delay of 125ms. His echocardiogram, 24-hour tape, and sleep study were all normal. Serum glucose and thyroid function tests were normal.

Genetic analysis of family members identified a very small expansion (51–100 CTG) in the father and a medium expansion (200–700 CTG) in the brother.

Learning point Inheritance and anticipation in DM1

DM1 is a disorder with autosomal dominant inheritance. As it can cause increased morbidity and mortality, it is important to screen other family members for the disease. It is caused by an abnormal expansion of the CTG microsatellite repeat in the 3′ untranslated region of the *DMPK* gene in chromosome 19q13.3 [11]. A healthy individual carries between 5 and 37 repeats. Patients who carry more than 50 repeats will develop the disease. The expansion length predicts both age of onset and severity of disease. Individuals who carry intermediate expansions (38–50 repeats) are usually asymptomatic and might only be diagnosed after their children develop clinical features.

CTG expansion	Repeat size	Type of disease
Intermediate	38–50	Asymptomatic
Very small	51–100	Late-onset disease with cataracts and mild myotonia
Small	100–200	Classic disease or childhood-onset DM1
Medium	200–700	Classic disease or childhood-onset DM1
Large	>700	Congenital DM1

DM1 classically shows anticipation where the disease increases in severity and has an earlier age of onset in successive generations. This occurs because *DMPK* alleles longer than 37 repeats are unstable in replication and therefore may increase in size during meiosis or mitosis of cells [12]. This instability is sex-specific. Paternal alleles are more unstable, potentially causing larger expansions, but these probably lead to non-viable gametes when the expansion is very large. Consequently, congenital DM1 is almost exclusively inherited from the maternal allele [13].

The phenomenon of anticipation is evident in this case where the patient's grandparents were unaffected, his father had a very small expansion and was mildly affected with onset in his late forties, but both the patient and his brother had medium-sized expansions and were affected in their teens (Figure 9.1b). It is important to counsel these patients appropriately, so that they are aware that their children are likely to be more severely affected.

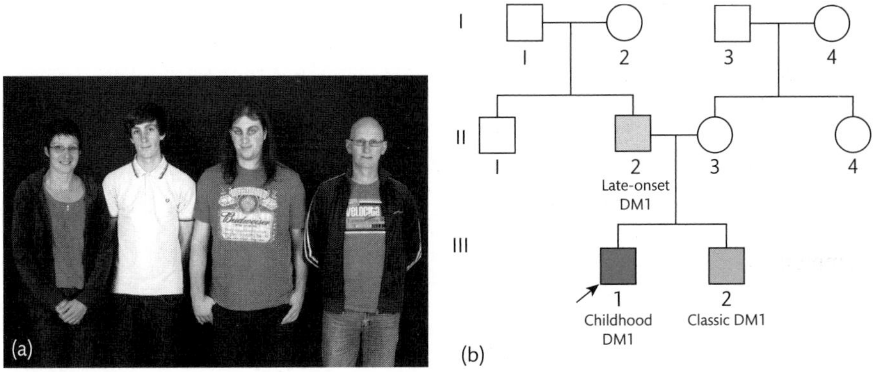

Figure 9. 1 (a) Photograph of the patient and his family. The patient is located centre right, and the ptosis and myopathic facies can be clearly seen. His father is on the right with balding and mild facial myopathy. The patient's brother is on the centre left with very mild myopathic facies. His unaffected mother is on the left. (b) Pedigree of the patient (indicated by the arrow). The affected family members are shaded according to severity.

Discussion

This case illustrates the variability of clinical presentation of DM1 within a family, the range of multisystem problems experienced by patients, and the importance of family testing. DM1 is one of the most common neuromuscular disorders with a prevalence of approximately 1 in 8000 [14] and can be associated with sudden death secondary to cardiac arrhythmias. Therefore it is vital that patients are diagnosed promptly and managed appropriately with long-term follow-up from a multidisciplinary team.

> **Expert comment**
>
> One can expect patients with myotonic dystrophy (DM) to develop a cardiomyopathy in a manner similar to other muscular dystrophies. If a cardiomyopathy occurs in myotonic dystrophy, it is often mild and usually does not require treatment in its own right. The main cardiac problem in DM1 is with the conduction tissue, leading to brady- and tachyarrhythmias which account for up to 30 per cent of premature mortality. We recommend that patients have at least an annual ECG where the most common abnormalities are prolongation of the QRS and PR intervals. If these or other abnormalities are found, patients should be referred to a cardiologist, preferably with a specialist interest in genetic cardiac muscle conditions, and there should be a low threshold for performing an electrophysiological study.

DM1 can present in four different ways (Table 9.1): childhood onset, which is how this patient presented (motor symptoms may be non-specific at this age); adult onset ('classical' DM1), which is how the brother manifested; asymptomatic late onset, which affects the father here; and congenital onset. Childhood-onset DM1 is often the most complex of these phenotypes to diagnose as it often presents with atypical features. As in this case, it frequently manifests with difficulties at school and low IQ, and is often misdiagnosed as behavioural problems. The only signs may be mild facial weakness, dysarthria, and handgrip myotonia. These patients can go on to develop cardiac abnormalities and other systemic symptoms of DM1 and need regular follow-up. Adult-onset DM1 usually manifests initially with myotonia, weakness,

Table 9.1 Varying clinical phenotypes in different forms of DM1

Type of DM1	Clinical phenotype
Late onset	Cataracts and mild myotonia Occasionally weakness and daytime somnolence
Classic DM1	Weakness, myotonia, and cataracts Cardiac conduction defects, daytime somnolence, respiratory failure Gastrointestinal symptoms, insulin insensitivity
Childhood onset	Behavioural psychosocial problems, reduced IQ Facial weakness, dysarthria, myotonia Cardiac conduction defects
Congenital	Infantile hypotonia, respiratory failure, difficulty feeding Delayed milestones, learning disability Cardiorespiratory failure in third and fourth decades

or cataracts. Patients may then develop systemic symptoms in later life due to cardiac conduction defects, gastrointestinal dysfunction, daytime somnolence, and respiratory failure. Asymptomatic late-onset DM1 is commonly discovered in the ancestor who transmitted the mutation and typically manifests with early onset of cataracts. Occasionally, late-onset patients may develop myotonia, weakness, and daytime somnolence, and very rarely may progress to severe disease [15]. Congenital-onset DM1 is the most severe of the four types. It presents prenatally with polyhydramnios and reduced fetal movements. After birth, congenital DM1 neonates may be 'floppy' with hypotonia and have difficulty feeding or breathing. They often require intensive care monitoring and the infant mortality from respiratory failure is high. These children may then develop delayed motor and cognitive milestones. In the third and fourth decades, patients can go on to develop severe cardiac and respiratory complications. The extensive variation in clinical presentation is primarily related to the variation in size of the CTG expansion between family members.

Management of patients with DM is multidisciplinary because of the extensive number of systemic problems that may develop. The most important areas of management are identifying and treating cardiac arrhythmias, which account for 30 per cent of mortality in DM1, and management of respiratory complications, which account for 40 per cent of mortality [5].

Expert comment

Even though respiratory complications account for over 40 per cent of mortality in DM1, the management of this aspect of the disease is often difficult. Patients tend not to tolerate NIV and may ignore swallowing problems. There is growing awareness that a proportion of patients will need to be considered for tube feeding and an emergency admission plan is preferable. EDS is a related problem and can be associated with sleep-disordered breathing; however, patients usually continue to have EDS even when NIV is successfully commenced. EDS can often be treated successfully with psychostimulants such as modafinil, although there is currently no licence for this indication.

Clinical tip Follow-up of patients

As a minimum, patients should have annual ECGs, a sleep study, fasting glucose, and annual cataract assessment alongside management of gastrointestinal symptoms, treatment of myotonia (if necessary), and access to therapy services [1].

There is no effective treatment of the underlying condition, but a number of experimental approaches to reduce the burden of the build-up of toxic CTG repeats that are associated with disease are under development. These include the use of antisense oligonucleotides that can bind to the abnormal CUG RNA expansion, inducing RNA degradation and preventing the formation of ribonuclei foci [16, 17].

There have also been other approaches to target the mis-splicing effects of the DM1 mutation [18] and alter the activity of splicing regulators MBNL and CELF1, whose activities are altered by mutant *DMPK* mRNA [19, 20]. These approaches are yielding early positive results in animal models, and are being translated into early clinical trials. Symptomatic management and monitoring of complications remain the mainstay of treatment in DM1 patients.

Final word from the expert

The management of DM requires an active approach to monitoring and treating complications. Although early mortality is mostly associated with cardiorespiratory complications, it is the muscle weakness and gastrointestinal disturbances which often have the greatest effect on quality of life. Physiotherapy and orthotic input may be helpful for treating foot drop and sometimes neck drop, but hand-grip weakness is difficult to treat and often requires practical measures with occupational therapy input. Persistent gastrointestinal disturbance should be reviewed by a gastroenterologist to exclude other pathologies, followed by consideration of a trial of antibiotics and/or bile acid sequestrants for the IBS-type symptoms.

References

1. Turner C, Hilton-Jones D. The myotonic dystrophies: diagnosis and management. *J Neurol Neurosurg Psychiatry* 2010; 81(4): 358–67.
2. Raja Rayan DL, Hanna MG. Skeletal muscle channelopathies: nondystrophic myotonias and periodic paralysis. *Curr Opin Neurol* 2010; 23(5): 466–76.
3. Wahbi K, Meune C, Porcher R, et al. Electrophysiological study with prophylactic pacing and survival in adults with myotonic dystrophy and conduction system disease. *JAMA* 2012; 307(12): 1292–1301.
4. Groh WJ, Groh MR, Saha C, et al. Electrocardiographic abnormalities and sudden death in myotonic dystrophy type 1. *N Engl J Med* 2008; 358(25): 2688–97.
5. Mathieu J, Allard P, Potvin L, et al. A 10-year study of mortality in a cohort of patients with myotonic dystrophy. *Neurology* 1999; 52(8): 1658–62.
6. Annane D, Moore DH, Barnes PRJ, Miller RG. Psychostimulants for hypersomnia (excessive daytime sleepiness) in myotonic dystrophy. *Cochrane Database System Rev* 2006; (3): CD003218.
7. Rönnblom A, Andersson S, Danielsson A. Mechanisms of diarrhoea in myotonic dystrophy. *Eur J Gastroenterol Hepatol* 1998; 10(7): 607–10.
8. Ronnblom A, Andersson S, Hellstrom PM, Danielsson A. Gastric emptying in myotonic dystrophy. *Eur J Clin Invest* 2002; 32(8): 570–4.
9. Logigian EL, Martens WB, Moxley RT, et al. Mexiletine is an effective antimyotonia treatment in myotonic dystrophy type 1. *Neurology* 2010; 74(18): 1441–8.
10. Trip J, Drost G, van Engelen BG, Faber CG. Drug treatment for myotonia. *Cochrane Database System Rev* 2006; (1): CD004762.
11. Brook JD, McCurrach ME, Harley HG, et al. Molecular basis of myotonic dystrophy: expansion of a trinucleotide (CTG) repeat at the 3' end of a transcript encoding a protein kinase family member. *Cell* 1992; 68(4): 799–808.
12. de Temmerman N, Sermon K, Seneca S, et al. Intergenerational instability of the expanded CTG repeat in the *DMPK* gene: studies in human gametes and preimplantation embryos. *Am J Hum Genet* 2004; 75(2): 325–9.

13. Rakocević-Stojanović V, Savić D, Pavlović S, et al. Intergenerational changes of CTG repeat depending on the sex of the transmitting parent in myotonic dystrophy type 1. *Eur J Neurol* 2005; 12(3): 236–7.
14. Harper PS. *Myotonic Dystrophy* (3rd edn), (London: Saunders); 2001.
15. Arsenault M-E, Prévost C, Lescault A, et al. Clinical characteristics of myotonic dystrophy type 1 patients with small CTG expansions. *Neurology* 2006; 66(8): 1248–50.
16. Wheeler TM, Sobczak K, Lueck JD, et al. Reversal of RNA dominance by displacement of protein sequestered on triplet repeat RNA. *Science* 2009; 325(5938): 336–9.
17. Mulders SAM, van Engelen BGM, Wieringa B, Wansink DG. Molecular therapy in myotonic dystrophy: focus on RNA gain-of-function. *Hum Mol Genet* 2010; 19(R1): R90–7.
18. Wheeler TM, Lueck JD, Swanson MS, et al. Correction of ClC-1 splicing eliminates chloride channelopathy and myotonia in mouse models of myotonic dystrophy. *J Clin Invest* 2007; 117(12): 3952–7.
19. Warf MB, Diegel JV, von Hippel PH, Berglund JA. The protein factors MBNL1 and U2AF65 bind alternative RNA structures to regulate splicing. *Proc Natl Acad Sci USA* 2009; 106(23): 9203–8.
20. Wang G-S, Kuyumcu-Martinez MN, Sarma S, et al. PKC inhibition ameliorates the cardiac phenotype in a mouse model of myotonic dystrophy type 1. *J Clin Invest* 2009; 119(12): 3797–806.

CASE

10 A painful oculomotor nerve palsy

Vino Siva

Expert commentary Marios C. Papadopoulos and Daniel C. Walsh

Case history

Mrs P, a 64-year-old right-handed woman, attended her local accident and emergency department with an intolerable persistent headache of sudden onset, commencing two days previously. She had put the headache down to a severe attack of migraine and had spent the last two days in bed taking over-the-counter analgesia with little effect. She complained of associated sensitivity to bright light and reduced appetite due to nausea. On further questioning, it was apparent that over the previous fortnight she had been suffering from episodic double vision associated with a right-sided fronto-parietal headache. Her friends noted drooping of her right eyelid, which she had put down to fatigue.

Learning point Thunderclap headache (TCH)

TCH is a sudden severe headache that, according to the International Classification of Headache Disorders version II diagnostic criteria, reaches maximal intensity within 1 minute. The term was first coined in reference to the sentinel headaches associated with an unruptured intracranial aneurysm. Since then, multiple other causes have been associated with TCH [1, 2].

Differential diagnosis of TCH

- Vascular aetiology:
  - subarachnoid haemorrhage (SAH)
  - sentinel bleed related to unruptured aneurysm
  - arterial dissection
  - reversible cerebral vasoconstriction syndrome
  - cerebral venous sinus thrombosis
  - intracranial haemorrhage
  - pituitary apoplexy
  - reversible posterior leucoencephalopathy
  - arterial hypertension.
- Non-vascular intracranial disorders:
  - spontaneous intracranial hypotension
  - third ventricle colloid cyst
  - intracranial infection.

The time to maximal intensity is pivotal in the history and differentiates TCH from other severe headaches (migraine, cluster) [1, 3]. Therefore it is not sufficient to ask if the headache is the 'worst ever headache' in the patient's life, but also to qualify timing to peak intensity by asking how long it takes to reach maximum intensity. Patients may volunteer information regarding timing to peak intensity by describing the headache as akin to being 'hit with a bat'.

(Continued)

Expert comment

This patient's presentation is very characteristic, suggesting not only a diagnosis but also a location for the pathology. A patient presenting with a sudden onset of severe headache for the first time should be considered to have aneurysmal subarachnoid haemorrhage until that diagnosis is excluded, by cerebrospinal fluid (CSF) examination if necessary.

Expert comment

If the history is suggestive of SAH (sudden-onset headache) but the CT scan shows no subarachnoid blood, consider two other important diagnoses that are often missed; their treatment and outlook are very different from that of SAH. One is pituitary apoplexy—if there is an expanded sella turcica on CT, proceed to emergency MRI. The other is venous sinus thrombosis—if there is a hyperdense venous sinus (often associated with brain oedema and sometimes venous haemorrhages), proceed to CT or MR venogram.

SAH is the most common cause of secondary TCH, accounting for up to 25 per cent of patients presenting with TCH. It should be the focus of initial investigations in vie w of the high morbidity and mortality associated with misdiagnosis, especially as it may be possible to treat a sentinel bleed before a potentially fatal bleed occurs. Sentinel headaches/bleeds or warning headaches occur in up to 50 per cent of patients with SAH. These headaches are sudden and severe, and resolve within 24 hours. They most commonly occur within two weeks of the SAH, peaking within the preceding 24 hours. They have been attributed to a small aneurysmal leak or dynamic physical changes within the aneurysmal wall.

Mrs P lived with her husband, and was an avid gardener. She had been a smoker since her late teenage years, recently cutting down to 10 cigarettes a day. She was generally fit and well, apart from being on medication for high blood pressure, diabetes mellitus, and high cholesterol. Her family history was unremarkable except that her father suffered from a fatal 'stroke' in his seventies.

Learning point Risk factors for aneurysmal SAH (aSAH)

Modifiable risk factors [4]

- Hypertension—studies report a relative risk up to 3.4 (CI 2.3–5.7).
- Smoking [5]—a significant risk factor that demonstrates a dose-dependent relationship between cigarettes smoked and risk of aSAH:
  - heavy smoker (>20 cigarettes/day) odds ratio (OR) 11.1 (CI 5.0–24.9)
  - current smoker (<20 cigarettes/day) OR 4.1 (CI 2.3–7.3)
  - ex-smoker odds ratio (OR) 1.8 (CI 1.0–3.2).
- Heavy alcohol consumption (>150g/week)—there is evidence to suggest that light drinking has a protective effect (possibly via antioxidant activity protecting against vessel inflammation), with a dose-dependent increase for higher alcohol consumption.
- Oestrogen preparations—there is evidence suggesting that oral contraceptives (OCPs) increase the risk of aSAH, with a meta-analysis [6] suggesting a greater risk associated with high-oestrogen OCPs than with low-oestrogen OCPs. In contrast, oestrogen replacement therapy appears to have a risk-reducing effect.
- Cocaine.

The mechanisms by which the above modifiable risk factors predispose to aSAH may be classified into those that cause vessel wall injury (Figure 10.1) and those that produce haemodynamic stress (Figure 10.2).

It is worth noting that many risk factors simultaneously lead to vessel wall damage and haemodynamic stress, and have a synergistic effect on aneurysm formation.

Non modifiable risk factors:

Conditions associated with an increased incidence of cerebral aneurysms include:
- autosomal dominant polycystic kidney disease (ADPKD)
- fibromuscular dysplasia (FMD)
- arteriovenous malformations (AVMs)—flow-related aneurysms
- connective tissue disorders
  - Ehlers-Danlos sydrome (especially type IV and deficient collagen type III)
  - -Marfan syndrome
  - -pseudoxanthoma elasticum.

Expert comment

One might add genetic factors which render an individual susceptible to the formation and rupture of a cerebral aneurysm as a non-modifiable risk factor. Knowledge is evolving in this area and work has emerged suggesting that first-degree relatives are at somewhat increased risk of forming intracranial

(Continued)

aneurysms and are at increased susceptibility to environmental factors such as smoking. It remains to be determined whether screening for aneurysms in such a population confers health benefit in the long term. It would seem appropriate to counsel relatives on the modification of lifestyle factors at the very least [7, 8].

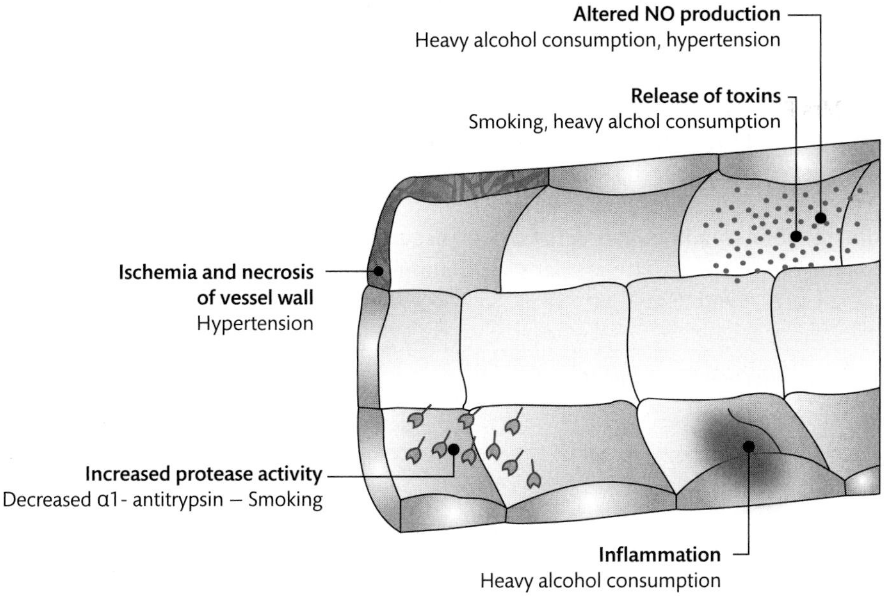

Figure 10.1 Mechanisms of vessel wall damage that contribute to aneurysm formation with the associated modifiable risk factors for each mechanism.

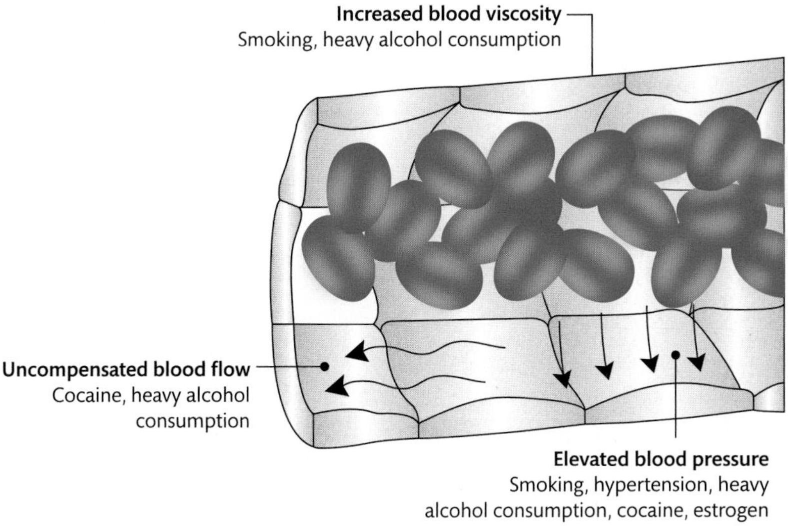

Figure 10.2 Mechanisms of haemodynamic stress that contribute to aneurysm formation with the associated modifiable risk factors for each mechanism.

Clinical tip Aneurysmal oculomotor palsy

The old 'rule of the pupil' (i.e. pupil sparing excludes the oculomotor nerve being compressed externally by an aneurysm) should only apply if there is a complete oculomotor nerve palsy. Relative sparing of the pupil is reported in 30–40 per cent of aneurysmal incomplete oculomotor nerve palsies.

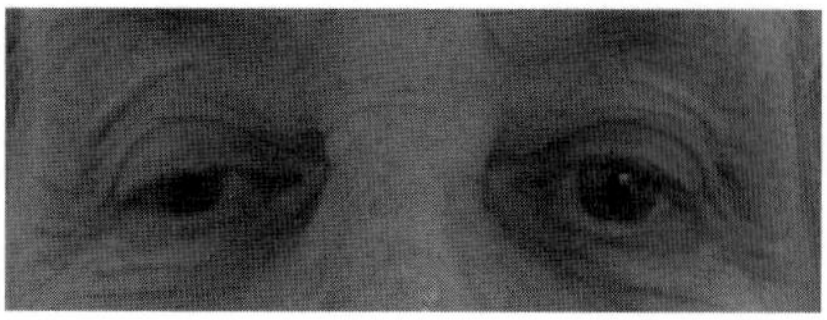

Figure 10.3 Partial right sided pupil-sparing oculomotor nerve palsy.

On hospital admission at day 2 post-ictus ('ictus' refers to onset of the presumed bleed), Mrs P was alert and orientated in time, place, and person. She was in obvious discomfort from her headache, and exhibited photophobia and nuchal rigidity on neck flexion. She had an incomplete right-sided ptosis and a sluggishly reactive right pupil, but no anisocoria. Eye movements were restricted, with diplopia. Examination findings were consistent with a partial right-sided pupil-sparing oculomotor nerve palsy. Her vital signs were unremarkable except for raised blood pressure of 172/89mmHg (Figure 10.3).

Learning point Signs of SAH

Meningism occurs as a result of meningeal irritation from blood products. It manifests as follows.

- Nuchal rigidity—more pronounced on flexion, often occurring 6–24 hours post-ictus.
- Photophobia and continuing headache are typical.
- Kernig's sign—pain in hamstrings following extension of the knee from a flexed position with the hip flexed to 90°.
- Brudzinski's sign—involuntary hip flexion on passive flexion of the patient's neck whilst in a supine position.
- Ocular haemorrhage may occur as a result of central retinal vein obstruction from a distended meningeal optic nerve sheath. Terson's syndrome refers to vitreous haemorrhage following SAH.

Subarachnoid blood products may impair CSF reabsorption by arachnoid granulations leading to a **communicating hydrocephalus**, or clots in the ventricles may lead to **obstructive hydrocephalus**. These manifest as symptoms and signs of raised intracranial pressure, which include nausea, vomiting, and a reduced conscious state.

Cerebral infarcts/ischaemia from regional or diffuse vasospasm can lead to focal neurological deficits. Aneurysmal SAH may also be associated with intracerebral haemorrhage with corresponding focal neurological deficits when in eloquent brain.

Expert comment

An associated intracerebral haematoma is related to the projection of the aneurysm. The most frequent rupture point is at the apex of the dome, and if this is projecting into the temporal lobe, as is the case in some middle cerebral artery (MCA) aneurysms, or toward the gyrus rectus, as in anterior communicating artery (ACom) aneurysms, intracerebral haematoma is more likely.

An urgent unenhanced CT head scan was performed to investigate for SAH. This was reported as unremarkable.

Expert comment

In many cases of a PCom aneurysm causing oculomotor nerve palsy, the nerve palsy will recover within six months. The chance of complete recovery with surgery (which removes the pressure of the aneurysm on the nerve) is about 90 per cent; it is about 60 per cent with coiling, even though coiling does not deflate the aneurysm. The reason why coiling allows the oculomotor nerve to recover is not understood, but may be because coiling removes the aneurysmal pulsation against the nerve.

Expert comment

The diagnosis of a painful oculomotor nerve palsy, even if aSAH is excluded by CSF analysis, **still** constitutes a neurosurgical emergency and mandates urgent neurovascular imaging to exclude a posterior communicating (PCom) artery aneurysm, or less commonly a superior cerebellar artery (SCA) aneurysm (Figure 10.4). Even in the absence of a bleed, the aneurysm should be treated as an emergency, as the oculomotor nerve palsy is probably due to expansion of an aneurysm at imminent risk of rupture.

She was seen by the on-call medical team, who performed a lumbar puncture (LP) after one unsuccessful attempt. The first attempt, by a junior doctor, collected a few drops of blood-stained fluid insufficient for analysis. The second lumbar puncture, performed 30 minutes later, was successful in collecting three sequential samples of CSF and demonstrated an opening pressure of 18cmH2O. On visual inspection the

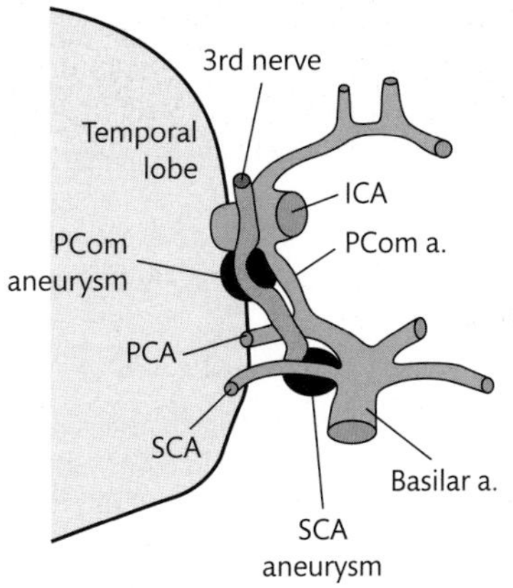

Figure 10.4 Diagram illustrating how a PCom or SCA aneurysm can compress the oculomotor nerve (view looking up at the circle of Willis).

first sample was blood-stained, becoming clearer with the sequential bottles. CSF spectroscopy confirmed both a bilirubin and an oxyhaemoglobin peak.

Learning point Investigation for SAH

CT

CT scanning (with a third-generation 'rotational' or 'helical' scanner) is 98 per cent sensitive in detecting SAH in the first 12 hours, but this drops to 80–85 per cent after 24 hours, and further to 70 per cent by three days after the haemorrhage. The exact percentage will vary according to the experience of the reporting radiologist and the scanner type.

CT is also useful for detecting ventriculomegaly, which may represent hydrocephalus and any areas of associated intracerebral or subdural haemorrhage, as well as estimating blood load (associated with risk of vasospasm). The distribution of blood may indicate the location of the aneurysm; this is particularly important in patients with multiple aneurysms.

Lumbar puncture

In patients with a normal CT scan, a lumbar puncture for analysis of CSF for xanthochromia is imperative [9]. Erythrocytes in the CSF undergo lysis to release oxyhaemoglobin approximately 2-4 hours after haemorrhage. Macrophages metabolize oxyhaemoglobin (oxyHb) to bilirubin, and sometimes methaemoglobin (metHb). Only bilirubin is produced in vivo, taking up to 12 hours, whereas both oxyHb and met Hb can occur in vitro.

Xanthochromia is almost 100 per cent sensitive by 12 hours after haemorrhage, falling to approximately 70 per cent at three weeks. There is ongoing controversy as to whether visual inspection of CSF or spectrometry is better. Evidence suggests that spectrometry is more sensitive, but lacks specificity. The presence of high levels of plasma bilirubin and CNS protein may give false-positive results.

MRI is not sensitive in the acute period because there is too little metHb. It is excellent for subacute to late presentation of SAH (after approximately 10 days), with FLAIR sequences being the most sensitive.

Following discussion with the on-call neurosurgeon, she was transferred as an emergency that night to her regional neurosurgery unit for further investigation and management of her SAH.

Expert comment

It has been argued that CSF examination is unnecessary with high-quality CT scanning services. The conditions under which CT scans are reported in emergency practice are suboptimal. The consequences of rebleeding from a ruptured aneurysm are much more severe than the morbidity of lumbar puncture [10]. If there is any doubt on CT, a lumbar puncture is mandatory.

Expert comment

About 15 per cent of aneurysms are multiple. In the context of a SAH, it is important to know which aneurysm bled in order to target treatment. This is determined from the distribution of blood on the CT. If the patient in this case had an aneurysm far from the optic nerve, then her headache was not aneurysmal. An alternative cause for her symptoms would need to be investigated, with counselling for the incidental aneurysm identified.

Clinical tip Identification of aneurysm

Once SAH has been diagnosed, the aim is to identify the underlying vascular anomaly. Digital subtraction angiography (DSA) remains the gold standard if an aneurysm is not identified by the less invasive CT angiography (CTA).

Expert comment

Proximal vascular access for coiling can be very difficult in elderly patients and in our experience surgical clipping can be very rewarding in this setting.

Expert comment

In cases of posterior communicating artery aneurysm, one of the things to study on the angiogram is whether the patient has a fetal circulation, in which the distal posterior cerebral artery is supplied from the posterior communicating artery rather than the basilar artery. If there is a fetal circulation, any iatrogenic damage to the posterior communicating artery (e.g. by incorporating the posterior communicating aneurysm in the clip) will cause a posterior cerebral artery infarct.

Expert comment

During surgery for a posterior communicating artery aneurysm, the surgeon identifies and preserves the anterior choroidal artery, which is a small branch of the ICA that arises proximal to the posterior communicating artery. Flow through the anterior choroidal artery should also be confirmed during intra-operative post-clipping indocyanine green video-angiography. Damaging the anterior choroidal artery may cause post-operative contralateral hemiplegia, contralateral sensory loss, and homonymous hemianopia.

Learning point Referring to neurosurgery

When referring to the neurosurgeon on-call, he/she will want to know the following details.

- Date/time of ictus (in this context, 'ictus' refers to the initial haemorrhage). The number of days post-ictus is important for evaluating whether the method of diagnosis (CT, LP) is sufficiently accurate and assessing the risk of further complications, such as delayed ischaemic neurological deficit (DIND), hydrocephalus, and rebleeding.
- Glasgow coma scale (GCS)—note that this scale refers to the patient's **best** eye, verbal, and motor scores. It is best to give a breakdown in words to avoid confusion. The motor component is the most important.
- The patient's baseline neurological and functional status.
- Focal neurological deficits.
- Comorbidities, and whether the patient is on any antiplatelet or anticoagulant medications.
- The timing of the LP if performed. If multiple attempts were required, the timing of the attempts and whether any CSF was accessed at each attempt. For example, if there was a traumatic tap and a subsequent attempt was made the next day, the CSF is likely to be positive for bilirubin, making the result inconclusive. Therefore the decision will depend on a thorough history.

On day 2 post-ictus, Mrs P was commenced on oral nimodipine, analgesia, stool softeners, and intravenous fluids, and placed on mechanical thromboprophylaxis. She was nursed in the neurosurgical high-dependency unit to closely monitor her neurological status (GCS as well as regular review for focal neurological deficits), serum electrolytes, fluid status, blood pressure, and cerebral vessel velocity using interval transcranial Doppler (TCD) ultrasonography.

Learning point Supportive management of an aneurysmal subarachnoid haemorrhage

- Nimodipine: there is level I evidence supporting the use of prophylactic oral nimodipine (60mg every four-hours for 21 days). It has been shown to reduce the incidence of cerebral ischaemia and infarction by a third in patients with aSAH.
- Intravenous fluids: the patient is kept well hydrated (euvolaemic or slight positive balance) to minimize the effects of vasospasm and cerebral salt-wasting. Fluids must be managed judiciously in patients with neurogenic pulmonary oedema or cardiac failure.
- Stool softeners: are used to prevent constipation and straining, which may raise intracranial pressure unnecessarily.

CTA on arrival revealed a 6mm lobulated aneurysm arising from the posterior wall of the distal right internal carotid artery (ICA) (Figure 10.5a). The aneurysm was orientated postero-inferiorly with a 2mm bleb at its tip. The next day, following discussion of her case in an ad hoc neurovascular multidisciplinary meeting consisting of an interventional neuroradiologist and a neurovascular surgeon, endovascular treatment was attempted, but stable access to the aneurysm could not be achieved owing to the tortuosity of the internal carotid artery (ICA).

Therefore Mrs P underwent an operation to perform surgical clipping of her right PCom aneurysm on the same day. In the procedure, a myocutaneous flap was raised and a lateral supra-orbital mini-craniotomy was performed (Figure 10.5b). After a curved durotomy had been fashioned, subfrontal dissection of the optic apparatus was performed to identify the vascular apparatus (Figure 10.5c). The right ICA was identified and followed to the neck of the aneurysm (Figure 10.5d), and after careful dissection an 8mm Yasargil clip was successfully applied (Figure 10.5e). Intra-operative indocyanine green video-angiography demonstrated arterial phase flow in the distal ICA with no flow in the aneurysm. The dome of the aneurysm was intentionally punctured to ensure satisfactory clipping (Figure 10.5f).

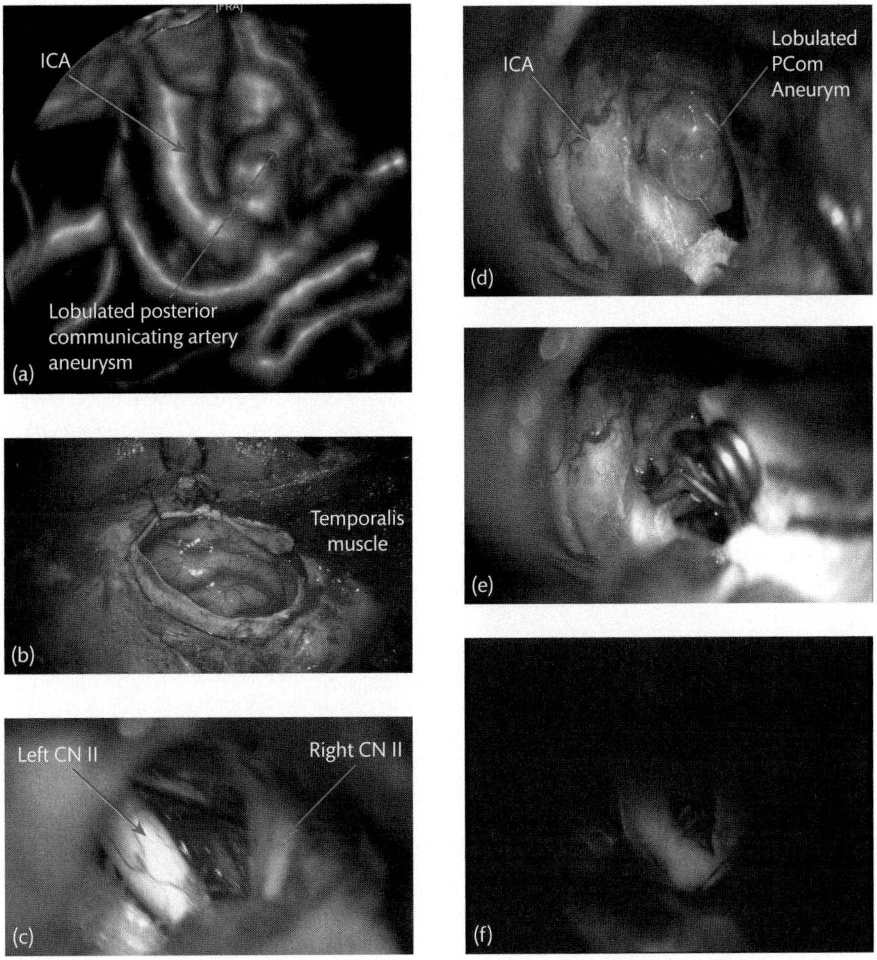

Figure 10.5 Surgical clipping of a PCom aneurysm: (a) CTA identifying a lobulated PCom aneurysm; (b) lateral supra-orbital mini-craniotomy; (c) subfrontal dissection of the optic apparatus; (d) right ICA followed to reach the PCom aneurysm; (e) neck dissected and ligated with an 8mm straight Yasargil titanium clip; (f) indocyanine green video-angiography demonstrating arterial phase flow in the distal ICA and no flow in the aneurysm.

Mrs P made good post-operative recovery with no new neurological deficit. Post-operative instructions were to ensure normotension, normovolaemia, normothermia, and normoglycaemia, and to provide deep vein thrombosis prophylaxis in the form of compression stockings and intermittent pneumatic compression devices from the time of surgery. She commenced enoxaparin after 24 hours.

Mrs P made a good recovery until day 5 post-ictus, when she was found to be slightly more confused and not her usual interactive self. A left-sided pronator drift was evident on examination. TCD ultrasound demonstrated a trend in increased velocities, and her serum sodium was normal. Sodium imbalances are a known complication of aSAH and may lead to cerebral oedema (see discussion).

Learning point Delayed cerebral ischaemia (DCI)/delayed ischaemic neurological deficit (DIND)/'clinical vasospasm'

The prevention of DCI/DIND is central to the medical management of aSAH. It is classically thought to be related to vasospasm, which is an angiographic or radiological finding of cerebral arterial narrowing. Angiographic vasospasm is distinguished from DCI/DIND/'clinical vasospasm', characterized clinically by a decreased level of consciousness, confusion, or focal neurological deficit such as hemiparesis or dysphasia. The terminology is confusing, and reflects our poor understanding of the pathophysiological mechanisms underpinning the delayed neurological deterioration in aSAH patients where no other attributable cause (such as hydrocephalus or seizure) is found. Current evidence suggests that it is multifactorial, with angiographic vasospasm being only one factor. The term 'clinical vasospasm' is misleading and is best avoided as vasospasm is not present in some patients who deteriorate in this manner. The term makes reference to the underlying pathophysiology, which is currently not well understood, and does not reflect the other pathophysiological mechanisms involved. DCI/DIND is a more general term and better reflects the numerous underlying mechanisms leading to cerebral ischaemia (see Discussion) in this patient group.

Angiographic vasospasm is reported to occur in 70–90 per cent of aSAH patients, with clinical (symptomatic) vasospasm occurring in up to 30 per cent. The high-risk period is 3–14 days post-ictus—hence the importance of knowing the time of the ictal headache. The ultimate aim is to prevent or reverse cerebral ischaemia in order to halt progression to the irreversible stage of cerebral infarction. Patients who present with a high-grade SAH and have a heavy blood load on CT are at higher risk of DIND. A history of known hypertension and current cigarette smoking have also been shown to be risk factors.

DSA is the gold standard for diagnosing radiological vasospasm, but TCD ultrasonography can be a useful non-invasive bedside diagnostic tool. CTA is also commonly used to demonstrate vasospasm. Other modalities such as those looking at alterations in cerebral blood flow (perfusion CT, MRI, SPECT) can be helpful.

Learning point Transcranial Doppler ultrasonography

Transcranial Doppler (TCD) ultrasonography is a non-invasive and relatively inexpensive method which can be used to measure cerebral blood flow velocities in the basal cerebral arteries [11]. This can be done at the bedside by an experienced technician using a low-frequency (2MHz) transducer probe to measure cerebral blood flow velocities via naturally thin bone windows in the skull (i.e. transtemporal, suboccipital/transforaminal, and transorbital) (Figure 10.6) [11, 12]. Blood flow velocity is determined indirectly by measuring the difference between the emitted and reflected wave frequency (Doppler shift frequency) from flowing red blood cells. The temporal bone window is most commonly used, and is able to detect the middle cerebral artery, as well as the anterior cerebral and internal carotid arteries. However, 10–20 per cent of patients have inadequate temporal bone windows.

An increase in velocity may be due to either an increase in blood flow (hyperaemia) or a decrease in vessel diameter (vasospasm) (Figure 10.7). The Lindegaard ratio, measured by dividing the flow velocity in the MCA by the velocity in the ipsilateral extracranial internal carotid artery, is used to identify vasospasm, with a value >3 signifying vasospasm (Table 10.1).

Detectable changes can precede clinical symptoms, so baseline studies are performed before vasospasm is likely to occur, and periodic measurements that suggest increases in velocities provide good supporting evidence of impending vasospasm.

A fluid status review demonstrated that she had a cumulative 1L negative fluid balance over the previous 48 hours. Her blood pressure was about 130/62mmHg compared with her baseline of approximately 145/80mmHg. Intravenous colloid fluid challenges and cessation of her usual antihypertensive medication improved her blood pressure so that it was closer to her baseline, with corresponding clinical

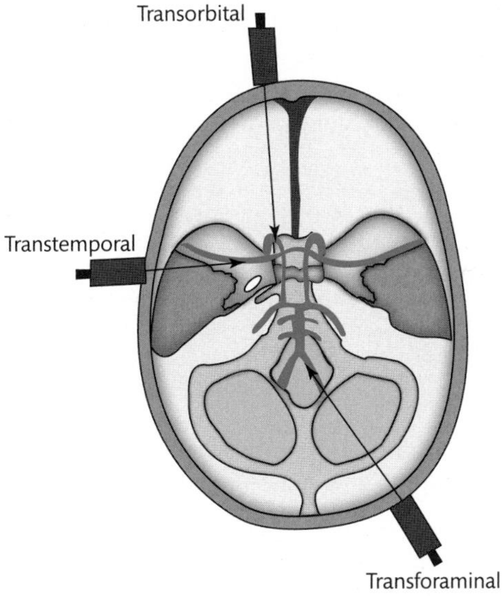

Figure 10.6 Commonly used bone windows for TCDs.

Reproduced from *Postgrad Med J*, 83(985), Sarkar SI, Ghosh S, Ghosh SK, Collier A., Role of transcranial Doppler ultrasonography in stroke, pp. 683–9, © 2007, with permission from BMJ Publishing Group Ltd.

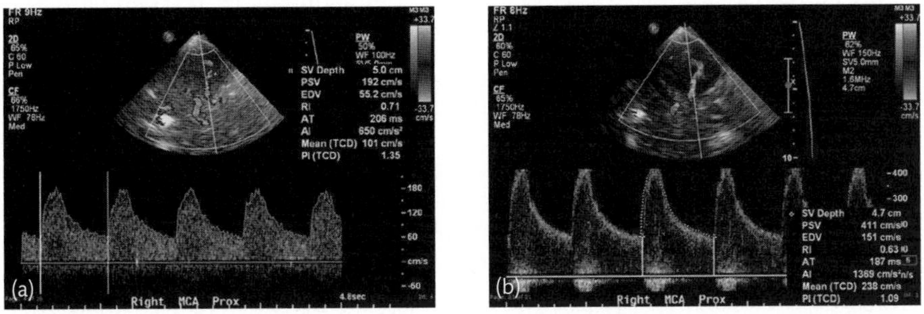

Figure 10.7 (a) Right MCA TCD waveform (bottom) with colour Doppler (top). (b) TCD demonstrates an increased peak systolic velocity (PSV) and mean flow velocity (MFV) in the right MCA, consistent with severe vasospasm.

Reproduced from *Int J Vasc Med*, 2013: 629378, Naqvi J, Yap KH, Ahmad G, Ghosh J, Transcranial Doppler ultrasound: a review of the physical principles and major applications in critical care, © 2013, reproduced under the Creative Commons Attribution License 3.0.

Table 10.1 Interpretation of MFV and the Lindegaard ratio

Mean flow velocity (cm/s)	Lindegaard ratio (MCA:ICA)	
<120	<3	Normal
120–200	3–6	Mild vasospasm
>200	6	Severe vasospasm

Adapted from Greenberg MS, *The Handbook of Neurosurgery*, p. 1048, © 2010, with permission from Thieme Medical Publishers, Inc.

improvement in her alertness and pronator drift. Over the next 24 hours her neurological status was very sensitive to her blood pressure, requiring a mean arterial pressure (MAP) >90mmHg. To maintain her MAP, she was transferred to the neurosurgical intensive care unit for vasopressor support (noradrenaline)

Clinical tip Management of delayed ischaemic neurological deficit (DIND)

Medical treatment is usually the initial step when DIND is suspected. It is usually performed by administration of intravenous fluids, albumin, inotropic agents, and vasopressors. Unfortunately, however, vasospasm is often refractory to these interventions.

Moreover, many patients do not tolerate induced hypertension (referring to attempts to reverse neurological deficits by increasing MAP), usually because of cardiac and pulmonary complications The well-documented 'triple-H' therapy (comprising hypertension, hypervolaemia, and haemodilution) is an almost obsolete term, and has not been shown to change the overall prognosis of DIND. Early endovascular treatment appears to be the best alternative for these patients. The most common modalities used in the endovascular treatment of cerebral vasospasm are mechanical dilatation with balloon angioplasty, pharmacological dilatation with intra-arterial drug infusion, or a combination of both.

Later, Mrs P reported worse headaches in the morning, and a repeat CT scan demonstrated more prominent ventricles with no evidence of any bleed. Therapeutic lumbar punctures were performed periodically for her evolving communicating hydrocephalus, demonstrating repeated high opening pressures >25cmH2O with transient improvement in her morning headaches before they relapsed the next day. Finally, a lumbar drain was inserted to help manage her intracranial pressure. This allowed a reduction in her vasopressor support to maintain her cerebral perfusion pressure and improvement in her headaches.

Learning point Hydrocephalus after SAH [13, 14]

Hydrocephalus is a common complication of SAH—it may be acute or chronic, with the former occurring within hours and the latter weeks to months after ictus. Acute obstructive hydrocephalus occurs in approximately 15–20 per cent of patients, requiring placement of an external ventricular drain whereby a catheter is inserted into the right frontal horn, draining CSF externally to a bag connected to a manometer so that the pressure at which fluid drains can be regulated. There is a school of thought that suggests that there is increased risk of rebleeding if CSF diversion procedure is implemented in a patient with an unprotected aneurysm, possibly due to a change in the transmural pressure across the wall of the aneurysm.

Where there is communicating hydrocephalus, interval lumbar punctures can be performed and, if required, a lumbar drain can be inserted for continual drainage.

There is evidence to suggest that drainage of CSF (via an external ventricular drain or a lumbar drain) reduces the risk of vasospasm, possibly by reducing the blood load in the subarachnoid space.

Mrs P was successfully weaned off her vasopressor support and transferred back to the high dependency unit three days later (day 8 post-ictus). After observation of no increased velocities on TCD, stable serum sodium levels, less labile blood pressure recordings, and a consistently good clinical status the lumbar drain was removed. Mrs P was discharged home on day 14 post-ictus after assessment by therapists and advised to stop driving temporarily and inform the DVLA. She attended the outpatient clinic six months later with complete resolution of her oculomotor palsy and regained independent function.

Discussion

Subarachnoid haemorrhage, although only accounting for 5 per cent of strokes, is a devastating disease resulting in significant morbidity and mortality for a relatively young population, with consequent loss of productive years comparable to ischaemic stroke [15]. This case highlights the multifaceted approach required to manage a patient with aSAH, with surgical or endovascular intervention forming only one part, albeit a crucial one, of the management pathway. The peri-operative medical management of such patients is pivotal not only in preventing fatalities, but also in delivering the patient as close to their neurological baseline as possible at the end of the disease process.

Once an aneurysm ruptures, the patient can be perceived as embarking on a journey with numerous pitfalls; securing the aneurysm only addresses one such pitfall, i.e. the risk of rebleeding. Even if the patient were to enter this journey neurologically intact with their aneurysm successfully secured, they remain at risk of death or significant disability as a result of the diverse neurological sequelae of aSAH. Therefore the medical management of such patients centres around anticipating and monitoring potential complications during the high-risk period, and managing them appropriately to prevent the patient developing further neurological deficits by the end of this disease journey.

A review of population-based studies estimated the case fatality to average 51 per cent [16], with up to 15 per cent of all patients dying before reaching hospital. The neurological status at presentation of the survivors covers a wide spectrum, ranging from being neurologically intact to suffering a focal deficit or being in a comatose state. Over the last few decades, the World Federation of Neurosurgical Societies (WFNS) scale has been widely used to determine a patient's prognosis after SAH [17]. The WFNS grade is determined by the conscious level of the patient and whether they have a focal deficit or not (Table 10.2).

Learning point World Federation of Neurosurgical Societies (WFNS) SAH grade

Because of the variability in applying the WFNS grade to patients who may sometimes have subtle neurological deficits and the fact that the difference in outcome may also be subtle, particularly for grades II and III, a modified WFNS grading system has been proposed whereby patients are graded according to their GCS, with grade II assigned to patients with GCS 14, and grade III to patients with GCS 13 independent of whether or not they have a neurological deficit [18]. This modified WFNS scale appears to be simpler and a better prognosticator of outcome, but requires further validation before it comes into general use.

Approximately 1 in 20 SAH patients are missed in the emergency department, with the majority misdiagnosed as migraine or another type of headache [19]. Diagnosis can be challenging, particularly in neurologically intact patients presenting with headache only where there may be a reluctance to perform a lumbar puncture. However, it is in this neurologically intact group where it is important not to miss the diagnosis, as one has the opportunity to preserve the patient's functional status with expeditious treatment before they suffer the potentially catastrophic consequences of a rebleed or another disabling complication of SAH.

Table 10.2 WFNS SAH grade

WFNS grade	GCS score	Neurological focal deficit
1	15	
2	13–14	Absent
3	13–14	Present
4	7–12	Absent or present
5	2–6	Absent or present

This case emphasizes the need for lumbar puncture in CT negative patients with a history suggestive of SAH, particularly in late presentations. Furthermore, it is important to clearly document the timing and success of any lumbar punctures performed, as a traumatic first lumbar puncture (commonly from damage to epidural veins) introduces blood into the CSF, which may produce xanthochromia in subsequent attempts if not performed immediately afterwards, hence a false-positive result. Even if an aneurysm is found on CTA, the question as to whether or not the aneurysm had ruptured is key to managing these patients. In CT negative patients with inconclusive lumbar punctures, the decision as to whether they are transferred to a neurosurgical unit for further investigation depends on a good history.

Expert comment Subtle features of a subarachnoid haemorrhage

A subarachnoid haemorrhage might be missed on CT. If no blood is apparent at first sight, one should look for the following subtle features.

1. The temporal horns: they are not normally visible, but often become visible after a subarachnoid haemorrhage.
2. The interhemispheric fissure, especially the CSF space between the cingulate gyri: subtle evidence of blood, which suggests a pericallosal aneurysm, may be missed.
3. Blood/CSF level in the occipital horns of the lateral ventricles with the patient lying supine.
4. Loss of a CSF space because of isodense blood in it, if the subarachnoid blood is a few days old.
5. Blood in a sulcus from a distal aneurysm (e.g. mycotic) or dural arteriovenous fistula.

When patients with aSAH are found to have multiple aneurysms, which can occur in 15–30 per cent of cases, radiological clues such as the distribution of blood, areas of focal vasospasm on angiogram, and irregularities in the aneurysm shape may be used to identify which aneurysm has bled.

With the use of CT and MRI becoming more prevalent in clinical practice, the diagnosis of incidental (i.e. unruptured) aneurysms is becoming more common. The patient and neurosurgeon face the dilemma of whether to treat the incidental aneurysm, with all the risks that it entails but with a potential cure if the aneurysm is successfully secured, or to let it be, foregoing risks of intervention but knowing that a future bleed may result in significant disability or fatality [20]. The natural history of unruptured incidental aneurysms is key in assessing the risk of rupture versus the risk of preventative treatment. A large prospective international study into unruptured incidental aneurysms (International Study of Unruptured Intracranial Aneurysms Investigators (ISUIA) [21]) showed that rupture rates depended on aneurysmal size and location. A history of previous subarachnoid haemorrhage from an unrelated aneurysm has also been shown to be a risk factor for rupture of small incidental aneurysms (<7mm).

Learning point Incidental aneurysm: assessing the risk of rupture

Table 10.3 shows the five-year cumulative haemorrhage rates by aneurysm site, size, and patients grouped into those without SAH from a separate aneurysm (group 1) and those with SAH from a separate aneurysm (group 2) (for aneurysms <7 mm).

The PHASES aneurysm risk score, based on the pooled analysis of patient data in over 8000 patients derived from six large prospective studies (including ISUIA), provides a practical method of accounting for patient and aneurysm factors to estimate the risk of rupture [22]. Six prognostic factors (age, hypertension, aneurysm size, aneurysm site, history of SAH, and geographical region) are used to derive a risk score which is used to assist the decision-making process. In young patients the cumulative risk of rupture over their remaining life may outweigh the risks associated with preventative treatment. It is worth noting that the risks of endovascular/surgical treatment are assessed up front at the time of the intervention, whereas the risk of rupture is assessed over the patient's lifetime.

Table 10.3 Five-year cumulative rupture rates according to size and location of unruptured aneurysm

	<7mm		7–12mm	13–24mm	>25mm
	Group 1	Group 2			
Cavernous carotid artery (*n* = 210)	0	0	0	3.0%	6.4%
AC/MC/IC (*n* = 1037)	0	1.5%	2.6%	14.5%	40%
Post-PCom (*n* = 445)	2.5%	3.4%	14.5%	18.4%	50%

AC, anterior communicating artery or interior cerebral artery; IC, internal carotid artery (not cavernous carotid artery); MC, middle cerebral artery; Post-PComm, vertebrobasilar posterior cerebral arterial system, or posterior communicating artery.

Learning point Incidental aneurysm rupture risk score: PHASES risk score [22]

The predictors comprising the PHASES aneurysm rupture risk score are as follows.

Table 10.4 PHASES aneurysm rupture risk score

Predictor	Points
Population	
North American, European (other than Finnish)	0
Japanese	3
Finnish	5
Hypertension	
No	0
Yes	1
Age	
<70 years	0
≥70 years	1
Size of aneurysm	
<7.0mm	0
7.0–9.9mm	3
10.0–19.9mm	6
≥20 mm	10
Earlier SAH from another aneurysm	
No	0
Yes	1
Site of aneurysm	
ICA	0
MCA	2
ACA/PCom/posterior	4

ICA, internal carotid artery; MCA, middle cerebral artery; ACA, anterior cerebral arteries (including the anterior cerebral artery, anterior communicating artery, and pericallosal artery); PCom, posterior communicating artery; posterior, posterior circulation (including the vertebral artery, basilar artery, cerebellar arteries, and posterior cerebral artery).

The PHASES risk score for an individual is obtained by adding up the number of points associated with each indicator. For example, if Mrs P, a 64-year-old English woman, were to hypothetically have an incidental 8mm MCA aneurysm identified at a later date, her risk score would be 0 + 1 + 0 + 3 + 1 + 2 = 7 points. According to Figure 10.8, this score corresponds to a five-year risk of rupture of 2·4%.

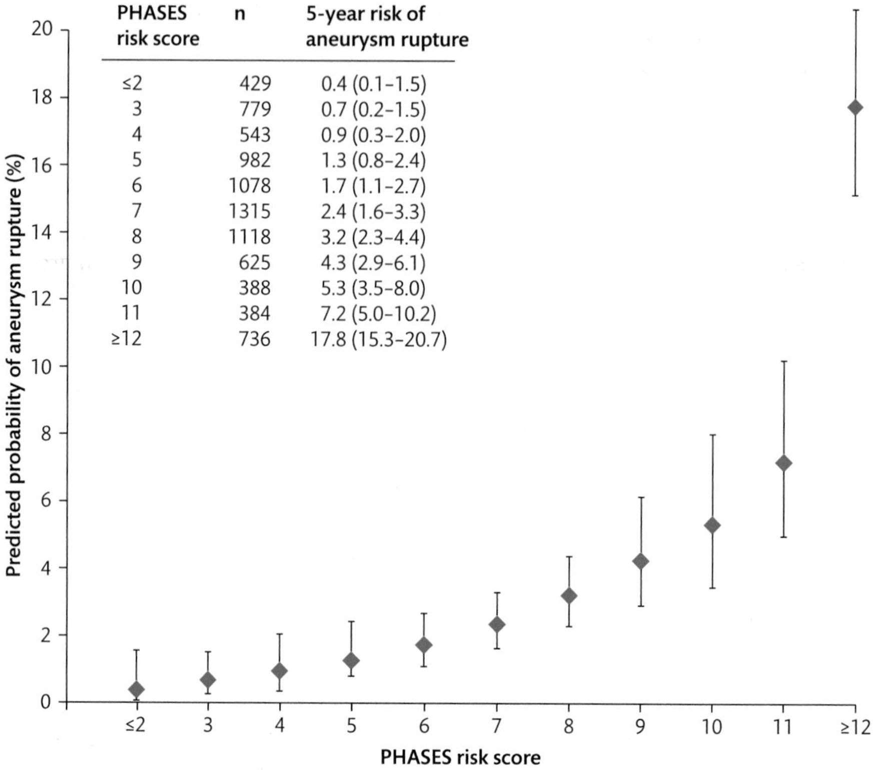

Figure 10.8 The predicted five-year risk of aneurysm rupture according to PHASES score.

Reproduced from *Lancet Neurol* 13(1), Greving JP, Wermer MJ, Brown RD Jr, et al., Development of the PHASES score for prediction of risk of rupture of intracranial aneurysms: a pooled analysis of six prospective cohort studies, pp. 59–66. © 2014, with permission from Elsevier.

When a patient arrives in a neurosurgical unit, one of the first priorities of the neurosurgeon is to identify the cause of the low conscious state or focal deficit which may be attributable to a reversible factor, such as hydrocephalus or seizure [23]. Apart from the effects of the initial haemorrhage, three main neurological complications can cause a poor outcome: rebleeding, DCI, and hydrocephalus. They are a major cause of disability and death in these patients. Seizures are also common, occurring in up to 25 per cent of aSAH patients, and require rapid loading of an anticonvulsant.

Treatable causes of an initially poor-grade SAH include large intracerebral extension of the aneurysmal haemorrhage causing mass effect and reduced conscious state—this will require immediate evacuation of the clot and, ideally, securing of the aneurysm. Extensive intraventricular extension of the haemorrhage (e.g. from an ACom aneurysm bleeding through the lamina terminalis) may require insertion of an external ventricular drain.

Rebleeding is the most important preventable cause of death, with 80 per cent of rebleeds resulting in fatality or significant disability. Surgical/endovascular treatment aims to address this risk. Bleeding risk is estimated to be 4 per cent in the first 24 hours, and 1–2 per cent per day thereafter for 13 days. Approximately 50 per cent of patients will rebleed within six months, with the risk falling to approximately 3 per cent per year thereafter. This estimate does not account for very early rebleeds that may occur before a patient is hospitalized [24].

Surgical or endovascular treatment aims to obliterate the aneurysm or exclude it from the cerebral circulation. The International Subarachnoid Aneurysm Trial (ISAT) has changed the landscape of neurovascular surgery, favouring endovascular treatment of aneurysms. The 2002 ISAT trial concluded that there was an absolute risk reduction of 6.9 per cent for dependency or death at one year for endovascular coiling versus surgical clipping [25]. The 2005 ISAT study suggested low rebleeding rates after coiling at one year, although rates were lower for the surgical group. Longer follow-up has demonstrated three times higher rebleeding rates in the endovascular coiling group (1.56 rebleeds per 1000 patient years in the endovascular group versus 0.49 per 1000 patient years in the surgical group) [26–28]. There have been numerous criticisms of ISAT, such as the inherent bias resulting from comparing specialist interventional neuroradiologists with the 'average' neurosurgeon (i.e. the skill level in the surgical arm ranges from the specialist neurovascular surgeon to the general neurosurgeon without specialist vascular interest), and the inclusion of patients who had rebled prior to surgical intervention and hence carry a worse prognosis not attributable to surgery. Nevertheless, ISAT remains one of the most rigorous studies looking at the management of aSAH. In most neurosurgical units, a multidisciplinary team of neurovascular surgeons and interventional neuroradiologists will work together to offer the most appropriate treatment option for the patient.

DCI/DIND is also a potentially devastating cause of patient deterioration days after the initial haemorrhage. It is recognized by the onset of a focal neurological deficit or deterioration in conscious level not attributable to another cause such as hydrocephalus, seizures, or infection [29]. It is a diagnosis of exclusion, but one where prompt treatment is required to prevent irreversible neurological deficit. Classically, delayed deficits were attributed to cerebral vasospasm leading to cerebral infarction and consequent neurological deficit; hence the common use of the term 'clinical vasospasm' in clinical practice.

Recent evidence goes against vasospasm being the only cause of DIND, with targeted treatment not translating to better neurological outcome. Angiographic vasospasm alone does not necessarily lead to DCI. The current view is that DCI is the result of a multitude of processes including microcirculatory constriction, microthrombosis, cortical spreading ischaemia, and failure of cerebral autoregulation [29, 30]. The brain's susceptibility to ischaemia, as determined by genetic factors (e.g. *APOE* alleles), physiological factors (e.g. adequacy of the circle of Willis), and clinical factors (e.g. MAP/CPP/ICP), determines whether a given degree of vasospasm causes cerebral infarction [30].

In addition to the primary effects of the initial haemorrhage and the secondary neurological complications, aSAH patients are predisposed to a host of medical complications that can lead to poor outcome [31]. One of the most common non-neurological complications is electrolyte abnormalities, especially of sodium. Sodium abnormalities can cause fluid shifts (intravascular and cerebral) resulting in exacerbation of cerebral vasospasm amongst other deleterious effects. Hyponatraemia is common and requires careful management. Common underlying causes in aSAH patients are the syndrome of inappropriate antidiuretic hormone (SIADH), cerebral salt wasting (CSW), and hypovolaemic hyponatraemia from administration of large fluid volumes. The pathophysiological mechanisms underlying hyponatraemia in

> **Clinical tip** Risk of delayed neurological deficit
>
> The risk of delayed ischaemic neurological deficit has been shown to correlate with the blood load (from estimation of blood volume on a CT scan of the brain) in the subarachnoid space after aSAH. It is worth reiterating that DCI and DIND are used interchangeably here.

this patient group is poorly understood, and difficulties arise as patients may suffer from any of the above causes at different times; furthermore, SIADH and CSW may occupy parts of the same clinical spectrum. Diagnosis requires strict monitoring of fluid status, electrolytes, and osmolalities (urine and plasma) to identify a trend. Treatment options include the use of hypertonic saline and vasopressin receptor antagonists. Fluid restriction is generally avoided in this patient group in view of its effects on vasospasm and mean arterial/cerebral perfusion pressure.

Cardiopulmonary complications are common and are a frequent cause of aSAH patients being misdiagnosed with an underlying cardiac disease in the emergency department. Neurogenic sympathetic hyperactivity can lead to transient arrhythmias. ECG changes are common and include ST depression and T-wave inversions. Patients of advanced age or poor-grade SAH may develop neurogenic pulmonary oedema requiring diuretics and positive end expiratory pressure (PEEP) ventilation.

Final word from the expert

Aneurysmal subarachnoid haemorrhage is a complex disease process with varied pathophysiological mechanisms and consequent implications for management. Clinical management is multifaceted with peri-operative medical care playing a pivotal role in preserving neurological function.

References

1. Schwedt TJ. Thunderclap headaches: a focus on etiology and diagnostic evaluation. *Headache* 2013; 53(3): 563–9.
2. Dilli E. Thunderclap headache. *Curr Neurol Neurosci Rep* 2014; 14(4): 437.
3. Schwedt TJ, Matharu MS, Dodick DW. Thunderclap headache. *Lancet Neurol* 2006; 5(7): 621–31.
4. Andreasen TH, Bartek J Jr, Andresen M, et al. Modifiable risk factors for aneurysmal subarachnoid hemorrhage. *Stroke* 2013; 44(12): 3607–12.
5. Longstreth WT Jr, Nelson LM, Koepsell TD, van Belle G. Cigarette smoking, alcohol use, and subarachnoid hemorrhage. *Stroke* 1992; 23:1242–9.
6. Johnston SC, Colford JM Jr, Gress DR. Oral contraceptives and the risk of subarachnoid hemorrhage: a meta-analysis. *Neurology* 1998; 51: 411–18.
7. Deka R, Koller DL, Lai D, et al. The relationship between smoking and replicated sequence variants on chromosomes 8 and 9 with familial intracranial aneurysm. *Stroke* 2010;41(6): 1132–7.
8. Rasing I, Nieuwkamp DJ, Algra A, Rinkel GJ. Additional risk of hypertension and smoking for aneurysms in people with a family history of subarachnoid haemorrhage. *J Neurol Neurosurg Psychiatry* 2012; 83(5): 541–2.
9. Cruickshank A1, Auld P, Beetham R, et al. Revised national guidelines for analysis of cerebrospinal fluid for bilirubin in suspected subarachnoid haemorrhage. *Ann Clin Biochem.* 2008; 45(Pt 3): 238–44.
10. Perry JJ, Stiell IG, Sivilotti MLA, et al. Sensitivity of computed tomography performed within six hours of onset of headache for diagnosis of subarachnoid haemorrhage: prospective cohort study. *BMJ* 2011; 343: d4277.

11. Sarkar S, Ghosh S, Ghosh SK, Collier A. Role of transcranial Doppler ultrasonography in stroke. *Postgrad Med J* 2007; 83(985): 683–9.
12. Naqvi J, Yap KH, Ahmad G, Ghosh J. Transcranial Doppler ultrasound: a review of the physical principles and major applications in critical care. *Int J Vasc Med* 2013; 2013: 629378.
13. Walcott BP, Iorgulescu JB, Stapleton CJ, Kamel H. Incidence, timing, and predictors of delayed shunting for hydrocephalus after aneurysmal subarachnoid hemorrhage. *Neurocrit Care* 2015; 23(1): 54–8.
14. Lewis A, Irvine H, Ogilvy C, Kimberly WT. Predictors for delayed ventriculoperitoneal shunt placement after external ventricular drain removal in patients with subarachnoid hemorrhage. *Br J Neurosurg* 2014; 9: 1–6.
15. Johnston SC, Selvin S, Gress DR. The burden, trends, and demographics of mortality from subarachnoid hemorrhage. *Neurology* 1998; 50: 1413–18.
16. Hop JW, Rinkel GJ, Algra A, van Gijn J. Case-fatality rates and functional outcome after subarachnoid hemorrhage: a systematic review. *Stroke* 1997; 28(3): 660–4.
17. Report of World Federation of Neurological Surgeons Committee on a Universal Subarachnoid Hemorrhage Grading Scale. *J Neurosurg* 1988; 68: 985–6
18. Sano H, Satoh A, Murayama Y, et al. Modified World Federation of Neuro surgical Societies subarachnoid hemorrhage grading system. *World Neurosurg* 2015; 83(5): 201–7.
19. Vermeulen MJ, Schull MJ. Missed diagnosis of subarachnoid hemorrhage in the emergency department. *Stroke* 2007; 38(4): 1216–21.
20. Brown RD Jr, Broderick JP. Unruptured intracranial aneurysms: epidemiology, natural history, management options, and familial screening. *Lancet Neurol* 2014; 13(4): 393–404.
21. Wiebers DO, Whisnant JP, Huston J 3rd, et al. Unruptured intracranial aneurysms: natural history, clinical outcome, and risks of surgical and endovascular treatment. *Lancet* 2003; 362: 103–10.
22. Greving JP, Wermer MJ, Brown RD Jr[3], et al. Development of the PHASES score for prediction of risk of rupture of intracranial aneurysms: a pooled analysis of six prospective cohort studies. *Lancet Neurol* 2014;13(1): 59–66.
23. van Gijn J, Kerr RS, Rinkel GJ. Subarachnoid haemorrhage. *Lancet* 2007; 369(9558): 306-18.
24. Ohkuma H, Tsurutani H, Suzuki S. Incidence and significance of early aneurysmal rebleeding before neurosurgical or neurological management. *Stroke* 2001; 32(5): 1176–80.
25. Molyneux A, Kerr R, Stratton I, et al. International Subarachnoid Aneurysm Trial (ISAT) of neurosurgical clipping versus endovascular coiling in 2143 patients with ruptured intracranial aneurysms: a randomised trial. *Lancet* 2002; 360: 1267–74.
26. Molyneux AJ, Kerr RS, Yu LM, et al. International Subarachnoid Aneurysm Trial (ISAT) of neurosurgical clipping versus endovascular coiling in 2143 patients with ruptured intracranial aneurysms: a randomised comparison of effects on survival, dependency, seizures, rebleeding, subgroups, and aneurysm occlusion. *Lancet* 2005; 366: 809–17.
27. Molyneux AJ, Birks J, Clarke A, et al. The durability of endovascular coiling versus neurosurgical clipping of ruptured cerebral aneurysms: 18 year follow-up of the UK cohort of the International Subarachnoid Aneurysm Trial (ISAT). *Lancet* 2015; 385 (9969); 691–7.
28. Li H, Pan R, Wang H, et al. Clipping versus coiling for ruptured intracranial aneurysms: a systematic review and meta-analysis. *Stroke* 2013; 44: 29–37.
29. Budohoski KP, Czosnyka M, Kirkpatrick PJ, et al. Clinical relevance of cerebral autoregulation following subarachnoid haemorrhage. *Nat Rev Neurol* 2013; 9(3): 152–63.
30. Macdonald RL. Delayed neurological deterioration after subarachnoid haemorrhage. *Nat Rev Neurol* 2014; 10(1): 44–58.
31. Wartenberg KE, Mayer SA. Medical complications after subarachnoid hemorrhage. Neurosurg Clin N Am 2010; 21(2): 325–38.

CASE

11 A complex sleep disorder

Joel S. Winston

Expert commentary: Sofia H. Eriksson

Case history

A 42-year-old woman was referred by her general practitioner to the sleep clinic at a university hospital. The patient's sleep-related problems had first been noted two years prior to referral when she complained of exhaustion on return from a summer holiday. She was diagnosed with depression, and fluoxetine was given with good effect on her mood but no benefit to her tiredness.

Approximately a year after first complaining of exhaustion, she started to fall asleep during the day, particularly in the early evening. These daytime sleeps ranged in length between two minutes and two hours; a striking feature was their sudden onset, whereby she would be rapidly overwhelmed by sleepiness. She could not recall dreaming during these sleeps.

A further more recent feature was of brief (15–20s) episodes in which her legs would buckle and her head drop, associated with slurring of speech. These episodes seemed to be provoked by laughter or possibly emotional upset; on one occasion she had been startled by a rat. Such episodes had increased in frequency and were experienced daily by the time of referral.

She reported going to bed at 10:30p.m. and waking at 7a.m. but not feeling refreshed by sleep. There was no history of snoring or limb movements in sleep, nor did she recall episodes of hypnogogic or hypnopompic hallucinations or sleep paralysis. Many years previously, she had experienced dream enactment, waking up to find herself tearful after emotionally upsetting dreams.

She had a nephew with epilepsy but there was no other relevant family history. She drank alcohol in moderation and did not smoke. She worked full-time as a lawyer and lived with her partner and two children. General and neurological examination was normal.

Clinically, the diagnosis of narcolepsy with cataplexy was made. Fluoxetine had been switched to clomipramine by her general practitioner prior to referral, and there was the suggestion that this had been associated with a reduction in frequency of cataplexy. It was suggested that clomipramine should be up-titrated as tolerated and needed, and modafinil could be introduced to help with somnolence. She was referred for investigations including actigraphy and sleep studies with multiple sleep latency testing (MSLT).

Clinical tip Importance of reflexes

If in doubt as to whether an event you are observing is a cataplexy attack, check tendon reflexes. These are absent during the attack but normal in between.

Clinical tip Symptoms to include in the history assessing a sleep disorder

- Somnolence—excessive sleepiness (to be differentiated from fatigue that is more related to lack of energy but not falling asleep)
- Snoring, pauses in breathing
- Hypnogogic/hypnopompic phenomena—movements or unusual sensory experiences associated with the moments of falling asleep or waking up
- Dream enactment—acting out things that they are dreaming about (note that people may say that they are acting out their dreams even in non-REM parasomnias although events described are often less complex than in REM sleep behaviour disorder)
- Sleep walking/night terrors—in childhood and/or now
- Movements during sleep—leg movements to suggest periodic limb movements or restless leg syndrome (before sleep onset)
- Nocturnal seizures

Note that a collateral history can be critical in eliciting some of these symptoms.

Learning point Other sleep disorders

Other concomitant sleep disorders such as RBD and obstructive sleep apnoea are common in patients with narcolepsy and may contribute to their symptoms. They may need separate treatment. Therefore investigations should include overnight polysomnography to evaluate the occurrence of these disorders.

Investigations

Actigraphy (Figure 11.1) revealed a regular sleep pattern but short sleep latency, reduced sleep duration, and occasional movements but no prolonged awakenings overnight. There were daytime naps lasting 30–90 minutes, the majority of which had been recorded by the patient.

Inpatient polysomnography (Figure 11.2) included 24-channel EEG, EOG, EMG (submentalis and tibialis anterior) and ECG recording with SpO_2 monitoring and continuous video surveillance. Review of the recordings revealed appropriate background changes during non-REM sleep, but abnormalities during REM sleep. Specifically, there was loss of atonia (demonstrated by EMG), and movement and vocalization during REM sleep. These findings were compatible with REM sleep behaviour disorder (RBD).

In addition, MSLT was conducted on day two of the inpatient stay. Mean sleep latency was 6.5min and REM sleep was recorded during two out of four naps, meeting the diagnostic criteria for narcolepsy.

Follow-up

At outpatient follow-up 5–6 months after she was initially seen, she was still troubled by somnolence despite modafinil 200mg bd. Clomipramine had been switched back to fluoxetine, which was felt to have improved the cataplexy. It was suggested that a hypnotic agent should be introduced to improve night-time sleep as well as to treat RBD, and clonazepam 0.5mg at night was started. Further dose increments of modafinil were trialled up to a total daily dose of 800mg. In addition, dexamfetamine was briefly tried, but was poorly tolerated. Twelve months after initial referral, the patient remained troubled by somnolence and was unable to work. At the most recent follow-up, a trial of sodium oxybate was planned as the next intervention.

Discussion

Given that humans spend approximately one-third of their lives asleep, it is unsurprising that sleep disturbance is a common medical complaint. More surprising is that doctors are taught so little about sleep, with one international study suggesting

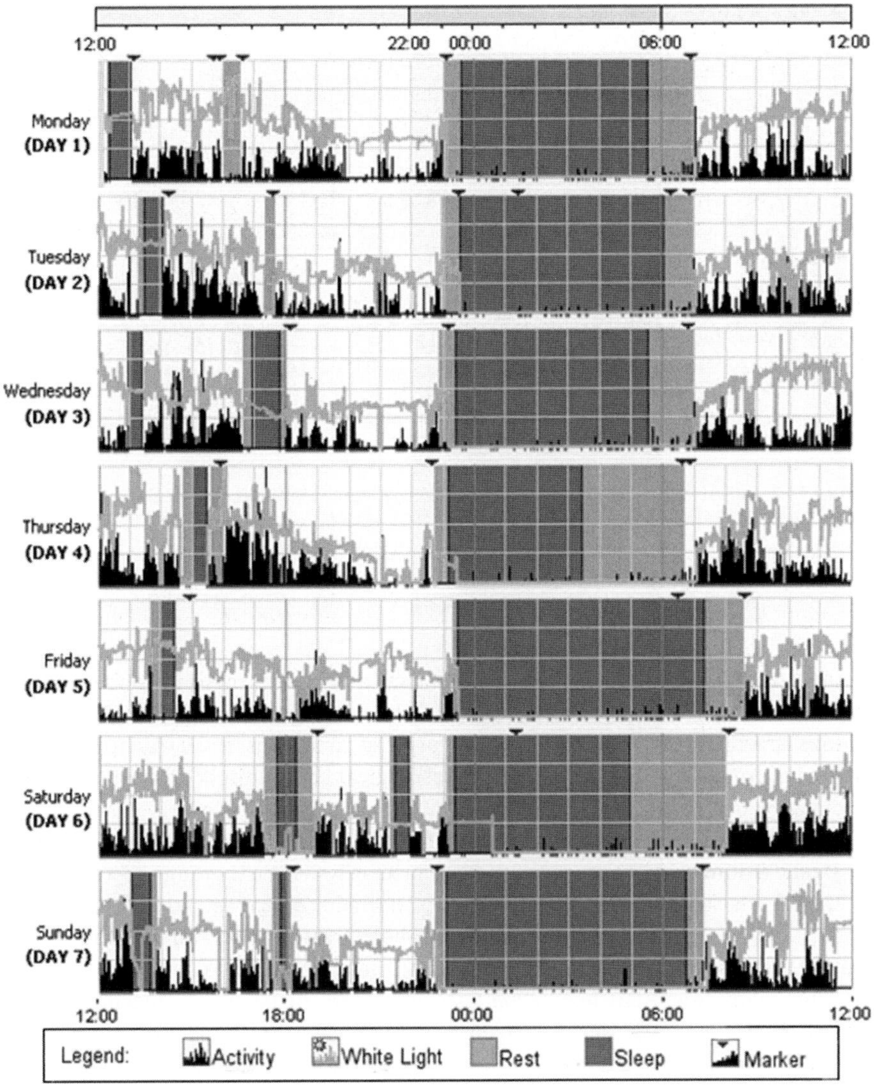

Figure 11.1 Actigraphy. The patient is asked to wear a watch ('actigraph') daily for a period of seven consecutive days. The watch contains an accelerometer which records low-frequency motion consistent with normal movement. Patients with narcolepsy show elevated and fragmented nocturnal motor activity and increased periods of sustained immobility during the day [1], which can be quantitatively assessed from the actogram. Please see colour plate section.

that medical students enjoy an average of 2.5 hours sleep-related education over their entire medical school careers [2]. Adult sleep-related problems are dealt with across a range of different medical specialties (including general practice, general medicine, psychiatry, geriatrics, and respiratory medicine), but where a primary cause is suspected, a neurologist's opinion is frequently sought.

Sleep problems are common in adulthood, with a prevalence (by self-report) of 20–30 per cent for insomnia or sleep disturbance and 5 per cent for excessive

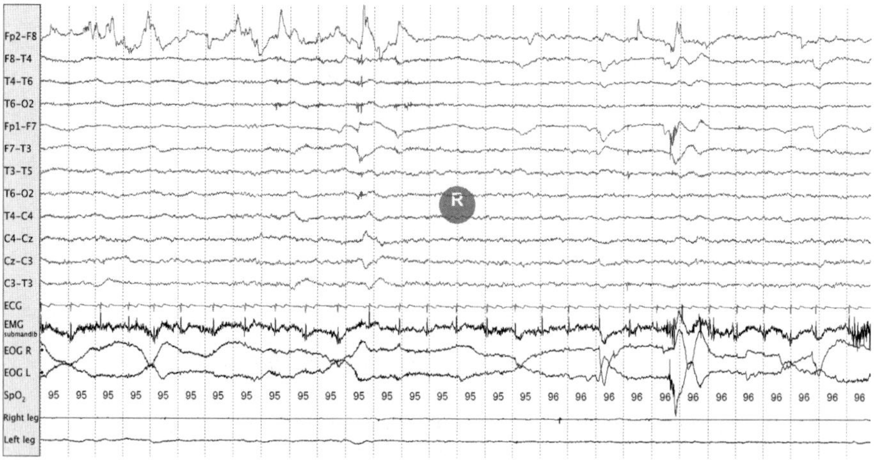

Figure 11.2 Screen shot of 30s epoch (EEG, EOG, EMG) REM sleep with loss of normal atonia. Recordings from the patient's overnight hypnogram. EEG (top 12 traces), ECG, EMG, and EOG are recorded for a 24-hour period including the patient's normal sleep. A 30s period of nocturnal REM is shown (ocular movement on the EOG traces is the easiest way to detect that this is REM) but there is ongoing muscle activity in the EMG, consistent with lack of the normal REM-associated atonia.

daytime somnolence [3]. In the initial clinical assessment, distinguishing fatigue from somnolence is important for stratifying likely diagnoses and planning investigations appropriately [4]. Fatigue as a presenting complaint in the absence of somnolence is frequently associated with psychological cause, rather than representing a primary sleep problem [5].

There is a broad differential diagnosis for daytime somnolence (Tables 11.1 and 11.2), and initial assessment of the patient, primarily with a thorough history, helps to eliminate some potential diagnoses (e.g. pharmacological causes, causes related to sleep quality/quantity, and mood disturbance). Examination can help to confirm that other causes (e.g. space-occupying lesion, general medical cause) are unlikely, and simple investigations (e.g. blood tests to confirm suspicions of anaemia or thyroid disease) may be appropriate. History should include assessment of somnolence, most commonly by means of the Epworth Sleepiness Scale [6] which is helpful for distinguishing somnolence from fatigue and characterizing symptom severity. A

Table 11.1 Classification and differential diagnosis of sleep disorders

Major categories
1. Insomnias
2. Sleep-related breathing disorders
3. Hypersomnias of central origin not due to a circadian rhythm sleep disorder, sleep-related breathing disorder, or other cause of disturbed nocturnal sleep
4. Circadian rhythm sleep disorders
5. Parasomnias
6. Sleep-related movement disorders
7 Isolated symptoms, apparent normal variants, and unresolved issues
8. Other sleep disorders

Data from *International Classification of Sleep Disorders* (2nd edn) (ICSD-2), © 2005, American Academy of Sleep Medicine.

Table 11.2 Common causes of hypersomnia

- Behaviorally inducedinsufficient sleep syndrome
- Hypersomnia due to disrupted nocturnal sleep or other sleep disorder (such as obstructive sleep apnoea or periodic limb movements of sleep)
- Hypersomnia due to a drug or substance
- Narcolepsy with/withoutcataplexy
- Idiopathic hypersomnolence
- Hypersomnia due to a medical condition

series of eight scenarios (e.g. watching TV, as a car passenger on an hour's journey, sitting inactive in a public place, sitting and talking to someone) are each rated on a 0–3 scale for the probability of falling asleep and the scores are summed. A total score >11 is considered abnormal, indicating significant somnolence.

The primary investigation if the initial clinical assessment is suggestive of a primary sleep disorder is a sleep study. This involves an overnight stay in a monitored hospital environment with electrophysiological recordings including EEG, EMG, EOG, ECG, respiratory flow measurement, and pulse oximetry. Continuous video surveillance is helpful for correlating apparent arousal on electrophysiological traces with associated behaviours. If somnolence is a clinically significant symptom, the overnight sleep study can be extended with MSLT the following day.

The MSLT comprises five nap opportunities during the day with 2 hours interval. The patient will be lying undisturbed in a quiet dark room and asked to fall asleep. The latency to sleep (defined strictly by EEG criteria) is measured in addition to the latency to REM sleep (from the onset of sleep). Mean latency to sleep of less than 8min is abnormal and more than two episodes of REM sleep during the day is highly suggestive of narcolepsy.

Preparation for the test includes maintenance of a sleep diary for two weeks prior to the test (or preferably actigraphy), a typical night's sleep preceding the test, the avoidance of caffeine or alcohol during or immediately before the test period (note that acute withdrawal confounds interpretation), and care to ensure an adequately darkened sound-proofed room [7]. It is also important to stop stimulants or antidepressant medication (this suppresses REM and may lead to a false-negative test) prior to admission.

An alternative to MSLT for the diagnosis of narcolepsy is to perform a lumbar puncture with analyses of CSF orexin. Levels of <110pg/ml are found in more than 90 per cent of patients with narcolepsy with cataplexy, but rarely in patients with other disorders. Currently, this is not done in routine clinical practice at most sleep centres.

In this patient's case, the diagnosis of narcolepsy was suspected clinically and confirmed by MSLT. The sleep study also showed evidence of REM sleep behaviour disorder, which had not been strongly suspected clinically.

Clinical tip Excessive daytime sleepiness

- It is important to distinguish between excessive daytime sleepiness and fatigue.
- Consider other, more common, causes for excessive daytime somnolence such as behaviourally induced insufficient sleep syndrome.

Learning point Multiple sleep latency testing

- Mean sleep latency of <8min is diagnostic for hypersomnolence, but in addition REM sleep in at least two naps is needed for a diagnosis of narcolepsy.
- As antidepressants are REM suppressants, these may contribute to a false negative MSLT and, if possible, should be stopped at least two weeks prior to the test.
- The MSLT results always need to be interpreted in the clinical context.

Narcolepsy

Narcolepsy is a syndrome comprising excessive daytime somnolence, episodes of cataplexy, sleep paralysis, and hypnogogic hallucinations. Further, nocturnal sleep is often considerably disrupted, contributing to somnolence. The pathophysiology remains incompletely understood, but destruction of a specific subtype of neuroendocrine cells that release orexin (also known as hypocretin) in the lateral

Expert comment

Narcolepsy is divided into type I (with cataplexy) and type II (without cataplexy). Patients without cataplexy may have only marginally reduced CSF orexin levels, and in this group of people CSF orexin is often less helpful for the diagnosis. This also implies that there may be different underlying mechanisms for the different types of narcolepsy.

Clinical tip Daytime naps

Patients with narcolepsy often find short daytime naps helpful and restorative, and taking regular naps of no more than 15 minutes as well as maintaining good sleep hygiene is important non-pharmacological parts of management.

Expert comment

Pharmacological treatment of narcolepsy is currently symptomatic, but in the future may include immune-modulating therapy and more specific treatment aimed at the orexin pathway.

hypothalamus is thought to be central to the disorder. The destructive process is presumed to be autoimmune in the majority of cases, but rarer aetiologies including structural lesions and vascular causes have been reported [8]. In health, orexin release is thought to modulate brainstem and mid-brain neurotransmitter and neuromodulator release (including all major monoaminergic systems), and additionally acts directly on the thalamus. Connections with these pathways suggest that orexin must be a central coordinator of arousal and REM-sleep-related behaviours [9]. In patients with narcolepsy, the destruction of orexin-secreting neurons results in dysfunctional arousal and REM-sleep-related behaviours. Strong emotional arousal normally elicits orexin release from the hypothalamus, which opposes direct emotional downregulation of noradrenaline release. After destruction of orexin neurons, unopposed noradrenaline suppression in response to emotional stimulation provokes loss of muscle tone and the symptoms of cataplexy [10]. It is proposed that antidepressant medications are beneficial for cataplexy via their actions on central noradrenergic transmission, although it is worth noting that high quality evidence for clinical benefit is limited [11].

Narcolepsy is strongly associated with a specific HLA allele (DQB1*0602 haplotype), giving support to the proposal of an autoimmune basis. Approximately 95 per cent of patients with narcolepsy with cataplexy are positive for DQB1*0602 compared with a baseline frequency of less than 30 per cent. The lack of specificity (i.e. high baseline frequency) means that positive HLA testing can at best be considered supportive evidence for the diagnosis. Environmental factors are also important, evidenced by low rates of concordance in monozygotic twins (about 30 per cent) [12]. There is some evidence at a population level and some circumstantial evidence for an inflammatory process [13, 14], but relatively few individual patients show markers of systemic infection or CNS inflammation. Case studies report mixed results in attempting immunomodulation with intravenous immunoglobulin [15]. A single case study shows a short-lived response to plasmapheresis (lasting a few days) [16] and others show no substantial success with steroids [17]. In patients showing a response, symptoms of cataplexy seem most amenable to treatment, but caution should be exercised given that cataplexy can be quite responsive to placebos [18]. It remains possible that there is a role for immunomodulatory therapy early after disease onset, but substantive evidence is currently lacking.

Orexin replacement treatment is not yet available. Therefore the mainstay of treatment for narcolepsy with cataplexy is symptomatic, and aimed at reducing the burden of cataplexy and increasing arousal levels to alleviate somnolent episodes.

Pharmacological therapies for somnolence include modafinil which is a short-acting 'wakefulness-promoting agent', thought to activate dopaminergic pathways. The potential for addiction seems low and it is generally well-tolerated, although it should be avoided in patients with a history of dysrhythmia. Methylphenidate is a CNS stimulant and a second-line drug for treatment of somnolence. Side effects are more problematic than for modafinil and include blood pressure increases and other autonomic disturbances. Dexamfetamine can also be used (as tried in the patient discussed here) but is prone to tolerance and abuse in addition to significant side effects.

Cataplexy is treated with antidepressant medications, particularly serotonin–noradrenaline reuptake inhibitors (SNRIs), such as venlafaxine, and selective serotonin reuptake inhibitors (SSRIs), such as fluoxetine. These are typically well tolerated and empirically benefit a majority of patients, although randomized controlled trial data is lacking. Less well tolerated, but also efficacious, are the tricyclic antidepressants; anticholinergic side effects can frequently be problematic at doses adequate to treat symptoms. Acute withdrawal of antidepressants is inadvisable and is associated with severe rebound cataplexy attacks.

More recently, gamma hydroxybutyrate (GHB or sodium oxybate) has been introduced to treat narcolepsy and in particular cataplexy. It may be associated with significant side effects such as dizziness and nausea, and also bedwetting, and there is a potential for abuse. There is evidence from randomized controlled trials of efficacy not only for cataplexy but also for excessive daytime sleepiness [19, 20], and a trial of treatment is worthwhile if cataplexy is poorly controlled by antidepressants. However, sodium oxybate treatment is expensive (approximately £25–50 per day in the UK for moderate to high doses) and special permission for prescriptions is currently needed from local clinical commissioning groups. The patient described here is currently awaiting such permission to undergo a trial of treatment.

Evidence base Xyrem International Study Group 2005

- Double-blind placebo-controlled multicentre trial recruiting 228 adults with narcolepsy with cataplexy.
- Mean age of included patients was 40.5 years (range 16–75 years); 149 (65 per cent) were women.
- Antidepressant therapy was withdrawn in an initial stage of the trial and patients were randomized to receive placebo (25 per cent) or one of three doses of sodium oxybate (25 per cent per maximum dose), with dose incremented over the trial period for those patients allocated to receive higher doses.
- Assessment was with standardized measures including Epworth Sleepiness Scale, maintenance of wakefulness test, and clinical global impression score at study baseline and study end. There was statistically significant ($p<0.001$) improvement in all measures for patients randomized to high-dose oxybate, with an apparent dose–response relationship between improvement and medication dose.

REM sleep behaviour disorder

REM sleep is a physiologically fascinating state. Brain activity is desynchronized compared with stage 3-4 sleep, and the EEG substantially alters to show high-frequency low-amplitude signals superficially similar to wakefulness. Eye movements are frequent but muscle tone is reduced (atonia). Autonomic systems show arousal, with greater variability of heart and breathing rates than during stage 3–4 sleep. This set of changes appears to be coordinated by small groups of neurons in the brainstem acting on the reticular activating system [21] (Figure 11.3).

In REM sleep behaviour disorder (RBD), there is a failure to manifest core features of REM sleep, typically atonia. In a simplistic sense, RBD can be considered the opposite of cataplexy; the former consists of failure to maintain atonia during REM sleep, and the latter is an inappropriate sudden onset of atonia during wakefulness [22]. There is limited suboptimal data on prevalence, which has been estimated to be 0.5 per cent. It can present as an isolated symptom or in association with other sleep or neurological disorders. A strong association with antidepressant therapy is apparent. In older adults it may prove prodromal to neurodegenerative disease, particularly Parkinson's disease, dementia with Lewy bodies, or multiple system atrophy, with a 10-year risk of >40 per cent [23]. In younger adults, it is frequently associated with narcolepsy (roughly one-third of patients with RBD also have narcolepsy). The aetiology remains unclear, but it is possible that different causes explain

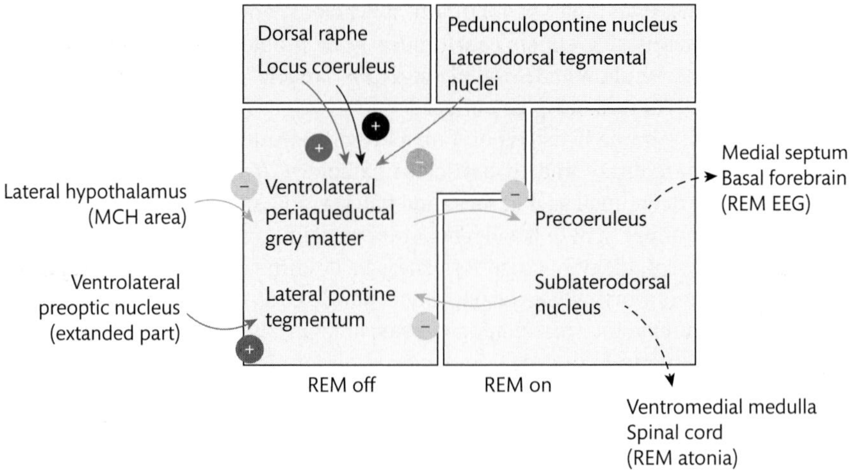

Figure 11.3 Proposed brainstem neuronal network underpinning the flip-flop model of REM sleep control. There is reciprocal GABA-ergic inhibition (yellow arrows) between REM-off and REM-on neurons located in clusters in the brainstem. Activity in the REM-off neurons is influenced by orexin (brown) and galanin/GABA from the lateral hypothalamus, as well as excitatory serotinergic and noradrenergic activation (purple/green) from the dorsal raphe/locus coeruleus and inhibitory influences from cholinergic populations (red) in pedunculopontine/laterodorsal tegmental nuclei. The mutually inhibitory populations of REM-on and REM-off neurons allow sharp transitions between REM states, but it is intuitively obvious from this circuitry why the physiology of sleep can be altered by many pharmacological agents, and why patients with narcolepsy have difficulty both staying awake and staying asleep.

Expert comment

Although RBD in the older population is often associated with neurodegenerative disorders, this does not appear to be the case in patients with narcolepsy and RBD, further strengthening the argument that there are different mechanisms involved in the development of RBD in this group of patients.

the different presentations of RBD; for example, in older adults, synucleinopathy may result in dysfunction of key sleep-related brainstem nuclei, whereas orexin dysfunction is thought to be important in RBD associated with narcolepsy [24].

Management of RBD must include ensuring safety for the patient and their bed partner. Barriers and additional mattresses may prevent injury; bed alarms that wake the patient on substantial movement may also be useful. Pharmacotherapy is primarily with hypnotic agents, and clonazepam (0.25–2mg at night) is typically the treatment of choice. Clonazepam may worsen cognitive impairment and obstructive sleep apnoea, so care must be taken with its use. Zopiclone may be an alternative, and melatonin (3–12mg) has also been used with success. In RBD associated with Parkinson's disease, dopamine agonists, including pramipexole, are sometimes found to be helpful. Clinically, patients treated with sodium oxybate for narcolepsy with cataplexy who also have RBD often have an improvement of their RBD symptoms. However, sodium oxybate is not licensed as a treatment for RBD.

The association of RBD with narcolepsy and treatment difficulties

As mentioned earlier and seen in the case discussed, there is an association between RBD and narcolepsy. Actively screening for RBD in patients diagnosed with narcolepsy suggests a high co-incidence [25]. Similarly, the incidence of narcolepsy in young patients with RBD is high [26]. This unfortunate association renders treatment of both conditions difficult. The treatment of narcolepsy symptoms with antidepressants can unmask or worsen symptoms of RBD. Adequate treatment of RBD symptoms with hypnotics can worsen daytime somnolence. A relatively limited evidence base, the relative youth of the diagnoses, and the complexity and incomplete understanding of the underlying neurobiology all compound the difficulties of treatment in these two associated conditions.

Final word from the expert

The current case highlights how narcolepsy affects both wakefulness and sleep owing to the brain's inability to regulate sleep-wake cycles normally, in particular REM sleep. Several of the symptoms in the classical tetrad are most likely caused by intrusion of REM phenomena into wakefulness, i.e. cataplexy and possibly also sleep paralysis due to loss of REM atonia occurring during wakefulness or sleep onset or offset. Hypnagogic and hypnopompic hallucinations are due to intrusion of REM dream contents at sleep onset and offset, respectively.

It is important to distinguish narcolepsy from the more common causes of excessive daytime somnolence, such as behaviourally induced insufficient sleep syndrome where the person simply does not get enough sleep. Actigraphy to study an individual's sleep pattern over two weeks is often helpful for the differential diagnosis.

As highlighted in the current case, concomitant sleep disorders such as RBD or obstructive sleep apnoea are common in patients with narcolepsy and may contribute to the symptoms. Treatment of these sleep disorders is an important part of management.

References

1. Middelkoop, HA, Lammers GJ, Van Hilten BJ, et al. Circadian distribution of motor activity and immobility in narcolepsy: assessment with continuous motor activity monitoring. *Psychophysiology* 1995; 32(3): 286–91.
2. Mindell JA., Bartle A, Wahab NA, et al. 2011. Sleep education in medical school curriculum: a glimpse across countries. *Sleep Med* 2011; 12(9): 928–31.
3. Soldatos CR, Lugaresi E. Nosology and prevalence of sleep disorders. *Semin Neurol* 1987; 7(3): 236–42.
4. Bodkin C, Manchanda S. Office evaluation of the 'tired' or 'sleepy' patient. *Semin Neurol* 2011; 31(1): 42–53.
5. Ridsdale L, Evans A, Jerrett W, et al. Patients who consult with tiredness: frequency of consultation, perceived causes of tiredness and its association with psychological distress. *Br J Gen Pract* 1994; 44(386): 413–16.
6. Johns MW. A new method for measuring daytime sleepiness: the Epworth Sleepiness Scale. *Sleep* 1991; 14 (6): 540–5.
7. Carskadon MA, Dement WC, Mitler MM, et al. Guidelines for the multiple sleep latency test (MSLT): a standard measure of sleepiness. *Sleep* 1986; 9(4): 519–24.
8. Silber MH, Rye DB. Solving the mysteries of narcolepsy: the hypocretin story. *Neurology* 2001; 56(12): 1616–18.
9. Kilduff TS, Peyron C. The hypocretin/orexin ligand-receptor system: implications for sleep and sleep disorders. *Trends Neurosci* 2000; 23(8): 359–65.
10. Siegel JM, Boehmer LN. Narcolepsy and the hypocretin system—where motion meets emotion. *Nat Clin Pract Neurol* 2006; 2(10): 548–56.

11. Vignatelli L, d'Alessandro R, Candelise L. 2008. Antidepressant Drugs for Narcolepsy. In *Cochrane Database System Rev* 2008; CD003724.
12. Mignot E. Genetic and familial aspects of narcolepsy. *Neurology* 1998; 50(2) (Suppl 1): S16–22.
13. Aran A, Lin L, Nevsimalova S, et al. 2009. Elevated anti-streptococcal antibodies in patients with recent narcolepsy onset. *Sleep* 2009; 32(8): 979–83.
14. Han F, Lin L, Warby SC, et al. 2011. Narcolepsy onset is seasonal and increased following the 2009 H1N1 pandemic in China. *Ann Neurol* 2011; 70(3): 410–17.
15. Plazzi G, Poli F, Franceschini C, et al. 2008. Intravenous high-dose immunoglobulin treatment in recent onset childhood narcolepsy with cataplexy. *J Neurol* 2008; 255(10): 1549–54.
16. Chen W, Black J, Call P, Mignot E. Late-onset narcolepsy presenting as rapidly progressing muscle weakness: response to plasmapheresis. *Ann Neurol* 2005; 58(3): 489–90.
17. Hecht M, Lin L, Kushida CA, et al. Report of a case of immunosuppression with prednisone in an 8-year-old boy with an acute onset of hypocretin-deficiency narcolepsy. *Sleep* 2003; 26(7): 809–810.
18. Fronczek R, Verschuuren J, Lammers GJ. Response to intravenous immunoglobulins and placebo in a patient with narcolepsy with cataplexy. *J Neurol* 2007; 254(11): 1607–8.
19. US Xyrem® Multicenter Study Group. A randomized, double blind, placebo-controlled multicenter trial comparing the effects of three doses of orally administered sodium oxybate with placebo for the treatment of narcolepsy. *Sleep* 2002; 25(1): 42–9.
20. US Xyrem® Multicenter Study Group. A double-blind, placebo-controlled study demonstrates sodium oxybate is effective for the treatment of excessive daytime sleepiness in narcolepsy. *J Clin Sleep Med* 2005; 1(4): 391–7.
21. Lu J, Sherman D, Devor M, Saper CB. A putative flip–flop switch for control of REM sleep. *Nature* 2006; 441(7093): 589–94.
22. Brown RE, Basheer R, J McKenna JT, et al. Control of Sleep and Wakefulness. *Physiological Reviews* 2012; 92(3): 1087–1187.
23. Postuma RB, Gagnon JF, Vendette M, et al. Quantifying the risk of neurodegenerative disease in idiopathic REM sleep behavior disorder. *Neurology* 2009; 72(15): 1296–1300.
24. Knudsen S, Gammeltoft S, Jennum PJ. 2010. rapid eye movement sleep behaviour disorder in patients with narcolepsy is associated with hypocretin-1 deficiency. *Brain* 2010; 133(2): 568–79.
25. Nightingale S, Orgill JC, Ebrahim IO. The association between narcolepsy and REM behavior disorder (RBD). *Sleep Med* 2005; 6(3): 253–8.
26. Bonakis A, Howard RS, Ebrahim IO, et al. 2009. REM sleep behaviour disorder (RBD) and its associations in young patients. *Sleep Med* 2009; 10(6): 641–5.

CASE

12 Symptoms come and go but the lesions get bigger

David Paling

Expert commentary: Declan Chard

Case history

A 25-year-old right-handed woman was referred to the neurology clinic for an opinion on three episodes of neurological dysfunction. Prior to these episodes she was fit and well with no previous medical history.

The first episode occurred 11 months prior to her first clinic appointment. Over the course of a day she had felt increasingly unsteady whilst walking. She went to work the next day but felt unsteady cycling, so walked instead. Whilst at work she noticed that she misjudged the left side of doors. These symptoms gradually worsened over two to three days, and she began noticing some blurring of the left hemi-field of her vision in both eyes. She did not have any double vision, other cranial nerve symptoms, limb numbness, or weakness. She was admitted to hospital via Accident & Emergency where it was noted that she had an unsteady gait. Unfortunately, further details of her neurological examination were not available to us. She had an MRI scan of the brain which showed a large lesion in the right parietal lobe with heterogeneous signal characteristics, and a smaller lesion in the left occipital lobe. She had a lumbar puncture which showed normal opening pressure; CSF cell counts, protein, and glucose were within normal limits; CSF culture proved negative. CSF oligoclonal bands were not looked for. After the lumbar puncture she developed a severe headache. This headache immediately worsened on sitting or standing, and improved on lying flat. Because of the severity of the headache she did not attempt to mobilize for five days. After five days her headache settled, and when she started to mobilize she felt that she had completely returned to normal. Her only medical treatments during her hospital stay were analgesic drugs and antiemetics.

Clinical tip Post lumbar puncture headache

Headache can be a complication of lumbar puncture in about a third of procedures [1]. The headache shows a characteristic postural variation, becoming worse on sitting up and better on lying flat, and tends to occur within the first three days of lumbar puncture [2]. Other features that may occur include tinnitus, hyperacusis, photophobia, and nausea [3]. Neck stiffness can be reported, although this may indicate infection. In over 95 per cent of patients the headache resolves within a week [3].

Whilst bed rest and increased fluid after lumbar puncture is often suggested, a recent Cochrane review found no evidence to suggest that these reduced headache [4]. Use of atraumatic needles which are postulated to separate rather than sever the dural fibres does significantly reduce the rate of post lumbar puncture headache, although they are more difficult to use and more likely to lead to procedure failure [1, 5].

She had a second episode, seven months prior to her first clinic appointment. One evening she noted some paraesthesia of the right leg. The next morning she noted that her right leg was dragging, but she was still able to cycle to work. Whilst at work she noted that she was having word-finding difficulties, and made some phonological word substitutions, i.e. 'shot' for 'shop' and 'boot' for 'blue'. She was aware that these were incorrect. Her handwriting deteriorated. In addition, her written output was grammatically incorrect, but she was able to read without difficulty. She was readmitted to hospital and had a further MRI scan, the results of which were not available to us. She was offered a further lumbar puncture, but opted against it because of the severity of her previous post lumbar puncture headache. She had a three-day course of intravenous methylprednisolone. She began to improve after two weeks, and after three weeks thought that she was entirely back to normal.

The third episode began five days prior to her clinic appointment when she began to notice some limb heaviness, initially affecting the right leg and three days later affecting the right arm. This was associated with paraesthesia of the right leg and the little and ring fingers of the right hand. This had worsened over the preceding three days.

On direct questioning she had no urinary, bowel, or cognitive symptoms. She recalled no other neurological episodes in the past, particularly no painful visual impairment, or Uhthoff's or Lhermitte's phenomena. She was taking the oral contraceptive pill but had stopped doing so after the first clinical episode. She took no other medications. There was no family history of neurological disease.

Clinical tip History-taking in a possible neuroinflammatory condition.

A distant history of neurological events can help clinch the diagnosis of multiple sclerosis (MS) and therefore it is worth spending time exploring previous symptoms. Whilst some symptoms (arm or leg weakness) are likely to be volunteered, the patient may not have attributed other symptoms to a neurological disease and they are worth investigating.

- Previous episodes of double vision, pain behind one eye, or impaired visual clarity or colour saturation may indicate brainstem or optic nerve inflammatory events. These may have been managed by ophthalmologists and therefore these records may not be in the hospital notes. While visual evoked potentials are not part of current consensus criteria for the diagnosis of MS [6], they can provide useful information about subtly symptomatic or asymptomatic demyelinating lesions within the optic pathways.
- A previous history (particularly in a young person) of 'vertigo'. Be particularly alert to a note of 'labyrinthitis' on the GP record sheet, particularly where the patient's account of the event is atypical.
- Unexplained urinary urgency or incontinence or erectile difficulties in a younger person.
- Previous sciatica with and without back pain in a younger person, particularly where an MRI scan of the lumbar spine has been performed and is normal.
- Lhermitte's phenomenon—the sensation of pins and needles down the neck and thoracic spine, arms, or legs on bending the head forward.
- Uhthoff's phenomenon—a worsening of neurological symptoms with heat (for example after exercise or having a hot bath).

Systemic examination was normal. On neurological examination higher mental function, speech, and writing were normal. Her cranial nerves, including visual fields to confrontation with a red pin, fundi, and extra-ocular movements were normal. She had a mild pyramidal pattern of weakness in the legs with power of 4+ +/5 of right hip and knee flexion. Reflexes were brisker on the right than the left in the arms and legs. The right plantar response was upgoing. Sensation was intact to pinprick, vibration, and joint position sense. Coordination was normal. She walked with slight right leg circumduction.

Blood tests for full blood count, renal function, liver function, autoimmune screen (ANA, ENA, ANCA), ESR, CRP, ACE, and HIV, hepatitis, and Lyme serology were all normal or negative. Repeat MRI scan of the brain and spinal cord showed extension of the lesion in the right parietal lobe into the corpus callosum and medial extension of the lesion in the left parieto-occipital lobe (Figure 12.1, scan 1). No enhancement was seen, no new lesions were seen, and no lesions were seen within the spinal cord. She had a repeat lumbar puncture. CSF examination showed three lymphocytes and four red blood cells, with normal protein, glucose, lactate, and ACE. CSF cytology was normal and PCR for HSV1+2, VZV, EBV, enterovirus, and parechovirus were negative. A CSF monoclonal band, which was not present in the serum, was detected in the CSF.

Learning point Monoclonal and oligoclonal bands in the CSF

Oligoclonal bands represent clones of antibodies produced by plasma cells, and their presence within the CSF, but not in the serum, can indicate an immune-mediated inflammatory process within the brain. They are seen in 95 per cent of patients with clinically definite MS, but are also seen in central nervous system infections and other neuroinflammatory and neoplastic conditions. A monoclonal band can be seen particularly early in the disease course in MS; however this has less specificity for the diagnosis of MS [7]. A high proportion of patients with a monoclonal band initially, but oligoclonal bands on repeat lumbar puncture, will eventually be diagnosed with MS. MS is much less common in patients where a repeat lumbar puncture shows resolution of the monoclonal band. A persistent monoclonal CSF band is seen in patients with MS, but has also been reported to occur in cerebral lymphoma [8], highlighting the importance of keeping patients with a monoclonal band under close review, particularly where the clinical history is unusual, as in this case.

Her symptoms settled fully within two weeks without any treatment. Our clinical impression was that she probably had MS; however, a few features were atypical, warranting further investigation. These were clinical features suggesting cortical involvement during her relapses, continuing enlargement of both lesions seen on MRI, and the finding of an isolated monoclonal band in the CSF.

Four months after her initial clinic appointment she was reviewed in clinic again as she had begun to develop new symptoms. These had begun 11 days previously, initially with weakness in her right leg which worsened over two days, followed by difficulty in speech with word-finding difficulties, particularly for low-frequency words. Over this time she also noted blurring of the right side of her vision, and numbness over the right side of her face. She had no symptoms suggestive of an infection.

On examination she had a clear new neurological deficit with an expressive dysphasia and acalculia, with otherwise intact comprehension. She had an incomplete right-sided hemianopia with macular sparing. Extra-ocular movements showed saccadic intrusion into smooth pursuit movements, more pronounced when looking to the right. She had no nystagmus or diplopia. Fundi left and right were normal. She had a reduction in right-sided facial sensation over all trigeminal dermatomes and a right upper motor neuron pattern facial weakness. Tone was increased in the right arm and right leg. Power was reduced in the right arm in a pyramidal distribution to MRC grade 3 for shoulder abduction, 2 for wrist extension, and 0 for finger extension, and in the right leg with grade 3 for hip flexion, 2–3 for knee flexion, and 1 for ankle dorsiflexion. Reflexes were brisker on the right than the left with an upgoing right plantar response. Her weakness was such that she was not able to walk more than a couple of steps without bilateral assistance.

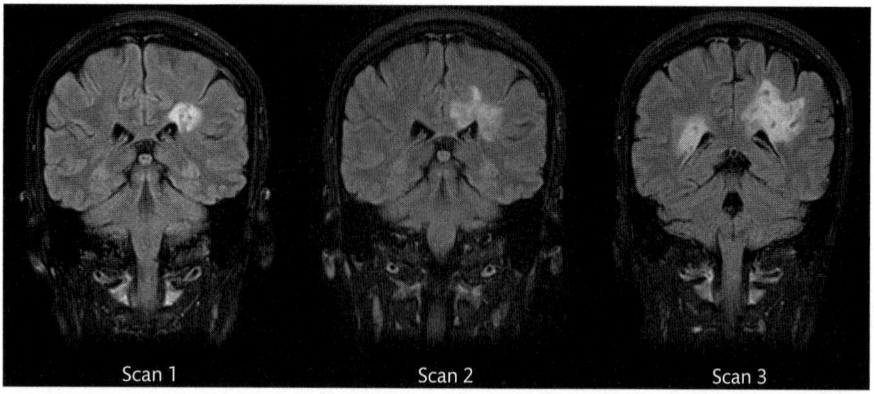

Figure 12.1 Serial coronal FLAIR sequences are shown, indicating the progression of the lesions. Scans 1, 2, and 3 were performed 3 weeks, 4 months, and 4.5 months, respectively, after the patient's first presentation to clinic.

Reproduced with thanks to Dr Zane Jaunmuktane, UCL Institute of Neurology, UK.

A repeat MRI scan showed a large extension of the left intracranial lesion with some peripheral diffusion restriction and contrast enhancement in the areas of enlargement (Figure 12.1, scan 2). There was also a small increase in the size of the right lesion. No new lesions were seen. The MRI findings were discussed with the neuroradiologists, who thought that they would be consistent with a tumefactive pattern of MS, but a neoplasm could not be ruled out. She was admitted to hospital for three days of intravenous methylprednisolone with an oral taper. Repeat lumbar puncture now showed the presence of oligoclonal bands in the CSF, not present in the serum. CSF cytology was normal. A CT PET scan to look for evidence of malignancy elsewhere was reported to be within normal limits. Repeat blood tests and a urine dipstick were normal.

She began to improve clinically on her second day of steroid infusion, and was reviewed two weeks later and had a repeat scan. At the time of her clinic review she had continued to improve, with resolution of the dysphasia and acalculia. Her weakness had improved markedly, to the extent that she had only subtle weakness in the right arm and leg. Reflexes were brisker on the right than the left but plantars were flexor. She was able to walk without assistance. However, her MRI scan showed an increase in the size of the two posterior lesions (Figure 12.1, scan 3), with the presence of a new contrast-enhancing lesion in the frontal region.

In view of the continuing increase in the size of the lesions she was counselled, and a joint decision was made with the neurosurgeons to proceed to brain biopsy to exclude a neoplastic process. Brain biopsy was performed using a frameless stereotactic technique guided by a pre-operative MRI scan, and she was discharged from hospital the next day.

Learning point Brain biopsy in neurological disorders

The aim of brain biopsy is to establish a tissue diagnosis, particularly where this will impact substantially on the likely prognosis or significantly affect treatment choices. Improvements in surgical technique, in particular the use of sterotactic guidance techniques, have increased the likelihood of tissue diagnosis and decreased the associated risks [9]. Despite the potential benefits of establishing a tissue diagnosis, this must still be carefully weighed on a case by case basis against the risks, which

(Continued)

include risks associated with the anaesthetic and focal brain haemorrhage or infection at the biopsy site which may lead to focal neurological deficits, seizures, and even death [10]. A tissue biopsy may also yield a non-diagnostic sample.

Brain biopsy for suspected tumours, as in this case, is well established in clinical practice. In neurological practice, brain biopsy can also be useful in the diagnosis of brain lesions in patients with HIV, and in the diagnosis of other neuroinflammatory disorders such as CNS vasculitis and neurosarcoidosis where non-invasive investigations have proved inconclusive [11].

Expert comment

The decision to undertake brain biopsy is challenging. The previous clinical course and response to steroids, the presence of multiple brain lesions at onset, and unmatched oligoclonal bands all point towards an inflammatory cause for symptoms, but the expansion of old lesions despite treatment with steroids is atypical and could indicate an underlying neoplasm. In addition, while MS is the most commonly recognized cause of large inflammatory brain lesions, they may also be seen in people with vasculitis and non-MS inflammatory conditions such as neuromyelitis optica (NMO) spectrum disorders. Differentiating these is important, as conventional treatments for MS may be ineffective in the case of people with CNS vasculitis and may paradoxically increase disease activity in people with NMO.

The biopsy demonstrated inflammatory demyelination and was supportive of a diagnosis of MS (Figure 12.2) and she was seen in clinic to discuss the advantages and disadvantages of either a first-line disease-modifying agent (beta-interferon or glatiramer acetate) or a second-line agent such as natalizumab.

Clinical tip: Disease-modifying treatments for multiple sclerosis

There are currently eight licensed disease-modifying drugs for MS in the UK (as of May 2014), and several more are in the late stages of development. These drugs have all be shown to reduce the frequency of relapses in the relapsing-remitting phase of the disease. There is currently no definitive evidence that any delay the onset of secondary progressive MS, or that they prevent disability not associated with relapses [12]; however, long-term follow up studies are limited.

Prior to 2006 there were two preparations of interferon beta-1a, two preparations of interferon beta-1b and glatiramer acetate. These drugs are all delivered by injection and in pivotal trials reduced relapse rates by about one-third compared with placebo. The beta-interferons are synthetic preparations of the endogenous cytokine interferon-beta and are thought to have anti-inflammatory effects upon T cells. In practice they frequently cause flu-like side effects that can usually be managed by taking paracetamol or non-steroidal anti-inflammatory agents prior to injection. Less frequently they can cause haematological and hepatic dysfunction which requires regular blood monitoring, and can worsen depression.

Glatiramer is a mixture of synthetic polypeptides composed of four amino acids resembling myelin basic protein. It binds to antigen-presenting cells which may activate regulatory T cells. In practice it causes injection site reactions which occur at least once in 70 per cent of patients; these range in severity from mild otherwise asymptomatic erythema to marked lipo-atrophy and discomfort.

In Englandthese drugs are funded by the NHS for patients with at least two clinically significant relapses in two years and who are able to walk at least 10m with assistance (100m without assistance for glatirimer acetate). What constitutes a clinically significant relapse is not specified, but is usually interpreted by clinicians as relapses leading to impairment in day-to-day activities or requiring steroid treatment. These drugs are commonly used first line in patients with MS.

Three further disease modifying agents are now available.

Teriflunomide is an oral treatment that was approved for use in the UK by NICE in 2014. It is the active metabolite of leflunomide which is used for rheumatoid arthritis, and inhibits synthesis of pyrimdine

(Continued)

for DNA replication and hence reduces the proliferation of activated lymphocytes. Pivotal trials have indicated a reduction in relapse rate of 31 per cent compared with placebo. Side effects include nausea, diarrhoea, paraesthesia, hair loss, liver enzyme abnormalities, and possible teratogenicity. Drug clearance is slow, taking eight months to two years, although this can be improved by use of oral colestyramine or activated charcoal for 11 days. In England teriflunomide is funded by the NHS for patients with two clinically significant relapses within the last two years.

Fingolimod is an oral sphingosine-1-phosphate receptor blocker which prevents egress of lymphocytes from lymph nodes. It has been shown to reduce relapse rates by 54–60 per cent compared witht placebo. Side effects include transient bradycardia and AV block which means that patients should be monitored for six hours after their first dose and when treatment is interrupted. Other side effects include macular oedema requiring ophthalmological monitoring, and lymphopenia and liver function test abnormalities requiring blood monitoring. In England fingolimod is funded by the NHS for patients with unchanged or increased relapse rate on treatment with interferon beta.

Natalizumab is discussed in detail in subsequent clinical tips and evidence base sections.

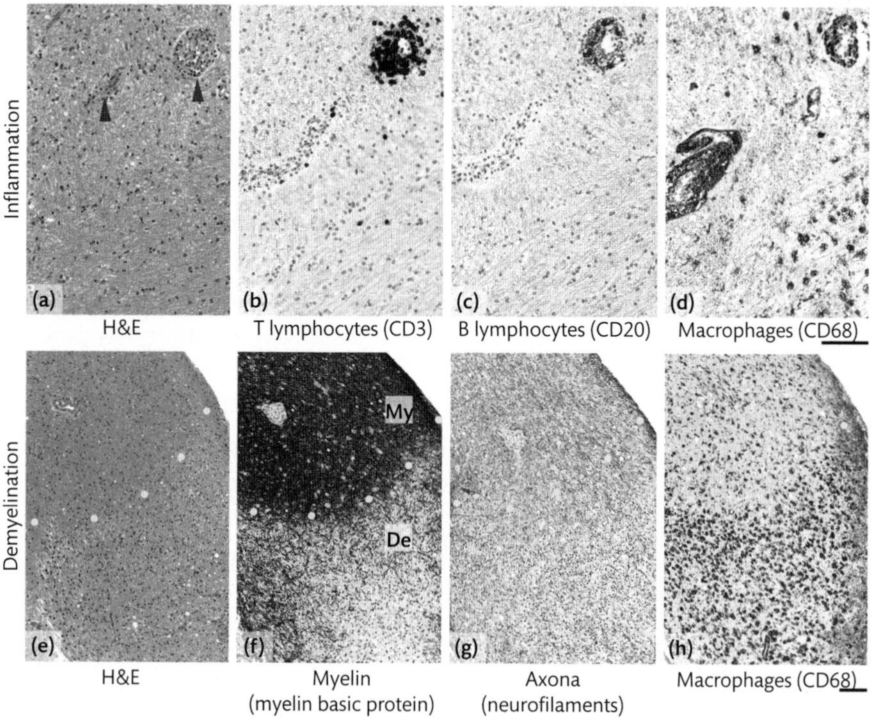

Figure 12.2 Brain biopsy specimen with stains specific for inflammation ((a)–(d)), demyelination ((e)–(h)), axonal integrity (g) and macrophages (h). (a)–(d) Inflammation: the haematoxylin-eosin (H&E) stained section (a) shows widespread perivascular infiltrates of mononuclear inflammatory cells; the majority of the lymphocytes are CD3+ T cells (b) with fewer CD20+ B cells (c); there are also numerous macrophages around the blood vessels and diffusely in the neural parenchyma (d). Demyelination ((e)–(h)): the H&E stained section (e) reveals a relatively sharp margin between the lesion and the surrounding neural parenchyma; immunostaining for myelin (f) with antibody for myelin basic protein (SMI94) accentuates the almost complete loss of myelin in the affected regions, while axons (g) immunostained with antibody for hyperphosphorylated neurofilaments (SMI31) are relatively preserved in the same areas. Immunostaining for CD68 (h) reveals numerous foamy macrophages in the demyelinated foci. Arrows indicate the perivascular inflammation. The dotted line indicates the border between myelinated (My) and demyelinated (De) regions. Scale bar: 100μm. Please see colour plate section.

Reproduced with thanks to Dr Zane Jaunmuktane, UCL Institute of Neurology, UK.

Clinical tip Practicalities of natalizumab treatment

Nataluzimab is a humanized IgG4 monoclonal antibody that binds the α4 subunit of the very late antigen-4 intergrin present on leucocytes, and prevents it from crossing the blood–brain barrier. It is administered as an infusion over one hour at a dose of 300mg every four weeks.

The most concerning side effect is the risk of developing progressive multifocal leucoencephalopathy (PML). Whilst infusions are usually tolerated well, allergic reactions can occur, typically during the first seven doses, most commonly on the second dose. These usually manifest as hives with or without other features of anaphylaxis. Delayed-type hypersensitivity reactions, which occur a few hours to days afterward and consist of fever, pruritus, and malaise, are also reported. Rare cases of liver impairment have been reported, so monitoring of liver function is recommended. Persistently positive anti-natalizumab antibodies are seen in 6 per cent of patients. These patients tend to have suboptimal clinical response and persistent infusion-related reactions [13].

She also had JC virus antibody screening to help stratify her risk of developing PML. Her JC virus antibody was positive, but in view of the severity of her relapses she opted to proceed with natalizumab treatment with clinical and radiological monitoring for PML.

Learning point The risk of developing progressive multifocal leucoencephalopathy with natalizumab

Two cases of PML, one of which was fatal, were noted in the SENTINEL trial [14] and the drug was temporarily withdrawn in 2005. PML is an opportunistic brain infection caused by the JC virus. The JC virus can be present normally in the body, and after an asymptomatic primary infection that occurs during childhood it may persist in a quiescent state in the kidneys, bone marrow, and lymphoid tissue. In the context of immunosuppression, which may be secondary to natalizumab, immunosuppressive drugs, HIV, or malignancy, a complex interaction occurs between the host immune response and the JC virus leading to the development of a mutated pathogenic form of the virus which reactivates [15]. This pathogenic virus infects and destroys oligodendrocytes, and leads to widespread demyelination and secondary neuronal damage. Natalizumab was re-introduced in 2006 with a global monitoring programme to monitor the risk of PML.

As of May 2014 about 123,000 people had been treated with natalizumab for MS worldwide (<http://www.biogenidec.co.uk>). Data from clinical trials and pharmacovigiliance programmes has enabled stratification of an individual's risk of developing PML [16]. Established risk factors for PML development are anti-JC virus antibody status, duration of treatment, and prior use of immunosuppressants such as mitoxantrone, methotrexate, cyclophosphamide, azathioprine, and mycophenolate. Approximate incidence of PML according to these risk factors in patients who are JC virus positive is shown in Table 12.1. Note that beyond six years of treatment there is still very little information, so it is difficult to stratify risk accurately.

Table 12.1 Incidence of PML stratified by previous immunosuppressant use in patients who are positive for the JC virus antibody

Natalizumab treatment duration	No prior immunosuppressant use	Prior immunosuppressant use
1–24 months	0.7 per 1000 (CI 0.5–1.0)	1.8 per 1000 (CI 1.1–2.7)
25–48 months	5.4 per 1000 (CI 4.4–6.2)	11.2 per 1000 (CI 8.6–14.3)
49–72 months	6.1 per 1000 (CI 4.8–7.8)	Insufficient data

Data from www.biogenidec.co.uk, accessed May 2014.

> **Learning point** Progressive multifocal leucoencephalopathy monitoring
>
> PML is a life-threatening complication of natalizumab treatment. Early estimates indicated a mortality of 30–50 per cent within three months of diagnosis. However, recent reports indicate that outcome is improved when it is diagnosed early, natalizumab therapy is discontinued, and plasmaphereisis employed to hasten reconstitution of immune function in the CNS [16, 17].
>
> The improvement in outcome with early identification highlights the importance of ongoing vigilance by the clinician, the patient, and their family for the clinical features suggestive of PML. Features seen commonly in PML, which would be atypical for MS relapses, include cognitive changes, neurobehavioural symptoms, disorders of language, visual symptoms, and seizures [15, 18]. Symptoms are typically progressive over weeks to months, and in comparison with MS relapses usually show little improvement following steroids. Any of these features should prompt urgent work-up with MRI scan of the brain and lumbar puncture for JC virus PCR.
>
> PML lesions appear as single or multifocal areas of T2 hyperintensity on brain MRI. They are distinct from MS lesions in that they typically appear diffuse, as opposed to MS lesions which tend to be well circumscribed. They additionally tend to be predominantly subcortical, and there is no mass effect even with large lesions [19].
>
> Positive CSF PCR for JC virus is strongly supportive of the diagnosis of PML. However, viral loads can be low, making detection difficult [18], and CSF PCR can be repeatedly negative in pathologically confirmed cases, indicating that a negative PCR result does not rule out PML [20].

The patient recently had her eighth monthly infusion of natalizumab without incident, and is now entirely symptom free from her MS, her neurological examination is normal, and she has returned to work.

Discussion

This woman presented with a clinical history of a relapsing and remitting neurological disorder with remissions occurring both spontaneously and in association with steroid treatment. Whilst a neuroinflammatory disorder was considered to be most likely on clinical grounds, a few features were sufficiently atypical to warrant further assessment. Although she did have objective clinical evidence of at least two lesions disseminated in time and space, we did not consider that a confident diagnosis of MS could be made via the MacDonald criteria [6] for the following reasons. The clinical features during the relapses were unusual, with the prominence of features suggestive of cortical dysfunction including dysphasia and acalculia. Such features can occur in MS but are less common [21]. Her neuroimaging features were also unusual with the presence of large lesions >2cm in size with some mass effect, oedema, ring enhancement, and cystic changes. Whilst these features can be seen rarely in the tumefactive forms of MS [22], they could indicate a tumour, particularly lymphoma in which multiple lesions can be seen in up to 50 per cent of patients [23] or multifocal glioma. In view of the continuing expansion and contrast enhancement of the lesions which persisted despite steroid treatment, and in consultation with the patient and the neurosurgeons, we opted to refer the patient for a brain biopsy. This enabled a tumour to be effectively excluded, a clear diagnosis established, and treatment initiated.

In view of the frequency and severity of her relapses, with two significant relapses within the preceding year indicating rapidly evolving severe MS we opted for treatment with natalizumab, one of the most efficacious treatments currently licensed for the treatment of MS [24,25]. One of the most worrisome side effects of natalizumab is the risk of PML, which can be stratified by clinical factors and a JC virus-antibody blood test. Given that she had not been on immunosuppressive agents previously, but was positive for the JC virus-antibody, her approximate risk of developing PML would be less than 1 per 1000 for the first two years of treatment, followed by 5.4 per 1000 for the next two years [16]. While on this treatment she will be closely followed clinically and with serial MRI scanning. Our institution's policy is to perform MRI scans yearly, and additionally if patients develop new neurological symptoms, particularly if they are atypical of an MS relapse.

Expert comment

There is no consensus on the optimal MRI screening protocol for PML in people with MS on natalizumab, but serial scans are usually recommended for those thought to be at higher risk (e.g. people who are JC virus antibody positive) with greater vigilance after two or more years of treatment and in those who have previously had immunosuppressants.

Serial scans serve two purposes: detecting PML lesions early, in the hope that this will improve clinical outcomes; and providing a refreshed baseline scan with which to compare imaging undertaking in light of new symptoms suggestive of PML.

There is some evidence that early detection of PML improves outcomes, albeit in people with symptoms suggestive of PML [16, 26, 27]. To date there have only been a few case reports, with favourable outcomes, in people with pre-symptomatic PML lesions [27]. With greater experience, the recognized radiological features of PML lesions are also expanding [28], but it is still to be determined which sequences best enable early asymptomatic lesions to be detected, and how frequently scans should be undertaken.

In view of the markedly increased risk of PML after two years, our institution's policy is to discuss treatment options again with patients after two years, and if the patient and physician agree to continue natalizumab, to explicitly seek consent again.

Lastly, whilst clinical instinct would suggest such a dramatic tumefactive presentation of MS would portend a grim long-term prognosis, studies suggest that this may not be the case, and follow-up studies have shown significantly less disability and progression than in age- and disease-duration-matched population cohorts [22, 29].

Evidence base Natalizumab for relapsing remitting multiple sclerosis

The effectiveness of natalizumab in MS has been established against placebo in the AFFIRM trial and in combination with interferon beta 1a in the SENTINEL trial.

In the AFFIRM trial natalizumab reduced annualized relapse rate by 68 per cent, reduced new or enlarging T2 lesions by 83 per cent, and reduced gadolinium-enhanced lesions by 92 per cent compared with placebo [24].

In the SENTINEL trial natalizumab and interferon beta 1a reduced annualized relapse rates by 55 per cent, reduced new or enlarging T2 lesions by 83 per cent and gadolinium-enhanced lesions by 89 per cent compared with interferon beta 1a alone [14].

The reduction in annualized relapse rates seen with natalizumab in these trials is significantly greater than was seen in previous trials of other disease-modifying treatments for MS including interferon beta and glatiramer acetate which are of the order of 33 per cent.

Following these trials, natalizumab was approved by the National Institute for Health and Clinical Excellence (NICE) for patients who have two or more disabling relapses within one year (rapidly evolving MS), and either a gadolinium-enhancing lesion on brain MRI scan or a significant increase in T2 lesion load.

Final word from the expert

While the spontaneous remission of early symptoms in this person's case makes an inflammatory cause much more likely than a neoplastic one, and recalling that MS is the most likely cause of an inflammatory CNS disorder in younger adults in the UK, establishing a diagnosis of MS can still be difficult, particularly after the first clinical episode. Serial clinical and radiological assessment may be required to clarify whether a neoplastic or inflammatory cause is most likely, and determine if early biopsy is indicated.

The presence of more than one lesion on brain imaging further reduces the likelihood of a primary neoplastic cause, but does not exclude it. Lesions in locations typical for MS (periventricular, juxtacortical, in the posterior fossa or spinal cord) would further increase the probability of the eventual diagnosis being MS, but again cannot be considered specific; for example, people with NMO or NMO spectrum disorders may fulfil current radiological criteria for MS (2010 McDonald criteria).

Where present on MRI, incomplete ring-like enhancement with gadolinium contrast (usually open towards grey matter) has been associated with demyelination more than neoplasia [30], although there have been reports of this rarely being seen in people with primary CNS lymphoma [31].

Disease-modifying treatment for MS may be ineffective or harmful when used in other CNS inflammatory conditions. When a person with a working diagnosis of MS, but atypical clinical features or investigation findings, appears not to respond toa disease-modifying treatment for MS, or has a paradoxical increase in disease activity while receiving such treatment, the diagnosis should be reconsidered.

References

1. Lavi R, Yarnitsky D, Rowe JM, et al. Standard vs atraumatic Whitacre needle for diagnostic lumbar puncture: a randomized trial. *Neurology* 2006; 67: 1492–4.
2. Turnbull DK, Shepherd DB. Post-dural puncture headache: pathogenesis, prevention and treatment. *Br J Anaesth* 2003; 91: 718–29.
3. International Headache Society. *International Headache Classification 2* 2004. Available at: <http://ihs-classification.org/en/ (accessed 21 April 2014).
4. Arevalo-Rodriguez I, Ciapponi A, Munoz L, et al. Posture and fluids for preventing post-dural puncture headache. *Cochrane Database Syst Rev* 2013; 7: CD009199.
5. Thomas SR, Jamieson DRS, Muir KW. Randomised controlled trial of atraumatic versus standard needles for diagnostic lumbar puncture. *BMJ* 2000; 321: 986–92.
6. Polman CH, Reingold SC, Banwell B, et al. (2011). Diagnostic criteria for multiple sclerosis: 2010 revisions to the McDonald criteria. *Ann Neurol* 2011; 69: 292–302.
7. Davies G, Keir G, Thompson EJ, Giovannoni G. The clinical significance of an intrathecal monoclonal immunoglobulin band: a follow-up study. *Neurology* 2003; 60: 1163–6.
8. Trip SA, Wroe SJ, Davies G, Giovannoni G. Primary CNS mantle cell lymphoma associated with an isolated CSF monoclonal IgG band. *Eur Neurol* 2003; 49: 187–8.
9. Yuen J, Zhu CX, Chan DT, et al. A sequential comparison on the risk of haemorrhage with different sizes of biopsy needles for stereotactic brain biopsy. *Stereotact Funct Neurosurg* 2014; 92: 160–9.

10. Air EL, Leach JL, Warnick RE, McPherson CM. Comparing the risks of frameless stereotactic biopsy in eloquent and noneloquent regions of the brain: a retrospective review of 284 cases. *J Neurosurg* 2009; 111: 820–4.
11. Rice CM, Gilkes CE, Teare E, et al. Brain biopsy in cryptogenic neurological disease. *Br J Neurosurg* 2011; 25: 614–20.
12. Shirani A, Zhao Y, Karim ME, et al. Association between use of interferon beta and progression of disability in patients with relapsing-remitting multiple sclerosis. *JAMA* 2012; 308: 247–56.
13. Calabresi PA, Giovannoni G, Confavreux C, et al. The incidence and significance of anti-natalizumab antibodies: results from AFFIRM and SENTINEL. *Neurology* 2007; 69: 1391–1403.
14. Rudick RA, Stuart WH, Calabresi PA, et al. Natalizumab plus interferon beta-1a for relapsing multiple sclerosis. *N Engl J Med* 2006; 354: 911–23.
15. Tan CS, Koralnik IJ. Progressive multifocal leukoencephalopathy and other disorders caused by JC virus: clinical features and pathogenesis. *Lancet Neurol* 2010; 9: 425–37.
16. Bloomgren G, Richman S, Hotermans C, et al. Risk of natalizumab-associated progressive multifocal leukoencephalopathy. *N Engl J Med* 2012; 366: 870–80.
17. Dahlhaus S, Hoepner R, Chan A, et al. Disease course and outcome of 15 monocentrically treated natalizumab-associated progressive multifocal leukoencephalopathy patients. *J Neurol Neurosurg Psychiatry* 2013; 84: 1068–74.
18. Clifford DB, De Luca A, DeLuca A, et al. Natalizumab-associated progressive multifocal leukoencephalopathy in patients with multiple sclerosis: lessons from 28 cases. *Lancet Neurol* 2010; 9, 438–46.
19. Sahraian MA, Radue E-W, Eshaghi A, et al. Progressive multifocal leukoencephalopathy: a review of the neuroimaging features and differential diagnosis. *Eur J Neurol* 2012; 19: 1060–9.
20. Kuhle J, Gosert R, Bühler R, et al. Management and outcome of CSF-JC virus PCR-negative PML in a natalizumab-treated patient with MS. *Neurology* 2011; 77, 2010–16.
21. Pardini M, Uccelli A, Grafman J, et al. Isolated cognitive relapses in multiple sclerosis. *J Neurol Neurosurg Psychiatry* 2014; 85(9); 1035–7.
22. Lucchinetti CF, Gavrilova RH, Metz I, et al. Clinical and radiographic spectrum of pathologically confirmed tumefactive multiple sclerosis. *Brain* 2008; 131: 1759–75.
23. Lolli V, Tampieri D, Melançon D, Delpilar Cortes M. Imaging in primary central nervous system lymphoma. *Neuroradiol J* 2010; 23: 680–9.
24. Polman CH, O'Connor PW, Havrdova E, et al. A randomized, placebo-controlled trial of natalizumab for relapsing multiple sclerosis. *N Engl J Med* 2006; 354: 899–910.
25. Lanzillo R, Quarantelli M, Bonavita S, et al. Natalizumab vs interferon beta 1a in relapsing-remitting multiple sclerosis: a head-to-head retrospective study. *Acta Neurol Scand* 2010; 126: 306–14.
26. Phan-Ba R, Belachew S, Outteryck O, et al. The earlier, the smaller, the better for natalizumab-associated PML. In MRI vigilance veritas? *Neurology* 2012; 79:1067–9.
27. Blair NF, Brew BJ, Halpern J-P. Natalizumab-associated PML identified in the presymptomatic phase using MRI surveillance. *Neurology* 2012; 78: 507–8.
28. Yousry TA, Pelletier D, Cadavid D, et al. Magnetic resonance imaging pattern in natalizumab-associated progressive multifocal leukoencephalopathy. *Ann Neurol* 2012; 72: 779–87.
29. Altintas A, Petek B, Isik N, et al. Clinical and radiological characteristics of tumefactive demyelinating lesions: follow-up study. *Mult Scler* 2012; 18: 1448–53.
30. Smith PD, Cook J, Trost NM, Murphy MA. Teaching NeuroImage: open-ring imaging sign in a case of tumefactive cerebral demyelination. *Neurology* 2008; 71: e73.
31. Zhang D, Hu LB, Henning TD, et al. MRI findings of primary CNS lymphoma in 26 immunocompetent patients. *Korean J Radiol* 2010; 11: 269–77.

CASE

13 Symptoms falling on deaf ears

Krishna Chinthapalli

Expert commentary: Graham Warner

Case history

A 36-year-old woman presented to the neurology clinic due to abnormal imaging findings of intracranial calcification.

Learning point Causes of intracranial calcification[1, 2]

Physiological

- Occurs with age in many brain structures.
- Pineal gland calcification occurs in two-thirds of adults (and calcification of the habenula, just anterior to it, occurs in 15 per cent).
- Choroid plexus calcification is also very common after 20 years, usually in the lateral ventricles.
- Meningeal calcification is seen in the elderly (falx cerebri, tentorium cerebelli, and arachnoid granulations).
- Faint punctate basal ganglia calcification occurs in 1 per cent of adults.

Neurocutaneous syndromes

- Tuberous sclerosis, with over 50 per cent of people having calcified tubers or subependymal nodules.
- Sturge–Weber syndrome, with linear cortical calcification in a minority.
- Rarely, neurofibromatosis type 1 may have calcification of intracranial tumours.
- Intracranial lipomata, with up to 50 per cent showing calcification.

Infectious

- Congenital infections that commonly cause calcification are TORCH (toxoplasmosis, rubella, cytomegalovirus, and herpes simplex virus) and HIV.
- Granulomatous infections:
  - identification of a travel history to endemic areas is important.
  - tuberculosis shows calcified tuberculomas in over 10 per cent of cases
  - neurocysticercosis may show calcified cysts.
- Rarely, chronic viral encephalitis or fungal infections may cause calcification.

Neoplastic

- The presence of calcification does not differentiate between benign and malignant tumours.
- Oligodendrogliomas calcify in 80 per cent of cases.
- Germ cell or pineal gland tumours calcify in 70 per cent of cases.
- Craniopharyngiomas calcify in 60 per cent of cases.
- Primitive or dysembryoplastic neuroepithelial tumours (PNET or DNET) in up to 50 per cent.
- Meningiomas and astrocytomas calcify in <20 per cent of cases.
- Metastases rarely calcify.

(Continued)

Vascular

- Arterial calcification is associated with atherosclerosis and age.
- Commonly affected arteries are the internal carotid (60 per cent), vertebral (20 per cent), and middle cerebral and basilar (5 per cent each).
- Arteriovenous malformations calcify in a quarter of cases.
- Aneurysms, in which calcification is often round and associated with intramural thrombosis.

Metabolic and endocrine

- Disorders of calcium metabolism, including hyperparathyroidism, hypoparathyroidism, and pseudo-hypoparathyroidism, cause calcification.
  - Hypothyroidism is occasionally associated with calcification.
  - Mitochondrial diseases.

Dystrophic

- Dystrophic calcifications occur at the site of damage after an insult such as trauma, surgery, infarction, or radiotherapy.

Idiopathic

- Fahr disease is a poorly defined rare condition of basal ganglia calcification, now thought to be genetically based.

Expert comment

CT is the imaging modality with highest sensitivity for intracranial calcification, but gradient echo sequences on MRI imaging can be a useful adjunct. Review of the images by a neuroradiologist may be valuable in producing a differential diagnosis.

She was referred by an ear, nose and throat surgeon who had ordered a CT scan of the head prior to cochlear implants for bilateral deafness.

She was born prematurely at 30 weeks gestation, for unknown reasons, along with her identical twin sister. Her birth weight was 1.310kg. Her family had noticed that she had slightly impaired hearing in both ears at the age of eight years. However, she was only diagnosed with hearing loss at the age of 20 years. From the age of 27 years, she was given bilateral hearing aids and followed up in audiology clinic. At 35 years, she had noticed worsening hearing loss such that she could not hear her mobile phone even on speaker setting with her hearing aids switched on. Her speech was normal. A repeat pure tone audiogram at this time showed profound bilateral sensorineural hearing loss (Figure 13.1), with a deterioration since the previous audiogram two years earlier (Figure 13.2).

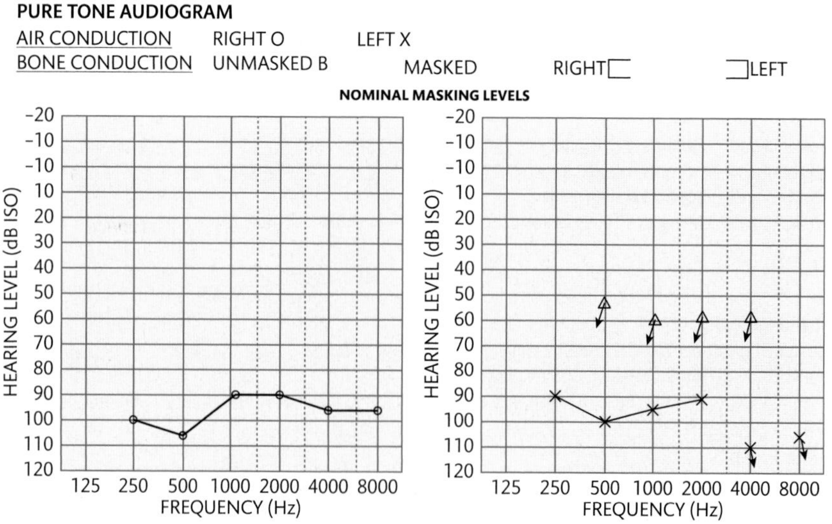

Figure 13.1 Most recent pure tone audiogram showing profound bilateral sensorineural hearing loss.

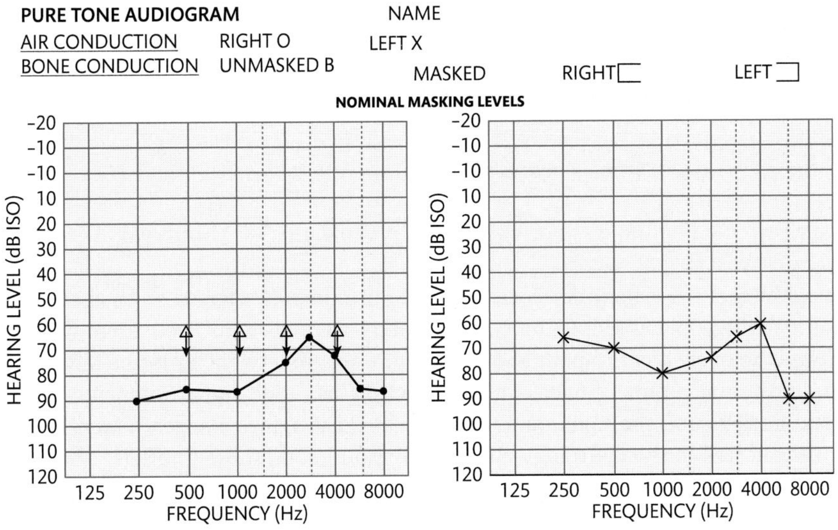

Figure 13.2 Audiogram two years before presentation showing less severe bilateral sensorineural hearing loss compared with the most recent audiogram, particularly in the left ear (graph on right).

Learning point Interpreting audiograms [3]

Testing

- Pure tone audiometry is performed using an audiometer, a device which can produce sounds at a single desired frequency ('pure tone') and at a particular volume.
- Sounds are presented at different volumes and frequencies in each ear. For each frequency, the softest volume ('threshold') that is heard by the subject is recorded.
- Testing is done in a quiet room after otoscopy, and requires the cooperation of the subject to signal when a stimulus has been heard.

Audiograms

- An audiogram is the representation of audiometry findings. It is a graph with sound frequencies in hertz (Hz) on the horizontal axis and sound pressure in decibels (dB) on the vertical axis.
- Conventionally, frequencies increase from left to right along the axis but sound volume decreases upwards on the vertical axis, with zero decibels hearing level (db HL) at the top.
- Normal hearing is at 0–20db HL at frequencies between 125 and 8000Hz. The normal threshold value is zero decibels; note that the scale is logarithmic, so a volume of 20db HL is 100 times louder than 0db HL.
- Air conduction is initially tested by presenting sound through earphones. Thresholds are represented on the audiogram using **O** for the right ear and **X** for the left ear (Figure 13.1).
- Bone conduction can be tested using a vibrating device applied to the mastoid process, which is recorded using **<** for the right ear and **>** for the left ear.
- If hearing is worse in one ear, masking the opposite ear with static noise can prevent sounds being heard by the opposite ear. For air conduction, this is recorded using **Δ** for the right ear and **□** for the left ear. For bone conduction, **[** is used for the right ear and **]** for the left ear.

Findings

- An air–bone gap, in which bone conduction is better than air conduction, is seen in conductive deafness. No air–bone gap suggests sensorineural deafness or normal hearing.
- Mild hearing loss (at a threshold of 20–40dB) means that soft sounds or whispers are not heard.
- Moderate hearing loss (at a threshold of 40–70dB) means that normal conversation is not heard.
- Severe hearing loss (at a threshold of 70–90dB) means only shouts are heard.
- Profound hearing loss (at a threshold of ≥90dB) means that only very loud noises, such as engines, are heard.

(Continued)

Implications

- According to National Institute for Health and Care Excellence (NICE) guidelines [4] cochlear implants are indicated in the NHS for profound hearing loss at frequencies of 2kHz and 4kHz.
- Unilateral cochlear implants are offered if hearing aids do not work.
- Simultaneous bilateral implants are only indicated in people with profound hearing loss *and* other disabilities, including blindness, which increase reliance on hearing.

An electrocardiogram was normal with no prolongation of QT interval. A CT scan of the ears was normal.

She now met the criteria for cochlear implants and was referred to an ear, nose, and throat surgeon. Otoscopy and tympanometry were normal. The patient wished to proceed with cochlear implantation. Therefore she underwent a routine MRI scan of the brain and petrous bones. This showed diffuse high-signal intensity in the caudate nucleus and the thalamus bilaterally on T1-weighted images (Figure 13.3). She was referred to the neurology clinic for an opinion on these findings. Ahead of clinic, a plain CT scan of the head was performed. This found bilateral symmetrical calcification within the caudate nucleus, putamen, globus pallidus, and thalamus (Figure 13.4).

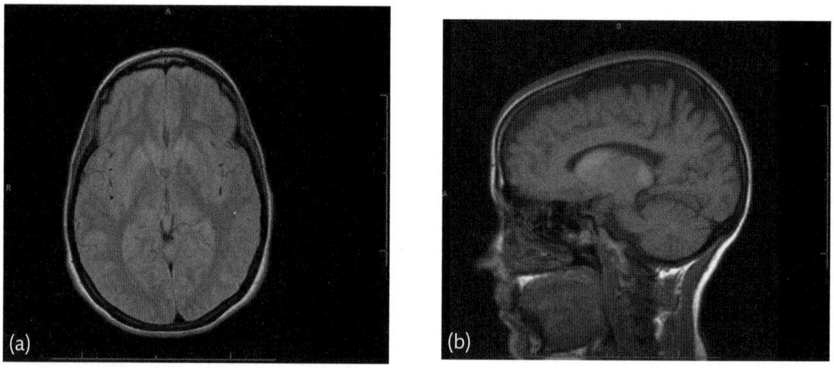

Figure 13.3 T1-weighted MRI scan of the brain with (a) an axial image and (b) a parasagittal image showing bilateral symmetric high-signal intensity in the basal ganglia, particularly the caudate nuclei and the thalami.

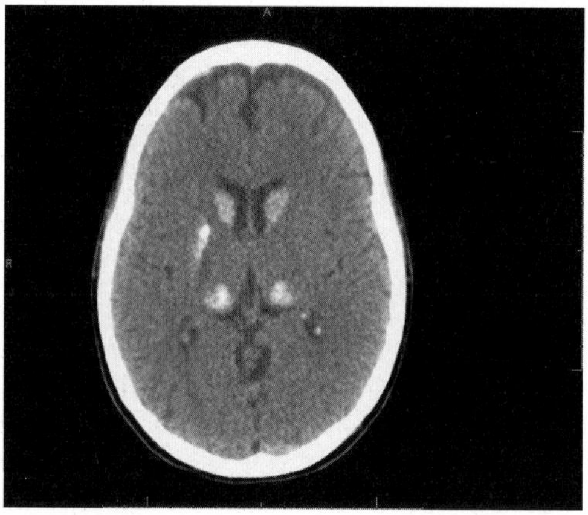

Figure 13.4 Axial image from a plain CT scan of the head showing high-attenuation lesions of the basal ganglia and thalami. There is clearly visible calcification in the right putamen and the posterior areas of both thalami.

In clinic, the patient reported feeling frustrated at not being able to communicate and that those she spoke to also became frustrated. She felt stressful in such situations and also found it difficult to communicate with her young son. This resulted in losing her independence and less interaction with other people. For example, she avoided family gatherings because she feared being left out of the conversations. Other than deafness, she had no neurological symptoms such as weakness or sensory disturbance. On questioning, she revealed that she had been underweight for most of her life. There was no other past medical history, particularly no diabetes mellitus or seizures. She took no medications except nutritional supplements. She did not smoke or drink alcohol. Her mother had diabetes mellitus and her maternal uncle had a possible muscular disease. Her twin sister also had mild hearing loss in both ears, but this started at the age of 26 years. Her sister had recently started to use bilateral hearing aids and was suffering from falls and unsteadiness.

On neurological examination, she was alert, orientated, and able to lip read. Cranial nerves were normal with a full range of eye movements. There were no involuntary movements, including jerks or tremor. However, her limbs were areflexic with normal power and sensation to light touch and proprioception. Coordination was also normal.

A nerve conduction study suggested a previously unrecognized mild sensory peripheral neuropathy. Routine blood tests including full blood count, urea and electrolytes, liver function tests, thyroid function tests, creatine kinase, glucose, calcium, phosphate, and parathyroid hormone were normal. Mitochondrial DNA mutation analysis was requested on a blood sample, and this revealed that the patient was heteroplasmic for the m.3243A>G mutation with an estimated proportion of 38 per cent.

She underwent cochlear implantation afterwards and was then referred to an adult genetics clinic for genetic counselling and further specialist referrals.

Discussion

Abnormal mitochondria were first associated with disease in two children with progressive proximal myopathy who underwent muscle biopsies [5]. The biopsies showed very large and very enzymatically active mitochondria. In 1988, it was shown that mitochondrial DNA mutations were present in these 'mitochondrial myopathies' [6]. Since then, a range of mitochondrial mutations and diseases have been described, and known phenotypes have both expanded and overlapped.

It is estimated that pathogenic mitochondrial DNA mutations are present in 1 in 5000 people [7]. Mitochondria produce energy by oxidative phosphorylation. Their structural proteins are encoded not only by nuclear DNA, but also by mitochondrial DNA inside the mitochondria themselves. Mutations in both types of DNA can cause mitochondrial disease. Nuclear DNA mutations that cause mitochondrial disease often show autosomal recessive inheritance, in common with many other inherited metabolic diseases. However, mutations in the *POLG* gene, which codes for the DNA polymerase gene in mitochondria but is located on chromosome 15, may cause an autosomal dominant chronic progressive external ophthalmoplegia. *POLG* mutations affect the transcription of mitochondrial DNA, and mutations can lead to depleted levels of mitochondrial DNA (as in Alpers syndrome) or deletions during transcription of mitochondrial DNA (as in sensory ataxic neuropathy with

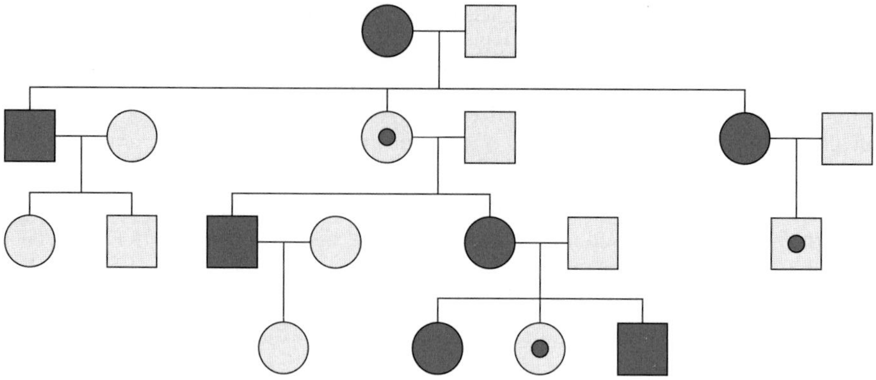

Figure 13.5 A typical inheritance pattern for pathogenic mitochondrial DNA mutations, which are inherited from the mother. Because of heteroplasmy, not all offspring may be affected.

Expert comment

Mitochondrial mutations are virtually never inherited from the father, although there are isolated case reports of paternal transmission [8]. Mothers may transmit it to both sons and daughters equally. Some mitochondrial diseases may in fact be due to nuclear DNA mutations (such as the *POLG* mutation in Alpers syndrome) and therefore could show autosomal dominant, autosomal recessive, or X-linked patterns of inheritance.

dysarthria and ophthalmoparesis). Since mitochondria are only present in the ovum and not sperm, mitochondrial DNA itself shows a characteristic pattern of maternal inheritance (Figure 13.5).

Unlike nuclear DNA, there are hundreds of copies of mitochondrial DNA in each cell and not just two. These copies may be different from each other; this is known as heteroplasmy. To assess the severity of mitochondrial disease, it is important to know the ratio of mutated DNA copies to normal DNA copies, as in the genetic test result for the patient above. Mitochondrial DNA mutations tend to cause loss of function and a certain threshold has to be reached before mitochondrial function is impaired. The heteroplasmy level of 38 per cent of mutated DNA in this patient is known to be sufficient to produce a clinical phenotype. In a study of 126 people with m.3243A>G mutations, there was a mean heteroplasmy level of 22 per cent [9]. The serum heteroplasmy level showed a significant positive correlation with disease severity, although heteroplasmy levels may vary in the brain.

Mitochondrial diseases are said to present in 'any symptom in any organ at any age', but, as one would expect, mitochondrial disease symptoms and signs are prominent in organ systems with high metabolic activity, such as the brain, muscles, and heart. Some classic mitochondrial syndromes have also been recognized for many years (Table 13.1). The variability of presentations means that neurologists have to maintain a high index of suspicion for mitochondrial disease, but there are characteristic 'red flag' features that should prompt baseline investigations. In particular, a family history or multi-organ involvement should raise suspicion (Table 13.2). Referral to a metabolic or mitochondrial disease specialist may be warranted at this stage.

McFarland et al. [13] propose an algorithm to follow for diagnosis if mitochondrial disease is suspected (Figure 13.6). First, baseline investigations and clinical assessment should determine if a person has a well-recognized mitochondrial syndrome, as outlined in Table 13.3. Serum lactate is raised in many mitochondrial diseases because impairment of the mitochondrial oxidative phosphorylation pathway leads to increased anaerobic respiration. In practice, serum lactate can also be raised due to exercise or the use of a tourniquet, limiting its specificity [14]. If so, genetic tests should be performed. Otherwise, a skeletal muscle biopsy may be needed to confirm mitochondrial disease by histochemical analysis. Further investigations then include biochemical analysis of respiratory chain enzymes involved in

Table 13.1 Mitochondrial syndromes and examples of genes that are implicated*

Syndrome	Features	Examples of genes (and mutations)
Alpers syndrome [10]	Developmental delay/regression Seizures Liver failure	*POLG* (nuclear) with mtDNA depletion
Kearns-Sayre syndrome	Progressive external ophthalmoplegia (PEO), ptosis Pigmentary retinopathy Cardiac conduction defects	>1kb mtDNA deletion
Leigh syndrome [11]	Neurodegenerative changes (hypotonia, spasticity, seizures, ataxia) Bilateral, symmetrical cerebral lesions	*SURF1* (nuclear) *MT-ATP6* (mtDNA)
LHON	Leber's **H**ereditary **O**ptic **N**europathy	*MT-ND4* (m.11778G>A)
MEGDEL [12]	**ME**thyl**G**lutaconic aciduria **D**eafness **E**ncephalopathy **L**eigh-like syndrome	*SERAC1* (nuclear)
MELAS	**M**itochondrial **E**ncephalomyopathy **L**actic **A**cidosis **S**troke-like episodes	*MT-TL1* (m.3243A>G)
MIDD	**M**aternally **I**nherited **D**iabetes **D**eafness	
MERRF	**M**yoclonic **E**pilepsy **R**agged **R**ed **F**ibres on muscle biopsy	*MT-TK* (m.8344A>G)
MNGIE	**M**itochondrial **N**euro-**G**astro-**I**ntestinal **E**ncephalomyopathy	*TYMP* (nuclear)
NARP	**N**europathy **A**taxia **R**etinitis **P**igmentosa	*MT-ATP6* (m.8993T>G)
MEMSA	**M**yoclonic **E**pilepsy **M**yopathy **S**ensory **A**taxia	*POLG* (nuclear) with mtDNA deletions
SANDO	**S**ensory **A**taxic **N**europathy with **D**ysarthria and **O**phthalmoparesis	

*For mitochondrial DNA (mtDNA) genes, the most common point mutations are described in parentheses.

oxidative phosphorylation and genetic testing using DNA sequencing or polymerase chain reaction (PCR).

In the case study here, there was a family history of sensorineural hearing loss in the twin sister and diabetes mellitus in the mother, consistent with maternal inheritance. Hence, maternally inherited diabetes and deafness (MIDD) syndrome was suspected and testing for common mitochondrial mutations was fruitful. MIDD is most commonly due to a point mutation from adenine to guanine at position 3243 in the mitochondrial gene *MT-TL1*, which encodes for tRNA leucine 1 protein. This is expressed as m.3243A>G and is found in up to 3 per cent of people with diabetes in the general population [15].

However, as with other mitochondrial mutations, people with m.3243A>G mutations show a large phenotypic spectrum [16]. In one study, whilst 30 per cent of those with the mutation have MIDD, 10 per cent fulfil criteria for MELAS (mitochondrial encephalomyopathy, lactic acidosis, stroke-like episodes) syndrome, 6 per cent for progressive external ophthalmoplegia, and 1 per cent for MERRF (myoclonic epilepsy with

Table 13.2 Key 'red flag' features that should raise suspicion of mitochondrial diseases

System	Features
Neurological	Cerebral stroke-like lesions, especially if not in one vascular territory
	Encephalopathy, especially after sodium valproate
	Epilepsy partialis continua, myoclonus, or status epilepticus
	Ataxia, cerebellar atrophy
	Sensorineural hearing loss, if early-onset or familial
	Intellectual disability, developmental delay, or cognitive decline
Ophthalmological	Optic atrophy
	Ophthalmoplegia
	Pigmentary retinopathy
	Ptosis
Other	Cardiomyopathy
	Diabetes mellitus
	Gastrointestinal dysmotility or obstruction
	Lactic acidosis
	Sensitivity to general anaesthesia

Data from *Pediatrics* 120(6), Haas RH, Parikh S, Falk MJ, et al., Mitochondrial disease: a practical approach for primary care physicians, pp. 1326-33,© 2007, with permission from American Academy of Pediatrics; *Dev Disabil Res Rev* 16(2), Parikh S, The neurologic manifestations of mitochondrial disease, pp. 120-8, ©2010, with permission from John Wiley & Sons.

ragged red fibres) syndrome. Looking at individual symptoms there is similar heterogeneity: 51 per cent have sensorineural hearing loss, 42 per cent have diabetes mellitus, 27 per cent have proximal myopathy, 24 per cent have ataxia, 23 per cent have migraines, 18 per cent have seizures, and 9 per cent are asymptomatic. The authors suggest that if there is no classic clinical mitochondrial syndrome or maternal family history of mitochondrial mutations, having multiple 'red flag' features may point to mitochondrial disease.

Management of mitochondrial disease should begin by completing baseline assessments for involvement of other organs. Swallowing assessment is useful for assessing dysphagia and the risk of aspiration, as well as for optimizing nutritional intake. Genetic counselling and discussion of prevention of transmission should be offered. Prenatal testing of embryos is not widely available and is difficult to interpret because of heteroplasmy.

Immunizations are safe, but a number of drugs should be avoided in mitochondrial disease (Table 13.4) [18]. Metabolic stressors, such as fever, dehydration, or starvation, should be avoided or treated aggressively to avoid decompensation. There is no high-quality evidence for any treatment in mitochondrial disease, but coenzyme Q10, riboflavin, arginine, and endurance training have been reported to be beneficial [13]. For many systemic features, treatment is symptomatic. This may include non-invasive positive pressure ventilation for respiratory failure or physiotherapy and baclofen for spasticity.

Cardiology, epilepsy, and ophthalmology guidelines for use in the NHS have been developed by the Newcastle Mitochondrial Centre [19–21]. All patients should undergo regular electrocardiography and echocardiography. Those with conduction defects or paroxysmal symptoms may need a prolonged ambulatory ECG and

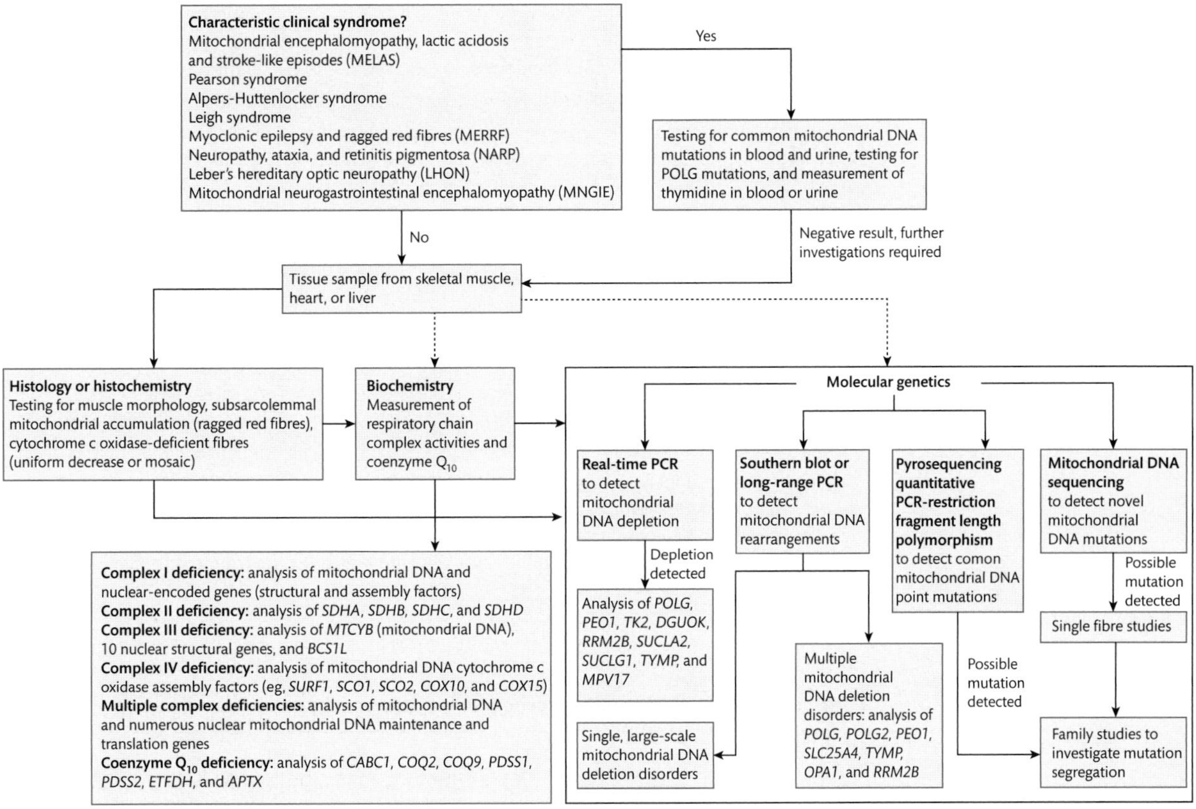

Figure 13.6 A diagnostic algorithm to follow for suspected mitochondrial disease.

Reproduced from *Lancet Neurol* 9(8), McFarland R, Taylor RW, Turnbull DM, A neurological perspective on mitochondrial disease, pp. 829–40, © 2010, with permission from Elsevier.

Table 13.3 Example baseline investigations and assessment

Investigation	Positive findings
Serum lactate, creatine kinase, glucose	Raised lactate, glucose, or slightly raised creatine kinase
CT scan of brain	Intracranial calcification
MRI scan of brain	Symmetrical deep grey matter hyperintensity or infarct-like lesions
Cerebrospinal fluid analysis, including lactate, protein, glucose, and cell count	Raised lactate
Electrocardiogram	Arrhythmias, heart block
Echocardiogram	Hypertrophic cardiomyopathy
Audiogram	Sensorineural hearing loss
Ophthalmology assessment	Optic atrophy Pigmentary retinopathy

Data from *Pediatrics*, 120(6), Haas RH, Parikh S, Falk MJ, et al. Mitochondrial disease: a practical approach for primary care physicians, pp. 1326-33,© 2007, with permission from the American Academy of Pediatrics

Evidence base [17]

Glover EI, Martin J, Maher A, et al. A randomized trial of coenzyme Q10 in mitochondrial disorders. *Muscle Nerve* 2010;42(5): 739–48.

Coenzyme Q10 is a cofactor for enzymes in the oxidative phosphorylation pathway and an antioxidant. It is not licensed as a drug, but instead sold as a supplement in many countries (including the USA and UK). A number of reports suggested that coenzyme Q10 may have benefit in mitochondrial disease and this trial assessed a range of biochemical, physiological, and clinical outcomes.

Thirty people with mitochondrial disorders (including 15 with MELAS) were recruited in Ontario, Canada, making it one of the largest trials in mitochondrial disease. It was a randomized double-blind crossover trial with participants taking either placebo or coenzyme Q10 600mg twice daily first for 60 days before crossover.

Muscle strength, markers of oxidative damage, lactate levels (in plasma and magnetic resonance spectrometry of cerebral cortex), activities of daily living, and quality of life did not differ when taking coenzyme Q10 or placebo, although plasma coenzyme Q10 levels increased fivefold.

The trial showed that there were no short-term benefits of taking coenzyme Q10 at the highest available daily dose. However, it is still commonly used in mitochondrial disease and fortunately has few adverse effects. It is unclear if there may be long-term advantages due to modulation of gene expression or adaptive changes, and further trials are under way using modified coenzyme Q10.

Table 13.4 Drugs with reported mitochondrial toxicity and the mechanism if known

Medication	Symptoms	Mechanism
Valproic acid	Hepatopathy; infrequently direct encephalopathy	Inhibition of fatty acid oxidation, the citric acid cycle, and oxidative phosphorylation
Antiretrovirals	Peripheral neuropathy, liver dysfunction, myopathy	Impairment of mtDNA replication causing mtDNA depletion, carnitine deficiency, lactic acidosis, lipodystrophy
Statins	Myopathy	Multiple postulated effects, including CoQ10 depletion
Aspirin	Reye syndrome	Inhibition and uncoupling of oxidative phosphorylation
Aminoglycoside antibiotics	Hearing loss, cardiac toxicity, renal toxicity	Impaired mtDNA translation
Aminoglycoside and platinum chemotherapeutics	Hearing loss, cardiac toxicity, renal toxicity	Impaired mtDNA translation
Paracetamol (acetaminophen)	Hepatopathy	Oxidative stress
Metformin	Lactic acidosis	Inhibition of oxidative phosphorylation, enhanced glycolysis
Beta-blockers	Reduced exercise tolerance	Oxidative stress
Steroids	Reports of deterioration in Kearns-Sayre syndrome	Unknown

CoQ10, coenzyme Q10; mtDNA, mitochondrial DNA.

Clinical tip **Avoid sodium valproate in mitochondrial disease**

Sodium valproate should be avoided in all patients with mitochondrial disease because of the risk of hepatotoxicity and encephalopathy.

subsequently a pacemaker or ablation therapy. Those with dilated or hypertrophic cardiomyopathy should be treated with beta-blockers and angiotensin-converting enzyme (ACE) inhibitors.

Although seizures may occur in people with mitochondrial disease, cardiac arrhythmias are also more common. In addition, baseline blood tests may show raised creatine kinase and raised serum lactate. Therefore diagnosing episodes of loss of consciousness may not be straightforward. Focal or non-convulsive status epilepticus and metabolic cerebral infarcts may also occur.

Sensorineural hearing loss is common in mitochondrial disorders but routine screening is often overlooked. If there is profound hearing loss, cochlear implants should be considered, as in this patient, and an ECG should also be performed to look for Jervell and Lange-Nielsen syndrome which can cause sudden death [22].

Clinical tip Edrophonium test

A Tensilon® (edrophonium) test may be dangerous if performed in people with mitochondrial disease as it may cause heart block. Be cautious if mitochondrial disease is a possible differential diagnosis in a patient presenting with ophthalmoplegia or ptosis.

Final word from the expert

Our patient was seen by a number of different specialists for her deafness, and the possibility of mitochondrial diseases was never explored. Pathogenic mitochondrial gene mutations are present in up to 0.5 per cent of the general population. The m.3243A>G mutation is associated with deafness and diabetes mellitus but routine screening is uncommon. Neurologists see it in MELAS syndrome but clearly other phenotypic presentations occur. Radiologically, it is associated with basal ganglia calcification, which is present in half of people tested; however, metabolic disturbance needs to be excluded and most cases of basal ganglia calcification are (as yet) idiopathic. Reaching a diagnosis allows the patient and family to understand their illness and prognosis, to undergo predictive testing if wished, and to undergo screening for other organ systems that may be affected as well as avoiding unnecessary investigations.

References

1. Kıroğlu Y, Callı C, Karabulut N, Oncel C. Intracranial calcifications on CT. *Diagn Interv Radiol Ank Turk* 2010; 16(4): 263–9.
2. Celzo FG, Venstermans C, De Belder F, et al. Brain stones revisited—between a rock and a hard place. *Insights Imaging* 2013; 4(5): 625–35.
3. Walker JJ, Cleveland LM, Davis JL, Seales JS. Audiometry screening and interpretation. *Am Fam Physician* 2013; 87(1): 41–7.
4. National Institute for Health and Care Excellence 2009. Cochlear implants for children and adults with severe to profound deafness. *NICE Technology Appraisal Guidance TA166*. Available at: <http://publications.nice.org.uk/cochlear-implants-for-children-and-adults-with-severe-to-profound-deafness-ta166/guidance>
5. Coleman RF, Nienhuis AW, Brown WJ, et al. New myopathy with mitochondrial enzyme hyperactivity. Histochemical demonstration. *JAMA* 1967; 199(9): 624–30.
6. Holt IJ, Harding AE, Morgan-Hughes JA. Deletions of muscle mitochondrial DNA in patients with mitochondrial myopathies. *Nature* 1988; 331(6158): 717–19.
7. Ylikallio E, Suomalainen A. Mechanisms of mitochondrial diseases. *Ann Med* 2012; 44(1): 41–59.
8. Schwartz M, Vissing J. Paternal inheritance of mitochondrial DNA. *N Engl J Med* 2002; 347(8): 576–80.

9. De Laat P, Koene S, van den Heuvel LPWJ, et al. Clinical features and heteroplasmy in blood, urine and saliva in 34 Dutch families carrying the m.3243A>G mutation. *J Inherit Metab Dis* 2012; 35(6): 1059–69. doi:10.1007/s10545-012-9465-2.
10. Saneto RP, Cohen BH, Copeland WC, Naviaux RK. Alpers–Huttenlocher syndrome. *Pediatr Neurol* 2013; 48(3): 167–78.
11. Baertling F, Rodenburg RJ, Schaper J, et al. A guide to diagnosis and treatment of Leigh syndrome. *J Neurol Neurosurg Psychiatry* 2014; 85(3): 257–65.
12. Wortmann SB, Vaz FM, Gardeitchik T, et al. Mutations in the phospholipid remodeling gene *SERAC1* impair mitochondrial function and intracellular cholesterol trafficking and cause dystonia and deafness. *Nat Genet*. 2012; 44(7): 797–802.
13. McFarland R, Taylor RW, Turnbull DM. A neurological perspective on mitochondrial disease. *Lancet Neurol* 2010; 9(8): 829–40.
14. Haas RH, Parikh S, Falk MJ, et al. Mitochondrial disease: a practical approach for primary care physicians. *Pediatrics* 2007; 120(6): 1326–33.
15. Schaefer AM, Walker M, Turnbull DM, Taylor RW. Endocrine disorders in mitochondrial disease. *Mol Cell Endocrinol* 2013; 379(1–2): 2–11.
16. Nesbitt V, Pitceathly RDS, Turnbull DM, et al. The UK MRC Mitochondrial Disease Patient Cohort Study: clinical phenotypes associated with the m.3243A>G mutation—implications for diagnosis and management. *J Neurol Neurosurg Psychiatry* 2013; 84(8): 936–8.
17. Glover EI, Martin J, Maher A, et al. A randomized trial of coenzyme Q10 in mitochondrial disorders. *Muscle Nerve* 2010; 42(5): 739–48.
18. Parikh S, Saneto R, Falk MJ, et al. A modern approach to the treatment of mitochondrial disease. *Curr Treat Options Neurol* 2009; 11(6): 414–30.
19. Newcastle Mitochondrial Centre. *Cardiac Involvement in Adult Mitochondrial Disease: Screening and Initial Management* 2010. Available at: <http://www.mitochondrialncg.nhs.uk/documents/Cardiology_Guidelines_2011.pdf>
20. Newcastle Mitochondrial Centre. *Epile Psy in Adult Mitochondrial Disease: Investigation and Management* 2010. Available at: <http://www.mitochondrialncg.nhs.uk/documents/Epilepsy_Guidelines_2011.pdf>
21. Newcastle Mitochondrial Centre. *Ocular Involvement in Adult Mitochondrial Disease: Screening and Initial Management* 2011. Available at: <http://www.mitochondrialncg.nhs.uk/documents/Ophthalmology_Guidelines_2011.pdf>
22. Yanmei F, Yaqin W, Haibo S, et al. Cochlear implantation in patients with Jervell and Lange-Nielsen syndrome, and a review of literature. *Int J Pediatr Otorhinolaryngol* 2008; 72(11): 1723–9.

CASE

14 Difficulty breathing and moving

Jennifer Spillane

Expert commentary: Dimitri M. Kullmann

Case history

A 64-year-old man presented to his general practitioner with a four-week history of malaise, general fatigue, and a feeling of heaviness in his legs. He had a background history of hypertension but had otherwise been well and was on no regular medication. He was an ex-smoker of 20 cigarettes a day for 30 years. General examination and routine blood test results were unremarkable.

Six weeks later, he became acutely unwell and was admitted to his local hospital. He was confused and had generalized weakness, most marked proximally. Shortly after admission, he became drowsy with a score of 11 on the Glasgow Coma Scale (GCS). Arterial blood gases showed pH 7.15, po_2 6.9 kPA, and pco_2 11.6 kPA. He was thought to have type 2 respiratory failure secondary to neuromuscular weakness. He was admitted to the intensive care unit (ICU) where he was intubated and ventilated. He was diagnosed with a left-sided pneumonia and was treated with antibiotics. A tracheostomy was performed and he was subsequently transferred to a specialist neurological intensive care unit (NICU).

Learning point Differential diagnosis of acute neuromuscular weakness in the ICU

The diagnosis of a patient with motor weakness in ICU is challenging, not least because neuromuscular weakness may not be appreciated initially in the setting of severe systemic illness. Neuromuscular diseases that present with acute-onset weakness can be divided into long-standing illnesses that acutely deteriorate and new presentations of disease. In the latter group, as was the case in this patient, subtle signs may have been present previously but overlooked. Moreover, latent neuromuscular weakness can be unmasked after surgery if there is difficulty weaning the patient from ventilation. CNS or spinal cord syndromes may be difficult to distinguish from neuromuscular causes of weakness in the ICU setting and must be considered in the differential diagnosis (see Table 14.1).

As patients with neuromuscular weakness in the ICU are often encephalopathic, sedated, and mechanically ventilated, clinical evaluation may be limited to testing reflexes. Electromyography is useful, and is usually necessary to identify the locus of neuromuscular weakness.

On arrival in the NICU he had a tracheostomy in situ and a GCS of 14. He was noted to have bilateral ptosis, worse on the left than the right. He had a full range of eye movements. Tongue movements were slow, but there were no fasciculations. On examination of his limbs, tone was normal throughout but he had severe proximal weakness in both upper and lower limbs. When his ventilator was disconnected, he tired quickly and was noted to have paradoxical inward movement of his abdomen during inspiration, indicating diaphragmatic weakness.

Expert comment

Although paradoxical breathing can point to diaphragmatic weakness, this is often overlooked especially if the patient requires urgent intubation and ventilation.

Table 14.1 Causes of acute neuromuscular weakness on ICU [1–4]

Anterior horn cell	ALS, poliomyelitis, post polio syndrome, SMA, Kennedy's disease, West Nile encephalitis
Peripheral neuropathy	GBS, CIDP, critical illness polyneuropathy, hereditary motor sensory neuropathies, porphyria, infectious polyneuropathy (CMV polyradiculopathy), acute vasculitic neuropathy
Disorders of the neuromuscular junction	myasthenia gravis, Lambert–Eaton myasthenic syndrome, congenital myasthenic syndromes, botulism
Myopathy and muscular dystrophy	Rhabdomyolysis, acute alcoholic myopathy, viral myopathy (eg HIV) Inflammatory myopathy (sporadic inclusion body myositis, dermatomyositis, polymyositis) Critical illness myopathy Hereditary muscular dystrophy (Duchenne's, Becker's, FSHD, LGMD especially LGMD 2C-2F, 2I myotonic dystrophy) Congential myopathy (central core myopathy, myotubular myopathy, nemaline myopathy, myofibrillar myopathy, multi-mini-core disease) Mitochondrial disease Metabolic myopathy (acid maltase deficiency) Toxic myopathy (organophosphate poisoning)
CNS	Stroke, encephalitis, central pontine myelinosis, brainstem infarct
Spinal cord	Trauma, infarction, transverse myelitis, acute ischaemia

ALS, amyotrophic lateral sclerosis; SMA, spinal muscular atrophy; GBS, Guillain–Barré syndrome; CIDP, chronic inflammatory demyelinating polyneuropathy; CMV, cytomegalovirus; FSHD, facioscapulohumeral muscular dystrophy; LGMD, limb girdle muscular dystrophy.

Reflexes were present in his upper limbs but absent in his lower limbs, with flexor plantar responses. Sensory examination was normal and the remainder of the general examination was unremarkable.

Detailed investigations were undertaken. Routine blood tests were unremarkable. Infectious and metabolic screens were both negative. CT and MRI scans of the brain were normal. Lumbar puncture revealed an opening pressure of $15cmH_20$, and the CSF was acellular with protein 0.78g/L, glucose 3.2mM/L (serum glucose 5.4), no growth on culture, and negative viral PCR. EEG was reported as showing moderate encephalopathy with no evidence of seizure activity.

Electrophysiological studies were performed in the NICU to help define the cause of his severe weakness. Sensory studies were normal but the compound muscle action potential (CMAP) amplitudes were small. Repetitive stimulation at 3Hz elicited a further reduction in amplitude. However, maximal exercise elicited an increase in CMAP amplitude of over 100 per cent, consistent with a presynaptic disorder of neuromuscular transmission (Figure 14.1).

Voltage-gated calcium channel antibodies were tested and found to be positive, confirming a diagnosis of Lambert–Eaton myasthenic syndrome (LEMS). Other antibody tests such as anti-*N*-methyl-D-aspartate receptor antibodies, anti-acetylcholine receptor antibodies, and anti-neuronal antibodies were all negative.

A search for an underlying neoplasm was undertaken. A CT scan of the thorax, abdomen, and pelvis showed mediastinal and hilar lymphadenopathy with bilateral pleural effusions but no definite solid lesion. A CT-guided biopsy of mediastinal lymph nodes showed malignant cells immunopositive for CD56, TTF-1, and

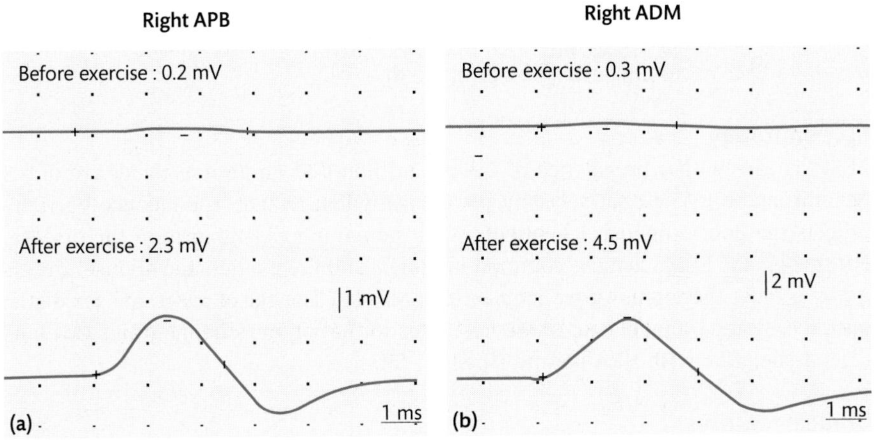

Figure 14.1 Pre- and post exercise stimulation mimicking high-frequency stimulation. Stimulation of (a) the abductor pollicis brevis and (b) the abductor digiti minimi was performed before (upper panel) and after (lower panel) 10 seconds of exercise. The amplitude increased significantly after exercise, consistent with presynaptic dysfunction.

synaptophysin, consistent with small-cell lung cancer (SCLC). Baseline tumour staging investigations showed that there were no distant metastases.

A diagnosis of SCLC with paraneoplastic LEMS was made. The patient was initially treated with five sessions of plasma exchange. He had a good response to this treatment and was gradually weaned from the ventilator. He was subsequently commenced on 3,4-diaminopyridine (3,4-DAP) at a dose of 10mg four times daily.

He was not deemed to be a surgical candidate and so underwent chemotherapy (six cycles of carboplatin–etoposide) and received adjunctive radiotherapy. He tolerated this well, but had an acute deterioration of his neurological syndrome with decreased proximal muscle strength. He was treated with intravenous immunoglobulin (2g/kg over four days) and was then commenced on oral prednisolone 30mg/day.

Nine months after discharge from the NICU he remains on a reducing dose of oral prednisolone and 3,4-DAP. Repeat imaging has shown a substantial reduction in tumour size. His strength has improved considerably, and he can now mobilize independently with only minimal proximal lower limb weakness.

Discussion

Lambert–Eaton myasthenic syndrome (LEMS)

LEMS is an autoimmune disorder of neuromuscular transmission that was first recognized clinically in the 1950s [5]. It was initially shown to be a distinct disorder from myasthenia gravis (MG) because of its distinctive electrophysiology, with a small baseline MAP and post-tetanic potentiation. It is characterized by reduced release of presynaptic acetylcholine-containing vesicles from the presynaptic motor nerve terminal. Antibodies against P/Q-type voltage-gated calcium channels (VGCCs) occur in 85 per cent of patients and are thought to lead to a reduction of action-potential induced calcium influx at the presynaptic nerve terminal, accounting for the decrease in vesicle release [6].

The largest case series have revealed that 50–60 per cent of patients with LEMS have an underlying malignancy, most often SCLC [7–9]. The remaining patients develop LEMS as an idiopathic autoimmune disease.

Epidemiology

LEMS is rare with a prevalence of 2.3 per million and an annual incidence of 0.5 per million [10]. The relatively low prevalence when related to incidence partially reflects the poor prognosis of patients with the paraneoplastic form of the disease. Paraneoplastic LEMS is more common in males, and the median age of onset in this group is older than in non-paraneoplastic LEMS [11]. The age of onset and sex distribution of non-paraneoplastic LEMS is similar to that of myasthenia gravis (MG), as is its association with HLA B8 and HLADR3 [6].

Clinical features

LEMS usually presents with proximal muscle weakness, affecting the legs in 80 per cent of cases, but upper limb weakness usually develops soon after [7]. Weakness typically spreads distally, and the speed of progression tends to be faster in patients with a malignancy [12]. MG also presents with proximal muscle weakness, although in MG the weakness tends to be more fatiguable, fluctuating throughout the day.

Facial weakness and extra-ocular muscle involvement are much less prominent in LEMS than in MG [6]. Although ocular symptoms do occur in LEMS, in contrast with MG they are rarely seen in isolation [7].

Respiratory failure in LEMS, as was seen in our patient, is uncommon but is recognized and has occasionally been reported as a presenting symptom [13]. It is more usually reported in association with malignancy, and in one-third of the reported cases occurred after administration of a neuromuscular blocking agent [8, 13–15].

Autonomic dysfunction is found in 80–96 per cent of patients with LEMS and may precede the onset of muscle weakness [16]. Autonomic symptoms may be more severe in patients with paraneoplastic LEMS [17]. Dry mouth is the most common symptom, followed by erectile dysfunction in men and constipation. Orthostatic hypotension, micturition difficulties, and dry eyes are seen less frequently [7].

On clinical examination, proximal weakness can usually be readily demonstrated and, in contrast with MG, patients often have depressed or absent reflexes. Post-exercise facilitation of reflexes can be demonstrated in approximately 40 per cent of LEMS patients [18].

Table 14.2 Distinguishing LEMS from MG

	MG	LEMS
Presenting symptom	Ocular in 85%	Proximal lower limb in 85%
Fatiguability	Common	Usually not demonstrable, weakness may improve after exercise
Reflexes	Normal	In 40% reflexes are absent but reappear after exercise
Electrophysiology	Normal CMAPS, decremental response to low frequency repetitive nerve stimulation	CMAPS have reduced amplitude, decremental response to low frequency stimulation but there is potentiation to high frequency stimulation or maximal voluntary contraction

(Continued)

Table 14.2 (Continued)

	MG	LEMS
Serology	85% of patients are positive for anti acetylcholine receptor antibodies. A variable proportion of the remainder have anti Muscle Specific Tyrosine Kinase antibodies (MuSK)	85–90% are positive for antibodies against the P/Q VGCC
Association with malignancy	15% of patients have an underlying thymoma and about 60% have thymic hyperplasia	50–60% of patients have an underlying malignancy, most often small cell lung carcinoma
Symptomatic treatment	Anti acetylcholinesterase inhibitors (pyridostigmine)	3,4 Diaminopyridine

Clinical tip Triad of symptoms in LEMS

The classical triad of proximal muscle weakness, areflexia, and autonomic dysfunction should prompt a high suspicion of LEMS, but not all patients will have all three features [8].

Diagnosis

The diagnosis of LEMS can be challenging, and the mean delay from first symptoms to correct diagnosis ranges from four months for paraneoplastic LEMS to 19 months for non-paraneoplastic LEMS [7]. Delay in diagnosis has been reported to be as high as 4.2 years in non-paraneoplastic LEMS in non-specialist centres [19].

Electrophysiology

The repetitive nerve stimulation (RNS) test is the main electrophysiological test for the diagnosis of LEMS. Classic findings include a low compound CMAP at rest, a decremental response at low-frequency stimulation (2–5Hz), and a short-lived incremental response at high-frequency stimulation (50Hz) or after brief exercise. An increment of 100 per cent has traditionally been used as the gold standard for the diagnosis of LEMS and is very specific. However, a lower increment of 60 per cent has been shown to have a sensitivity of 97 per cent for the diagnosis of LEMS and a specificity of 99 per cent in excluding MG [20], although other disorders that affect presynaptic neuromuscular transmission, such as botulism, can give similar findings.

Single-fibre EMG is generally also abnormal in LEMS with increased jitter and block. However, this finding is not specific and does not help distinguish LEMS from MG.

In mild cases of LEMS the electrical findings can resemble those of MG with normal amplitude, decrement at low rates of repetitive stimulation, and little facilitation [21].

Serology

Antibodies to P/Q-type VGCCs are detected in approximately 90 per cent of patients with LEMS and are seen in close to 100 per cent of patients with LEMS and SCLC [22, 23].

Antibodies to N-type VGCC have been found in up to 33 per cent of LEMS patients, but these patients also had antibodies against P/Q channels [23]. The pathogenicity of antibodies in LEMS has been established by passive transfer experiments in mice [24–26]. LEMS antibodies have also been shown to reduce calcium currents through P/Q-type VGCCs in SCLC cells and motor neurons [27, 28].

However, antibodies against P/Q-type VGCC are not exclusive for LEMS. Up to 3–5 per cent of patients with SCLC who do not have clinical or electrophysiological features of LEMS may have positive antibodies [29]. In particular, patients with

Clinical tip Seronegativity in LEMS

Approximately 10–15 per cent of patients with LEMS are seronegative and so the absence of detectable antibodies does not exclude LEMS. The clinical phenotype of these patients is similar to that of seropositive patients with the exception that SCLC is less common [31].

paraneoplastic cerebellar degeneration in association with SCLC may have positive LEMS serology in the absence of clinical evidence of neuromuscular junction dysfunction. VGCC antibodies have occasionally been described in pure cerebellar ataxia [30].

Screening for neoplasia

A diagnosis of LEMS should spark a thorough and systematic search for an underlying neoplasm as 50–60 per cent of cases are paraneoplastic; the most common malignancy associated with LEMS is SCLC [7, 8]. LEMS represents the most common paraneoplastic manifestation of SCLC and occurs in up to 1–3 per cent of patients with this tumour [32]. However, other tumours, including non-small-cell lung cancers, as well as breast, bladder, renal, and lymphproliferative malignancies, have all been reported in association with LEMS [32]. The neurological disorder generally presents before the underlying malignancy, and the tumour may not be detectable initially.

Screening by chest radiograph in insufficient to exclude a lung malignancy, and patients require CT and FDG-PET scans, and often bronchoscopy as well. If the initial search is negative, investigations should be repeated. However, most malignancies are detected within 12 months and discovery of a tumour after 24 months is very unusual [32].

There are certain clinical clues, such as associated cerebellar ataxia, the presence of other paraneoplastic antibodies, and a fast progression of neurological symptoms, that may suggest the presence of an underlying tumour [32]. Antibodies against SOX 1 protein have also been shown to represent a serological marker of SCLC in LEMS patients, with 95 per cent specificity and 65 per cent sensitivity [33].

Clinical tip Screening for small-cell lung cancer

Data from two national cohorts of LEMS patients were recently used to develop a screening score—the DELTA-P score for predicting the presence of an underlying SLCC in LEMS patients (see Table 14.3).

The DELTA P score is calculated as a sum score according to the different categories and ranges from 0 to 6. A score of 0–1 corresponds to a chance of SLCC below 3 per cent, whereas scores of 4 or more correspond to a probability of SCLC above 90 per cent [34]. It is recommended that all newly diagnosed patients undergo a thoracic CT and, if this is normal, an FDG-PET. If this is also normal, the DELTA-P score is calculated and further screening is dictated by this. (see Figure 14.2).

Table 14.3 The DELTA-P score

		Score
	<3 months since symptom onset	
D	Dysarthria, dysphagia, bulbar and neck weakenss	1
E	Erectile dysfunction	1
L	Loss of weight >5%	1
T	Tobacco use at onset	1
A	Age of onset >50 years	1
P	Karnofsky Performance score <60 (patients need at least some assistance with activities of daily living)	1

Reproduced from *Lancet Neurol* 10(12), Titulaer MJ, Lang B, Verschuuren JJ, Lambert-Eaton myasthenic syndrome: from clinical characteristics to therapeutic strategies, pp. 1098–1107, © 2011, with permission from Elsevier.

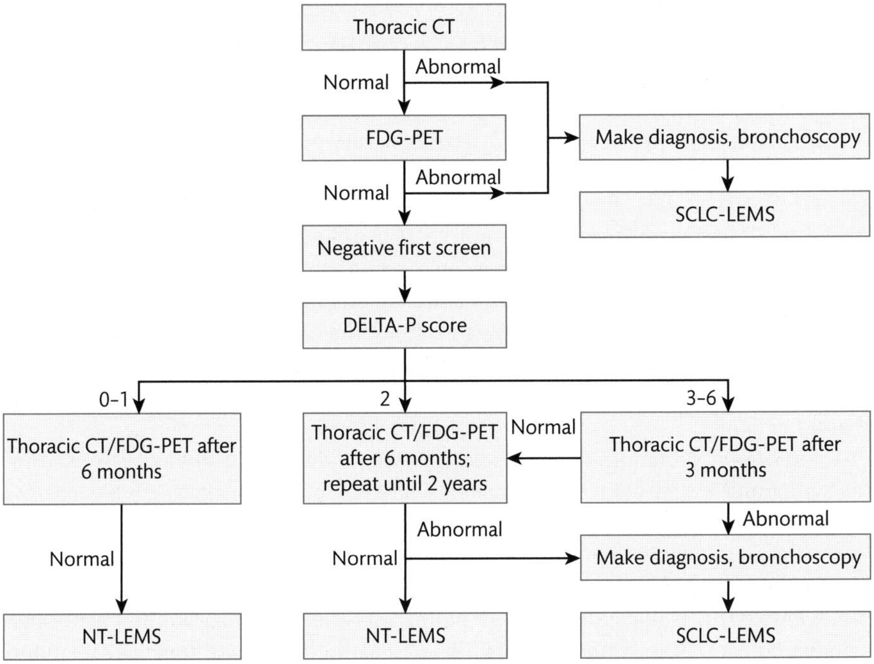

Figure 14.2 Flowchart of recommended screening of SCLC in patients with LEMS.

Reproduced from *Lancet Neurol* 10(12), Titulaer MJ, Lang B, Verschuuren JJ, Lambert–Eaton myasthenic syndrome: from clinical characteristics to therapeutic strategies, pp. 1098–1107, © 2011, with permission from Elsevier.

Treatment

Treatment of tumour

The treatment of LEMS depends on the presence of an underlying tumour. If SCLC is present, treatment must be directed toward this. The neurological symptoms have been shown improve if the malignancy that caused the syndrome is treated [35]. SCLC treatment typically involves combination chemotherapy, such as cisplatin and etoposide, rather than surgery. Anthracycline-based regimens with cyclophosphamide, doxorubicin, and vincristine have also been widely used [36]. Occasionally, patients are also treated with radiotherapy.

Interestingly, there are reports that patients with paraneoplastic LEMS hav
improved tumour prognosis compared with patients with a malignancy but
the neurological deficit. Preliminary results of an ongoing prospective st
that antibody-positive SCLC patients with LEMS have a longer mediar
patients without LEMS [37]. However, larger numbers of patients are
roborate this finding.

Symptomatic treatment

Symptomatic treatment for LEMS includes drugs that prolong the ne
action potential and so increase acetylcholine release at the neuromu
tion. The potassium channel blocker fampridine (4-aminopyridine) has
in LEMS, but its use is limited by central nervous system effects as it rea
the blood–brain barrier [38].

3,4 Diaminopyridine (3,4-DAP) is used more widely and is the first -line symptomatic treatment as recommended by the Task Force of the European Federation of Neurological Societies (EFNS) for both paraneoplastic and non-paraneoplastic LEMS [6]. There have been four double-blind randomized controlled trials investigating the effectiveness of 3,4-DAP in LEMS in 54 patients, and the evidence for its use was recently reviewed in a Cochrane database systematic review [39–42]. 3,4-DAP was shown to result in a significant improvement in muscle strength, CMAP amplitude, Quantitative Myasthenia Score (QMG), LEMS classification, and subjective symptom score compared with placebo. Peri-oral paraesthesia is a frequent but often transient side effect. At high doses, 3,4-DAP can cause seizures and it is contraindicated in patients with epilepsy. Prolongation of the QT interval is also occasionally mentioned as a side effect, and clinical and electrographic monitoring is recommended at initiation of the drug and yearly thereafter [43].

Guanidine hydrochloride also blocks potassium channels and has been used for the symptomatic treatment of LEMS [36]. Severe side effects, including bone marrow suppression, renal tubular acidosis, chronic interstitial nephritis, cardiac arrhythmias, and liver toxicity, have precluded its widespread use [21]. A small open-label study outlined the use of low-dose guanidine in combination with pyridostigmine in nine LEMS patients [44]. Although guanidine was effective in controlling neurological symptoms, a third of the patients discontinued it because of severe gastrointestinal side effects. It is not licensed in the UK.

Pyridostigmine, which is the main symptomatic treatment for MG, has been shown to be no more effective than placebo when prescribed in isolation in LEMS, and confers no additional benefit when prescribed with 3,4-DAP [41].

Immunomodulatory treatment

If, 3,4-DAP satisfactorily controls symptoms, no further treatment may be needed. However, immunomodulatory therapy may be required if symptoms do not respond to symptomatic therapy. Prednisolone and azathioprine are the most frequently used immunomodulatory agents and were prescribed in combination in 70 per cent of patients with autoimmune LEMS in one series [45]. Although this combination was effective in a retrospective study, these agents have not been tested in prospective randomized controlled clinical trials [46]. The rationale for the use of azathioprine as a steroid-sparing agent is extrapolated from evidence in MG, where it reduces the number of treatment failures and allows lower steroid doses to be used than in treatment with prednisolone alone [47]. Successful use of rituximab has also been reported in a small number of LEMS patients with severe weakness [48, 49]. There is one case report describing the use of ciclosporin in LEMS that was associated with a resolution of symptoms [50].

Plasma exchange and intravenous immunoglobulin (IVIG) are reserved for acute treatment of severe weakness. Plasma exchange showed a short-term clinical and electromyographic benefit in a small group of paraneoplastic and non-paraneoplastic LEMS patients [51]. The clinical benefits may not be seen for up to 10 days, longer than is typical in MG [52]. A randomized double-blind placebo-controlled crossover trial showed that IVIG resulted in significant improvement in muscle strength and a decline in VGCC antibody titres [53]. The benefit peaked at 2–4 weeks and declined by 8 weeks. Other data regarding the benefit of IVIG are scant, but case reports have suggested that it is beneficial [54, 55].

Final word from the expert

This case illustrates the diagnostic difficulties when a patient presents with generalized weakness and type II respiratory failure. Proximal weakness can be attributed to numerous causes other than a neuromuscular junction defect, and although the deep tendon reflexes are not documented at presentation in this case, areflexia can also be dismissed or attributed to critical care neuromyopathy. The demonstration of an increase in MAP following tetanic stimulation or forced maximal contraction was a clue to the diagnosis of LEMS, although this too may be missed because it is not part of a routine EMG. It is thought to result from a gradual accumulation of presynaptic calcium ions, which allow more acetylcholine vesicles to be released, overcoming the threshold for post-synaptic action potential initiation. 3,4-DAP also increases presynaptic calcium entry by blocking potassium channels and thereby broadening the presynaptic action potential. This patient was found to have a small-cell lung cancer, and responded to immunosuppression. The suggestion that antibodies against presynaptic P/Q-type calcium channels have an anti-tumour role remains speculative, and should not hold back immunosuppressive treatment if 3,4-DAP is insufficient.

References

1. Dhand UK. Clinical approach to the weak patient in the intensive care unit. *Respir Care* 2006; 51(9): 1024–1040.
2. Gorson KC. Approach to neuromuscular disorders in the intensive care unit. *Neurocrit Care* 2005; 3(3): 195–212.
3. Hutchinson D, Whyte K. Neuromuscular disease and respiratory failure. *Pract Neurol* 2008; 8(4): 229–37.
4. Lacomis D, Petrella JT, Giuliani MJ. Causes of neuromuscular weakness in the intensive care unit: a study of ninety-two patients. *Muscle Nerve* 1998; 21(5): 610–17.
5. Eaton LM, Lambert EH. Electromyography and electric stimulation of nerves in diseases of motor unit: observations on myasthenic syndrome associated with malignant tumors. *JAMA* 1957; 163(13):1117–24.
6. Titulaer MJ, Lang B, Verschuuren JJ. Lambert–Eaton myasthenic syndrome: from clinical characteristics to therapeutic strategies. *Lancet Neurol* 2011; 10(12): 1098–1107.
7. Titulaer MJ, Wirtz PW, Kuks JBM, et al. The Lambert–Eaton myasthenic syndrome 1988–2008: a clinical picture in 97 patients. *J Neroimmunol* 2008; 201–2: 153–8.
8. O'Neill JH, Murray NM, Newsom-Davis J. The Lambert–Eaton myasthenic syndrome: a review of 50 cases. *Brain* 1988; 111(Pt 3): 577–96.
9. Wirtz PW, Smallegange TM, Wintzen AR, Verschuuren JJ. Differences in clinical features between the Lambert–Eaton myasthenic syndrome with and without cancer: an analysis of 227 published cases. *Clin Neurol Neurosurg* 2002; 104(4): 359–63.
10. Wirtz PW, Nijnuis MG, Sotodeh M, et al. The epidemiology of myasthenia gravis, Lambert–Eaton myasthenic syndrome and their associated tumours in the northern part of the province of South Holland. *J Neurol* 2003; 250(6): 698–701.
11. Titulaer MJ, Verschuuren JJGM. Lambert–Eaton myasthenic syndrome: tumor versus nontumor forms. *Ann NY Acad Sci* 2008; 1132: 129–34.
12. Wirtz PW, Wintzen AR, Verschuuren JJ. Lambert–Eaton myasthenic syndrome has a more progressive course in patients with lung cancer. *Muscle Nerve* 2005; 32(2): 226–9.
13. Smith AG, Wald J. Acute ventilatory failure in Lambert–Eaton myasthenic syndrome and its response to 3,4-diaminopyridine. *Neurology* 1996; 46(4): 1143–5.

14. Sanders DB, Kim YI, Howard JF Jr, Goetsch CA. Eaton–Lambert syndrome: a clinical and electrophysiological study of a patient treated with 4-aminopyridine. *J Neurol Neurosurg. Psychiatry* 1980; 43(11): 978–85.
15. Gracey DR, Southorn PA. Respiratory failure in Lambert–Eaton myasthenic syndrome. *Chest* 1987; 91(5): 716–18.
16. Waterman SA. Autonomic dysfunction in Lambert–Eaton myasthenic syndrome. *Clin Auton Res* 2001; 11(3): 145–54.
17. O'Suilleabhain P, Low PA, Lennon VA. Autonomic dysfunction in the Lambert–Eaton myasthenic syndrome: serologic and clinical correlates. *Neurology* 1998; 50(1): 88–93.
18. Odabasi Z, Demirci M, Kim DS, et al. Postexercise facilitation of reflexes is not common in Lambert-Eaton myasthenic syndrome. *Neurology* 2002; 59(7): 1085–7.
19. Pellkofer HL, Armbruster L, Krumbholz M, et al. Lambert–Eaton myasthenic syndrome differential reactivity of tumor versus non-tumor patients to subunits of the voltage-gated calcium channel. *J Neuroimmunol* 2008; 204(1-2): 136–9.
20. Oh SJ, Kurokawa K, Claussen GC, Ryan HF. Electrophysiological diagnostic criteria of Lambert-Eaton myasthenic syndrome. *Muscle Nerve* 2005; 32(4): 515–20.
21. Sanders DB. Lambert–Eaton myasthenic syndrome: diagnosis and treatment. *Ann NY Acad Sci* 2003; 998: 500–8.
22. Lennon VA, Kryzer TJ, Griesmann GE, et al. Calcium-channel antibodies in the Lambert–Eaton syndrome and other paraneoplastic syndromes. *N Engl J Med* 1995; 332(22): 1467–74.
23. Motomura M, Lang B, Johnston I, et al. Incidence of serum anti-P/O-type and anti-N-type calcium channel autoantibodies in the Lambert–Eaton myasthenic syndrome. *J Neurol Sci* 1997; 147(1): 35–42.
24. Lang B, Molenaar PC, Newsom-Davis J, Vincent A. Passive transfer of Lambert–Eaton myasthenic syndrome in mice: decreased rates of resting and evoked release of acetylcholine from skeletal muscle. *J Neurochem* 1984; 42(3): 658–62.
25. Lang B, Newsom-Davis J, Prior C, Wray D. Antibodies to motor nerve terminals: an electrophysiological study of a human myasthenic syndrome transferred to mouse. *J Physiol* 1983; 344: 335–45.
26. Fukunaga H, Engel AG, Lang B, et al. Passive transfer of Lambert–Eaton myasthenic syndrome with IgG from man to mouse depletes the presynaptic membrane active zones. *Proc Natl Acad Sci USA*, 1983; 80(24): 7636–40.
27. Roberts A, Perera S, Lang B, et al. Paraneoplastic myasthenic syndrome IgG inhibits 45Ca2+ flux in a human small cell carcinoma line. *Nature* 1985; 317(6039): 737–9.
28. García KD, Beam KG. Reduction of calcium currents by Lambert–Eaton syndrome sera: motoneurons are preferentially affected, and L-type currents are spared. *J Neurosci* 1996; 16(16): 4903–13.
29. Titulaer MJ, Klooster R, Potman M, et al. SOX antibodies in small-cell lung cancer and Lambert–Eaton myasthenic syndrome: frequency and relation with survival. *J Clin Oncol* 2009; 27(26): 4260–7.
30. Gilhus NE. Lambert–Eaton myasthenic syndrome: pathogenesis, diagnosis, and therapy. *Autoimmune Dis* 2011; 2011: 973808.
31. Nakao YK, Motomura M, Fukudome T, et al. Seronegative Lambert–Eaton myasthenic syndrome: study of 110 Japanese patients. *Neurology* 2002; 59(11): 1773–5.
32. Titulaer MJ, Wirtz PW, Willems LNA, Vet al. Screening for small-cell lung cancer: a follow-up study of patients with Lambert–Eaton myasthenic syndrome. *J Clin Oncol* 2008; 26(26):4276–81.
33. Sabater L, Titulaer M, Saiz A, et al. SOX1 antibodies are markers of paraneoplastic Lambert–Eaton myasthenic syndrome. *Neurology* 2008; 70(12): 924–8.
34. Titulaer MJ, Maddison P, Sont JK, et al. Clinical Dutch–English Lambert–Eaton myasthenic syndrome (LEMS) tumor association prediction score accurately predicts small-cell lung cancer in the LEMS. *J Clin Oncol* 2011; 29(7): 902–8.

35. Chalk CH, Murray NM, Newsom-Davis J, et al. Response of the Lambert–Eaton myasthenic syndrome to treatment of associated small-cell lung carcinoma. *Neurology* 1990; 40(10): 1552–6.
36. Verschuuren JJGM, Wirtz PW, Titulaer MJ, et al. Available treatment options for the management of Lambert–Eaton myasthenic syndrome. *Expert Opin Pharmacother* 2006; 7(10): 1323–36.
37. Maddison P, Lang B. Paraneoplastic neurological autoimmunity and survival in small-cell lung cancer. *J Neroimmunol* 2008; 201–2: 159–62.
38. Keogh M, Sedehizadeh S, Maddison P. Treatment for Lambert–Eaton myasthenic syndrome. Cochrane Database Syst Rev. 2011; 2: CD003279.
39. McEvoy KM, Windebank AJ, Daube JR, Low PA. 3,4-Diaminopyridine in the treatment of Lambert–Eaton myasthenic syndrome. *N Engl J Med* 1989; 321(23): 1567–71.
40. Sanders DB, Massey JM, Sanders LL, Edwards LJ. A randomized trial of 3,4-diaminopyridine in Lambert–Eaton myasthenic syndrome. *Neurology* 2000; 54(3): 603–7.
41. Wirtz PW, Verschuuren JJ, Van Dijk JG, et al. Efficacy of 3,4-diaminopyridine and pyridostigmine in the treatment of Lambert–Eaton myasthenic syndrome: a randomized, double-blind, placebo-controlled, crossover study. *Clin Pharmacol Ther* 2009; 86(1): 44–8.
42. Oh SJ, Claussen GG, Hatanaka Y, Morgan MB. 3,4-Diaminopyridine is more effective than placebo in a randomized, double-blind, cross-over drug study in LEMS. *Muscle Nerve* 2009; 40(5): 795–800.
43. Lindquist S, Stangel M. Update on treatment options for Lambert–Eaton myasthenic syndrome: focus on use of amifampridine. *NeuroPsychiatr Dis Treat* 2011; 7: 341–9.
44. Oh SJ, Kim DS, Head TC, Claussen GC. Low-dose guanidine and pyridostigmine: relatively safe and effective long-term symptomatic therapy in Lambert–Eaton myasthenic syndrome. *Muscle Nerve* 1997; 20(9): 1146–52.
45. Maddison P, Lang B, Mills K, Newsom-Davis J. Long term outcome in Lambert–Eaton myasthenic syndrome without lung cancer. *J Neurol Neurosurg Psychiatry* 2001; 70(2): 212–17.
46. Newsom-Davis J, Murray NM. Plasma exchange and immunosuppressive drug treatment in the Lambert–Eaton myasthenic syndrome. *Neurology* 1984; 34(4): 480–5.
47. Palace J, Newsom-Davis J, Lecky B. A randomized double-blind trial of prednisolone alone or with azathioprine in myasthenia gravis. Myasthenia Gravis Study Group. *Neurology* 1998; 50(6): 1778–83.
48. Maddison P, McConville J, Farrugia ME, et al. The use of rituximab in myasthenia gravis and Lambert–Eaton myasthenic syndrome. *J Neurol Neurosurg Psychiatr* 2011; 82(6): 671–3.
49. Pellkofer HL, Voltz R, Kuempfel T. Favorable response to rituximab in a patient with anti-VGCC-positive Lambert–Eaton myasthenic syndrome and cerebellar dysfunction. *Muscle Nerve* 2009; 40(2): 305–8.
50. Yuste Ara JR, Beloqui Ruiz O, Artieda Gonzalez-Granda J, et al. [Cyclosporin A in the treatment of Eaton–Lambert myasthenic syndrome]. *An Med Interna* 1996; 13(1): 25–6 (in Spanish).
51. Newsom-Davis J, Murray NM. Plasma exchange and immunosuppressive drug treatment in the Lambert–Eaton myasthenic syndrome. *Neurology* 1984; 34(4): 480–5.
52. Newsom-Davis J. A treatment algorithm for Lambert–Eaton myasthenic syndrome. *Ann NY Acad Sci* 1998; 841: 817–22.
53. Bain PG, Motomura M, Newsom-Davis J, et al. Effects of intravenous immunoglobulin on muscle weakness and calcium-channel autoantibodies in the Lambert–Eaton myasthenic syndrome. *Neurology* 1996; 47(3): 678–83.
54. Bird SJ. Clinical and electrophysiologic improvement in Lambert–Eaton syndrome with intravenous immunoglobulin therapy. *Neurology* 1992; 42(7): 1422–3.
55. Takano H, Tanaka M, Koike R, et al. Effect of intravenous immunoglobulin in Lambert–Eaton myasthenic syndrome with small-cell lung cancer: correlation with the titer of anti-voltage-gated calcium channel antibody. *Muscle Nerve* 1994; 17(9): 1073–5.

CASE

15 Paroxysmal sensory and motor events

Ross W. Paterson

Expert commentary: Laszlo K. Sztriha

Case history

A 74-year-old woman presented with an episode of tingling and numbness and loss of function of her arm that lasted approximately 15 minutes. She was an ex-smoker (40 pack-years) and had been diagnosed with, and treated for, hypertension and hyperlipidaemia in her fifties.

This patient was suspected to have had a transient ischaemic attack (TIA), and was referred to the rapid access neurovascular clinic.

Expert comment

A TIA is traditionally defined as a sudden-onset focal neurological deficit of presumed vascular origin, lasting less than 24 hours [1] This duration is somewhat arbitrary, especially as most events resolve in less than an hour. Interestingly, many also have evidence of infarction on brain imaging. Instead of the traditional 'time-based' description, the American Stroke Association have proposed the use of a 'tissue-based' definition, identifying TIA as a transient episode of neurological dysfunction caused by focal ischaemia without acute infarction [2]. This obviously requires early brain imaging, preferably an MRI scan with diffusion-weighted imaging (DWI). In practice, however, investigations and management will be broadly similar regardless of how quickly or slowly recovery occurs and whether or not there is evidence of brain injury on imaging.

Learning point Risk of stroke after TIA

A TIA is frequently followed by a stroke, and the ABCD2 score (Table 15.1) is a helpful clinical tool for estimating this risk and guiding the urgency of specialist assessment. The Royal College of Physicians National Clinical Guideline for Stroke recommends that suspected TIA patients with an ABCD2 score of 4 or above should receive specialist assessment and investigation within 24 hours of onset of symptoms, whereas those with a score of 3 or below should be seen and investigated as soon as possible, but definitely within a week [3]. In addition to clinical parameters, imaging is also helpful for the assessment of stroke risk in patients with rapidly resolving symptoms. The presence of acute infarction, stenosis, or occlusion of a cerebral vessel may indicate a higher risk of subsequent stroke[4]. Table 15.2 provides an approach for the investigation of TIA patients, and Table 15.3 lists common treatment options.

Clinical tip Diffusion-weighted imaging

Diffusion-weighted imaging (DWI) is a form of MRI that measures the random motion of water. Cytotoxic oedema in acute ischaemia results in decreased diffusivity of water—this appears bright on the DWI and dark on the apparent diffusion coefficient (ADC) map. DWI will become positive as little as a few minutes after onset of ischaemia, and may remain positive for 7–14 days. Tissue with

(Continued)

increased water content, such as an old brain infarct, may produce an area of brightness on DWI known as 'T2 shine-through'; however, the ADC map will correctly separate the acute lesion (lower intensity) from the old infarct (higher intensity).

Other pathology that may have a high DWI signal includes severe hypoglycaemia, status epilepticus, active multiple sclerosis plaque, brain abscess, or prion disease (typically causing cortical brightness known as 'cortical ribboning').

Table 15.1 The ABCD2 score and associated risk of stroke

Symbol	Parameter	Criterion	Score
A	Age	≥60 years	1
B	Blood pressure	≥140mmHg systolic or ≥90mmHg diastolic	1
C	Clinical presentations	Unilateral weakness	2
		Speech disturbance without weakness	1
D1	Duration of symptoms	≥60min	2
		10–59min	1
D2	Diabetes	Diagnosis of diabetes	1
Total			0–7

	Risk of stroke (per cent)		
Total score	2 days	7 days	90 days
0–3	1.0	1.2	3.1
4–5	4.1	5.9	9.8
6–7	8.1	11.7	17.8

Reproduced from *Lancet* 369(9558), Johnston SC, Rothwell PM, Nguyen-Huynh MN, et al., Validation and refinement of scores to predict very early stroke risk after transient ischaemic attack, pp. 283–92, © 2007, with permission from Elsevier

Table 15.2 Investigations for transient ischaemic attack [2]

Investigation	First line	Second line
Brain imaging	MRI	CT
Vascular imaging	Carotid ultrasound	MRA, CTA, DSA, TCD
Cardiac tests	ECG	24-hour tape, TTE, TOE, bubble study
Laboratory tests	FBC, U&E, ESR, glucose, lipids, coagulation	Thrombophilia, autoimmune, homocysteine, haemoglobin electrophoresis, CSF analysis, genetic testing (e.g. CADASIL, Fabry's disease)

MRA, magnetic resonance angiography; CTA, CT angiography; DSA, digital subtraction angiography; TCD, transcranial Doppler; TTE, trans-thoracic echocardiography; TOE, trans-oesophageal echocardiography; CSF, cerebrospinal fluid; CADASIL, cerebral autosomal-dominant arteriopathy with subcortical infarcts and leucoencephalopathy.

Data from Warlow CP, Dennis MS, Wardlaw JM, et al., *Stroke: Practical Management* (3rd edn), © 2008, with permission from John Wiley & Sons; *Stroke* 40(6), Easton JD, Saver JL, Albers GW, et al., AHA/ASA Scientific Statement. Definition and evaluation of transient ischemic attack, pp. 2276–93, © 2009, with permission from Wolters Kluwer Health, Inc.

When seen in the neurovascular clinic this patient had a blood pressure of 150/100mmHg. Her ABCD2 score was calculated as 5. She received a brain CT scan which was normal. A carotid Doppler test did not reveal any plaques or significant stenosis, and an ECG showed sinus rhythm. Fasting blood glucose and lipids were not elevated. She was started on aspirin with a loading dose of 300mg and continued on a daily dose of 75mg. She continued to take simvastatin 40mg.

The patient returned to the emergency department two days later having experienced repeated 'turns'. The events were stereotyped, starting with altered sensory

Table 15.3 Management of TIA

Lifestyle	Smoking cessation, regular exercise, weight control, healthy diet, alcohol consumption within safe limits
Blood pressure lowering	ACE inhibitor, angiotensin II receptor blocker, diuretic, calcium-channel blocker
Lipid lowering	Statin
Antiplatelet therapy	Clopidogrel, aspirin plus modified-release dipyridamole, aspirin monotherapy
Carotid stenosis (50–99%)	Carotid endarterectomy, carotid stenting
Atrial fibrillation	LMWH, warfarin, apixaban, dabigatran, rivaroxaban, device occlusion of left atrial appendage

LMWH, low molecular weight heparin.

Data from *National Clinical Guideline for Stroke* (4th edn), Intercollegiate Stroke Working Party, 2012, © 2012, Royal College of Physicians; *N Engl J Med* 366(20), Davis SM, Donnan GA., Clinical practice: secondary prevention after ischemic stroke or transient ischemic attack, © 2012, with permission from Massachusetts Medical Society; *Stroke* 42(1), Furie KL, Kasner SE, Adams RJ, et al., Guidelines for the prevention of stroke in patients with stroke or transient ischemic attack: a guideline for healthcare professionals from the American Heart Association/American Stroke Association, pp. 227–76, © 2011, with permission from Wolters Kluwer Health, Inc.

perception of the hand or foot, described as 'tingling', that spread slowly (over minutes) to involve contiguous body parts until the left face, arm, and leg were involved. The patient reported no loss of awareness of her surroundings, although her son reported her speech to be 'mumbling' during attacks. After 15–20 minutes she would return quite quickly to feeling normal.

Discussion

Given the repeated, stereotyped nature of the attacks, does the differential diagnosis change?

Yes. It is still possible for transient ischaemic attacks to cause repeated and stereotyped events, but this scenario is relatively rare. One possible vascular cause is the 'capsular warning syndrome', a rare cause of repeated stereotyped motor, sensory, or sensorimotor symptoms probably as a result of transient ischaemia of the internal capsule due to angiopathy of the lenticulostriate arteries. The risk of subsequent stroke is high: 42–60 per cent of patients develop a completed stroke within seven days [5, 6]. Attacks typically increase in duration and severity with time [5] and may be perfusion-dependent and therefore susceptible to fluctuations in blood pressure. Conversely, recurrent TIAs caused by non-small vessel disease pathology carry no greater risk of stroke than single TIAs [6]. However, a history of repeated events calls for the differential diagnosis to be revised and for other non-vascular aetiologies to be considered. A detailed history/collateral history will help to differentiate other causes (summarized in Table 15.4).

The time taken for symptoms to evolve and the pattern of evolution can be diagnostically helpful. In this case, sensory symptoms spread slowly, over minutes, between contiguous body parts. Usually the onset of ischaemic stroke is abrupt. Seizures arising from the somatosensory cortex may spread over minutes, as epileptic discharges spread, but most seizures evolve more rapidly. The aura of migraine characteristically spreads slowly, over at least five minutes (IHCD-II).

The nature of symptoms can be helpful: positive symptoms (an excess of function, such as paraesthesia or visual aura) are more likely in epilepsy, migraine, or

Table 15.4 Features of the history and examination that differentiate TIA from other transient neurological events

	Transient ischaemic attack	Migraine aura	Seizure	Functional	Metabolic encephalopathy	Transient aura attack
Prodrome	None	1. Premonitory phase hours/days before 2. Aura: focal neurological phenomena (Sensory aura of the mouth and arm is second most frequently reported symptom of migraine after visual aura)	Frequently, type of aura depends on localization of seizure onset	No prodrome per se, but psychosocial stressors may precipitate an event	Non-specific; anxiety, restlessness; personality change; drowsiness	No
Onset	Over seconds	Over minutes, rarely sudden	Over seconds	Variable	Insidious	Over seconds to minutes
Evolution	Localization of deficit rarely alters significantly	Followed by headache in 60–70% cases. 'Acephalgic' aura more common with increasing age	Typically over 1–2 minutes	Variable and often inconsistent	Relapsing and remitting course	Over minutes
Loss of awareness	No	No. Basilar migraine may be an exception	Yes, if dialeptic seizure	No, but disproportionate lack of concern or *la belle indifference* supports diagnosis	Yes	Possibly
Duration	Less than 24 hours; typically less than 30 minutes	Typically 5–60 minutes	1–5 minutes	Variable	Variable but often hours to days	5–60 minutes
Frequency	Isolated event	May be frequent, repeated, and stereotyped	Variable	Variable	Variable	May be frequent, repeated, and stereotyped

Adapted from *Pract Neurol* 14(1), Nadarajan V, Perry RJ, Johnson J, Werring DJ, Transient ischaemic attacks: mimics and chameleons, pp. 23–31, © 2014, reproduced under the Creative Commons Attribution License 3.0; *Cephalalgia* 33(7), Viana M, Sprenger T, Andelova M, Goadsby PJ, The typical duration of migraine aura: a systematic review, pp. 483–90, © 2013, with permission from SAGE Publications.

transient aura attack, whereas TIAs are more commonly characterized by negative symptoms at onset (a loss of function, such as numbness or weakness [7].

Learning point Stereotyped TIAs

TIAs occurring as a consequence of penetrating or branch artery disease are more stereotyped than in other ischaemic aetiologies, and may occur many times during the day. The occurrence of repeated episodes of hemiplegia preceding a pure motor stroke was labelled the 'capsular warning syndrome', but this can occur in subcortical lesions in other areas and in the brainstem and is not limited to the internal capsule [8]. The capsular warning syndrome is rare (1.5 per cent of TIA presentations) but has a poor prognosis with a seven-day stroke risk of up to 60 per cent [6].

Expert comment

In addition to discussing TIA mimics it is worth remembering that there are rare situations where TIAs may look like something else. These TIA 'chameleons' include limb-shaking TIA, which always spares the face and is caused by brain hypoperfusion due to a critical stenosis of the carotid or middle cerebral artery. These, as well as the convulsive-like movements sometimes seen in brainstem ischaemia, may resemble a seizure. Altered level of consciousness is not characteristic of a TIA; however, it may rarely arise with transient ischaemia of the thalami or brainstem. Headache is not impossible with brain ischaemia, and is more likely to be seen in younger females and those with posterior circulation involvement or a previous history of migraine; these vascular events may potentially be misinterpreted as migraine.

Clinical tip Investigating recurrent stereotyped attacks

- **EEG** Can be used to 'rule in' rather than 'rule out' a diagnosis of epilepsy if an ictal or interictal EEG demonstrates evidence of epileptiform activity.
- **Vascular imaging** A CT or MR angiogram may help to identify cerebral large-vessel pathology but it is rarely useful in diagnosing small-vessel disease. Rarely, angiography can be used to detect evidence of vasculitis as a cause of capsular warning syndrome.

Structural imaging

In this situation an MRI scan would allow:

- detection of a structural lesion that could give rise to epilepsy
- detection of 'old' strokes, particularly lacunar infarcts, or evidence of leucoaraiosis, which might demonstrate evidence of small-vessel pathology
- Detection of a convexity subarachnoid haemorrhage or cortical superficial siderosis as a cause of transient aura attacks.

In this case the patient's susceptibility-weighted imaging (SWI) showed superficial cortical siderosis (Figure 15.1).

Learning point Susceptibility-weighted imaging

Susceptibility-weighted imaging (SWI) is a unique gradient echo MRI tool that is exquisitely sensitive to venous blood, haemorrhage, and iron deposition. SWI is sensitive for detecting microhaemorrhages (small punctate hypointensities usually less than 5mm), superficial cortical siderosis, and focal subarachnoid haemorrhage, some of the radiological features that can help to support a diagnosis of cerebral amyloid angiopathy.

Clinical tip Microhaemorrhages on MRI

There are two commonly used MRI tools to detect microhaemorrhage: the T2*-weighted gradient-recalled echo (GRE) technique and susceptibility-weighted imaging (SWI), which is a variant of T2*-weighted MRI that includes phase information. Microhaemorrhages appear as small (<5mm) hypointense (dark) rounded lesions. They can easily be mistaken for normal blood vessels ('vascular flow voids') or cerebral cavernous malformations [9]. Microhaemorrhages appear much larger on the scan than their actual size (which can be<1mm) because of the 'blooming effect' of the MRI signal at the border of these lesions.

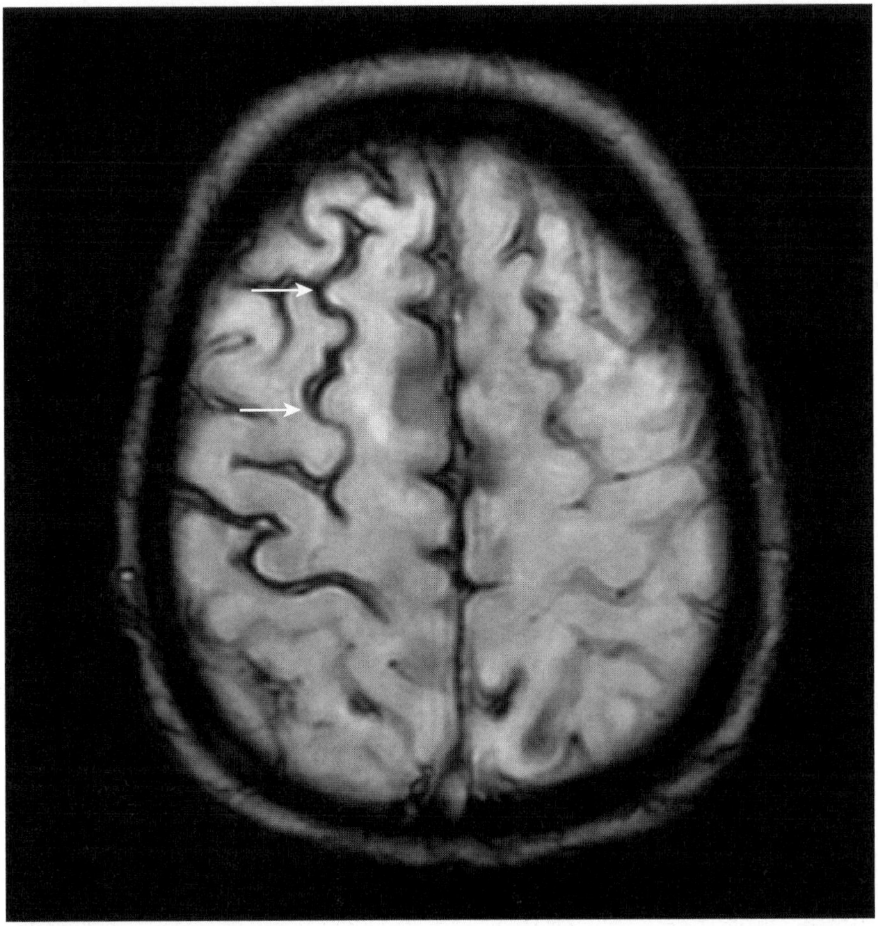

Figure 15.1 MRI SWI demonstrating an area of superficial siderosis.

The clinical history of slowly evolving positive sensory symptoms taken together with these MRI findings led the treating neurologist to make a diagnosis of **transient aura attacks** (TAA)[10], also known as **amyloid spells** [11], due to cerebral amyloid angiopathy.

Learning point Cerebral amyloid angiopathy as a cause of transient aura attacks

- Cerebral amyloid angiopathy (CAA) is a post-mortem diagnosis but the probability can be predicted during life using the Boston criteria [12].
- CAA is characterized pathologically by an accumulation of beta-amyloid 40 within the adventitia of small and mid-sized blood vessels (as opposed to extracellular beta-amyloid 42 found in the senile plaques of Alzheimer's disease [13].
- The prevalence of transient aura attacks due to CAA is unknown as there are no population-based studies
- The pathophysiology of transient aura attacks is unknown, but they are more likely to occur in brain areas where there is evidence of superficial siderosis or focal subarachnoid haemorrhage [14].
- Positive or negative sensory or visual symptoms may occur, and multiple stereotyped episodes are common. [15]
- The risk of symptomatic lobar haemorrhage after transient focal neurological episodes is high—approximately 50 per cent within 1 year[15].
- The pathophysiology of microhaemorrhage formation is unclear, but microhaemorrhages are more likely to occur in areas of the brain with radiological evidence of amyloid deposition [16].
- The presence of lobar microbleeds is associated with an increased risk of future intracerebral haemorrhage as well as ischaemic stroke. The prevalence of microbleeds in subjects with spontaneous intracerebral haemorrhage is 68 per cent [17].

Expert comment

Transient aura attack is not the only clinical manifestation of cerebral amyloid angiopathy. The clinical spectrum also includes symptomatic intracerebral haemorrhage, cognitive impairment/dementia, and rarely a rapidly progressive cognitive and neurological decline caused by inflammation (amyloid angiitis). The most important neuroimaging (MRI) correlates of cerebral amyloid angiopathy include cerebral microbleeds (GRE/SWI), leucoaraiosis (T2/FLAIR), convexity subarachnoid haemorrhage (GRE/SWI), cortical superficial siderosis (GRE/SWI), and microinfarcts (DWI).

Clinical tip Probability of cerebral amyloid angiopathy

The Boston Criteria (shown below) can be useful for determining the probability of CAA. However, in practice it is rarely justified for patients to have a pathological examination during life.

- Definite cerebral amyloid angiopathy:
  - full post-mortem examination reveals lobar, cortical, or cortical/subcortical haemorrhage and pathological evidence of severe cerebral amyloid angiopathy.
- Probable cerebral amyloid angiopathy with supporting pathological evidence:
  - clinical data **and** pathological tissue (evacuated haematoma or cortical biopsy specimen) demonstrate a haemorrhage as mentioned above and some degree of vascular amyloid deposition.
  - does not have to be post-mortem.
- Probable cerebral amyloid angiopathy:
  - pathological confirmation not required
  - patient >55 years
  - appropriate clinical history
  - MRI findings demonstrate **multiple** haemorrhages of varying sizes/ages with no other explanation.
- Possible cerebral amyloid angiopathy:
  - patient >55 years
  - appropriate clinical history
  - MRI findings reveal a **single** lobar, cortical, or cortical/subcortical haemorrhage without another cause, multiple haemorrhages with a possible but not a definite cause, or some haemorrhage in an atypical location.

Clinical tip Distinguishing amyloid spells from seizures and migraine

Be wary of new-onset stereotyped visual disturbance in the elderly—although these events could represent migraine, this is less likely in those without any antecedent migraine history and they could represent amyloid spells. Look for evidence of superficial siderosis, subarachnoid blood products, or lobar microhaemorrhages around the occipital lobes on suitable MRI sequences. Amyloid spells are typically longer than seizures and shorter than TIAs, and are almost certainly under-reported by doctors. They may occur several times a day or be much less frequent. A careful history may well be sufficient to confirm the diagnosis beyond reasonable doubt.

Antiplatelets were stopped and treatment with simvastatin and amlodipine (at an increased dose) continued. The patient continued to experience regular attacks (up to five a day) over the next two weeks. Therefore topiramate was trialled on pragmatic clinical grounds and the attacks terminated.

Expert comment

The need for statin therapy in this patient may be questioned, as it may potentially increase the risk of intracerebral haemorrhage. In the absence of specific randomized clinical trial data, one may only speculate that in patients with a recent amyloid-related lobar haemorrhage, avoiding statin therapy may be preferable. However, in patients suspected to have cerebral amyloid angiopathy on grounds of brain imaging but without a symptomatic macrohaemorrhage, as in our case, the risks and benefits of statin therapy are uncertain. Blood-pressure-lowering treatment is certainly beneficial in terms of preventing a symptomatic intracerebral haemorrhage in cerebral amyloid angiopathy, regardless of the presence of hypertension. Transient aura attacks frequently respond to antiepileptic medications.

Bleeding risk in CAA with antiplatelets

This leads us to consider the safety of antithrombotic and thrombolytic treatments which might increase the risk of intracerebral haemorrhage in patients with CAA pathology. Patients with cerebral microbleeds may be at increased risk of symptomatic intracerebral haemorrhage following thrombolysis for acute ischaemic stroke; however, current data are insufficient to justify withholding thrombolytic therapy solely on the basis of presence of cerebral microbleeds [18]. Some evidence suggests that CAA is a risk factor for anticoagulation-related intracerebral haemorrhage. Reliable detection of lobar cerebral microbleeds could in future serve as a tool for treatment decisions on anticoagulation [19]. Cerebral microbleeds are associated with intracerebral haemorrhage related to antiplatelet use. In patients with a large number of lobar microbleeds, the risk of intracerebral haemorrhage could outweigh the benefits of antiplatelet therapy[20]

We illustrate the potentially catastrophic effects of antiplatelet therapy in cerebral amyloid angiopathy in Figure 15.2.

Conclusions

The differential diagnosis of transient neurological episodes can be challenging because the symptoms and signs have usually resolved by the time of assessment. Therefore the diagnosis relies heavily on the patient's account of their history and on expert interpretation of that history. Up to 60 per cent of patients referred to a TIA clinic do not have a final diagnosis of TIA [21]. Even amongst stroke-trained neurologists diagnosing TIA on clinical grounds alone can be unreliable [22]. Therefore it is

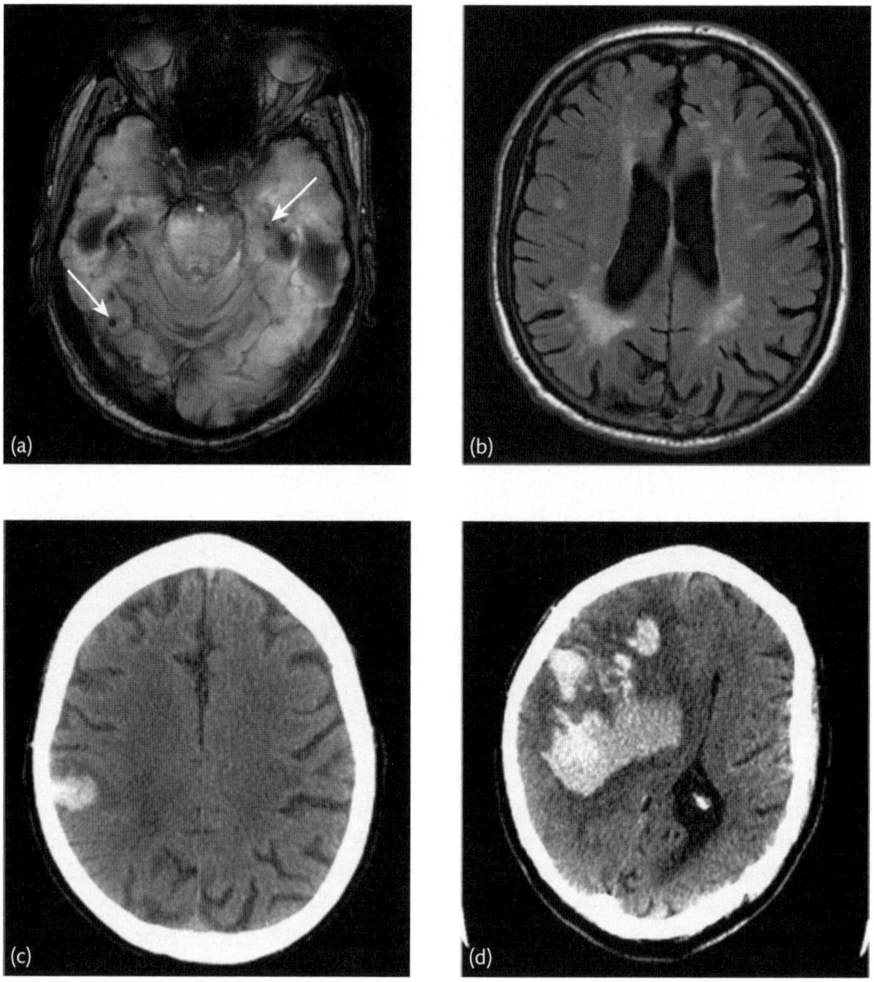

Figure 15.2 This 77-year-old man presented with recurrent episodes of altered sensation and weakness of the left arm. His brain MRI demonstrated (a) microhaemorrhages (arrows) as well as (b) white matter ischaemic change. He was treated with clopidogrel. Ten months later he was admitted with with sudden-onset left hemiparesis. His head CT revealed (c) a right frontal intracerebral haematoma which (d) increased in size within 24 hours, leading to midline shift and herniation.

reasonable to make use of clinical investigations, most importantly MRI with appropriate sequences to refine diagnosis. This may reduce the risk of completed stroke in those with a genuine TIA, and prevent those without TIA from being exposed to inappropriate secondary prevention such as antithrombotic treatment.

Final word from the expert

Common causes of transient neurological symptoms that can mimic TIA include migraine aura, seizure, and functional presentation, although many other causes are recognized [7]. Patients with transient unilateral paresis are more likely to have a TIA than those with other transient neurological signs or symptoms [23]. When attacks are repeated and stereotyped in nature 'amyloid spells' or epilepsy should be considered in addition to rare vascular presentations such as capsular warning syndrome. The second case (Figure 15.2) emphatically illustrates the potential to cause harm if cerebral amyloid angiopathy is not identified—more work is required to identify patients at greatest risk of thrombolytic, anticoagulant, or antiplatelet treatment.

References

1. Albers GW, Caplan LR, Easton JD, et al. Transient ischemic attack—proposal for a new definition. *N Engl J Med* 2002;347 (21): 1713–16.
2. Easton JD, Saver JL, Albers GW, et al. AHA/ASA Scientific Statement. Definition and evaluation of transient ischemic attack. *Stroke* 2009; 40(6): 2276–93.
3. Intercollegiate Stroke Working Party. *National Clinical Guideline for Stroke* (4th edn) (London: Royal College of Physicians); 2012.
4. Giles KA, Hamdan AD, Pomposelli FB, et al. Stroke and death after carotid endarterectomy and carotid artery stenting with and without high risk criteria. *J Vasc Surg* 2010; 52(6): 1497–1504.
5. Donnan GA, O'Malley HM, Quang L, et al. The capsular warning syndrome: pathogenesis and clinical features. *Neurology* 1993; 43(5): 957–62.
6. Paul NL, Simoni M, Chandratheva A, Rothwell PM. Population-based study of capsular warning syndrome and prognosis after early recurrent TIA. *Neurology* 2012; 79(13): 1356–62.
7. Nadarajan V, Perry RJ, Johnson J, Werring DJ. Transient ischaemic attacks: mimics and chameleons. *Pract Neurol* 2014; 14(1): 23–31.
8. Davis SM, Donnan GA. Clinical practice. Secondary prevention after ischemic stroke or transient ischemic attack. *N Engl J Med* 2012; 366(20): 1914–22.
9. Viswanathan A, Chabriat H. Cerebral microhemorrhage. *Stroke* 2006; 37(2): 550–5.
10. Izenberg A, Aviv RI, Demaerschalk BM, et al. Crescendo transient Aura attacks: a transient ischemic attack mimic caused by focal subarachnoid hemorrhage. *Stroke* 2009; 40(12): 3725–9.
11. Greenberg SM, Vonsattel JP, Stakes JW, et al. The clinical spectrum of cerebral amyloid angiopathy: presentations without lobar hemorrhage. *Neurology* 1993; 43(10): 2073–9.
12. Smith EE, Greenberg SM. Clinical diagnosis of cerebral amyloid angiopathy: validation of the Boston criteria. *Curr Atheroscler Rep* 2003; 5(4): 260–6.
13. Verbeek MM, Kremer BP, Rikkert MO, et al. Cerebrospinal fluid amyloid beta(40) is decreased in cerebral amyloid angiopathy. *Ann Neurol* 2009; 66(2): 245–9.
14. Charidimou A, Peeters A, Fox Z, et al. Spectrum of transient focal neurological episodes in cerebral amyloid angiopathy: multicentre magnetic resonance imaging cohort study and meta-analysis. *Stroke* 2012; 43(9): 2324–30.
15. Charidimou A, Law R, Werring DJ. Amyloid 'spells' trouble. *Lancet* 2012; 380(9853): 1620.
16. Dierksen GA, Skehan ME, Khan MA, et al. Spatial relation between microbleeds and amyloid deposits in amyloid angiopathy. *Ann Neurol* 2010; 68(4): 545–8.
17. Koennecke HC. Cerebral microbleeds on MRI: prevalence, associations, and potential clinical implications. *Neurology* 2006; 66(2): 165–71.
18. Shoamanesh A, Kwok CS, Lim PA, Benavente OR. Postthrombolysis intracranial hemorrhage risk of cerebral microbleeds in acute stroke patients: a systematic review and meta-analysis. *Int J Stroke* 2013; 8(5): 348–56.
19. Fisher M. MRI Screening for chronic anticoagulation in atrial fibrillation. *Front Neurol* 2013; 4: 137.

20. Gregoire SM, Jager HR, Yousry TA, et al. Brain microbleeds as a potential risk factor for antiplatelet-related intracerebral haemorrhage: hospital-based, case–control study. *J Neurol Neurosurg Psychiatry* 2010; 81(6): 679–84.
21. Prabhakaran S, Silver AJ, Warrior L, et al. Misdiagnosis of transient ischemic attacks in the emergency room. *Cerebrovasc Dis* 2008; 26(6): 630–5.
22. Castle J, Mlynash M, Lee K, et al. Agreement regarding diagnosis of transient ischemic attack fairly low among stroke-trained neurologists. *Stroke* 2010; 41(7): 1367–70.
23. Amort M, Fluri F, Schafer J, et al. Transient ischemic attack versus transient ischemic attack mimics: frequency, clinical characteristics and outcome. *Cerebrovasc Dis* 2011; 32(1): 57–64.

CASE

16 Picking out an inherited disease

Ignacio Rubio-Agusti

Expert commentary Robin Lachmann

Case history

A 39-year-old male computer programmer was referred to clinic complaining of tremor, poor coordination, and forgetfulness.

About three or four years earlier, he had developed a bilateral arm tremor when performing voluntary movements, such as when typing on the computer, writing, or holding a cup of tea. Over time, this tremor spread to involve the legs, particularly when standing. He also became clumsier, with his hands and tending to veer to either side when walking, with some instability and occasional falls. He found it particularly difficult to climb down stairs. He had trouble when reading a book, but not reading on his computer monitor or on television. During this time, he had developed mild slurring of his speech, which did not impair communication. He had no swallowing difficulties. He thought that he was not as mentally sharp as he used to be, and that his short-term memory and ability to perform calculations had worsened.

He had been born without complications after a normal pregnancy. Childhood development was normal and he had obtained a degree in information technology. He was one of three children from a non-consanguineous marriage. His younger brother had developed similar symptoms at age 33 years.

On examination, downward voluntary vertical saccades were slow with reduced range. However, range was normal when assessing the vestibulo-ocular reflexes. Horizontal saccades and smooth pursuit were normal. He had a mild dysarthria. Facial expression was reduced. He had bilateral jerky irregular postural and kinetic arm tremor, with occasional superimposed myoclonus and bilateral rest tremor of the hands. There was dystonic posturing of the fingers. He had dysmetria when performing finger-to-nose and heel-to-shin manoeuvres. When standing, he had an irregular jerky low-frequency tremor of the legs. Myotatic reflexes were brisk, with a few beats of ankle clonus. Plantar responses were flexor. There was no weakness or spasticity. He had enhanced rigidity and mild bradykinesia when performing rapid alternating movements with the fingers. On walking, he veered to the sides with a wide-based gait and was unable to tandem walk. While walking he had a bilaterally reduced arm swing. Sensation to pinprick, vibration sense, and position sense was normal. His postural reflexes were impaired. Abdominal examination revealed a palpable spleen 5cm below the costal margin. In summary, he had a combination of neurological disease, with cerebellar signs, cognitive symptoms, movement disorders (tremor, dystonia, parkinsonism, and myoclonus), and visceral involvement (splenomegaly).

Learning point Inborn errors of metabolism: clinical clues

- Inborn errors of metabolism (IEMs) are a group of inherited conditions in which the genetic defect alters a metabolic pathway. Although each individual condition is rare, collectively they are common, accounting for a third of all genetic disorders [1].
- Because of its complex and demanding metabolism, involvement of the central nervous system (CNS) is common. Patients often present with neurological and/or psychiatric symptoms.
- Since many of these conditions are treatable, the possibility of an IEM should always be considered when there are [2]:
  - fluctuations in the severity and/or type of symptoms
  - symptoms which appear to be related to a metabolic trigger (such as drugs, fasting, intercurrent illness, or other catabolic states)
  - widespread distribution of symptoms, involving multiple neurological systems (such as cerebellar, pyramidal, extrapyramidal, cognitive)
  - associated systemic symptoms or signs, including ocular signs, skin problems, bone abnormalities, visceromegaly
  - atypical clinical presentation, including unexpected symptoms/signs or lack of response to usual treatments (e.g. seizures may be refractory to anti-epileptic drugs)
  - a family history of consanguinity, neonatal deaths, or unexplained neurological symptoms in siblings.

Most IEMs are inherited as autosomal recessive traits. However, bear in mind, that most cases will appear to be sporadic.

Clinical tip Saccades and metabolic disorders[3].

- Voluntary saccades are rapid conjugate eye movements allowing quick changes of visual fixation. They bring the fovea of both eyes quickly from one point in the visual field to another.
- Saccades can be examined by asking the patient to look alternately between two distant targets (e.g. the tip of a pen and the examiner's nose). Targets should not be separated by more than 30° (otherwise two different saccades might be needed). The test can be performed in the vertical and horizontal planes.
- Four components of saccades should be assessed.
  - Latency: is there a pause before the eyes start moving?
  - Accuracy: do the eyes stop on target or do they need to refixate to the target after an initial movement?
  - Velocity: are the movements slower than normal?
  - Conjugacy: do both eyes move at the same speed?
- If the patient is unable to look voluntarily in one direction of gaze (gaze palsy), pursuit and the vestibulo-ocular reflexes should be assessed. They are both normal in early supranuclear gaze palsy. However, the reduction in gaze excursion may prevent pursuit testing.
- The supranuclear structures governing vertical saccades are located in the rostral midbrain close to the oculomotor and trochlear nuclei. Those controlling horizontal saccades are located in the pons, close to the abducens nuclei. A lesion or dysfunction of these structures may be caused by a number of pathologies, such as tumours, strokes, demyelination, or infections. An MRI scan of the brain should be obtained in patients with abnormal saccades to exclude a structural cause.
- Abnormal vertical saccades are a characteristic sign of Niemann–Pick disease type C (NPC), often occurring early in the course of the disease. Initially saccades will appear slow and reduced in range. Later on they will be abolished (vertical supranuclear gaze palsy). Clues from the history suggesting vertical gaze impairment include difficulties descending stairs and problems when looking down (such as when reading a book, but not a computer monitor). Unless saccades are specifically examined, this useful sign might easily be overlooked, as pursuit, which is more often assessed, will still be preserved. Later in the course of the disease, horizontal saccades will also be affected.
- Other lysosomal storage disorders (LSDs) can also affect visual saccades. Gaucher disease affects horizontal saccades and hexosaminidase-A deficiency may affect horizontal and vertical saccades.

An MRI scan of the brain showed non-specific white matter signal changes in the frontal lobes bilaterally. There were no abnormalities of the basal ganglia or cerebellum.

Formal psychometric testing showed minor impairments in executive function and memory tasks. His verbal IQ and performance IQ were still within normal levels, but below his premorbid estimates.

Basic blood tests, including blood cell count, liver function tests, renal function tests, thyroid function tests, lipid profile, vitamin B12, vitamin E, copper studies, electrolytes, and autoimmune panel, were normal. A skin biopsy was performed to look for Niemann-Pick disease.

Learning point Niemann-Pick disease type C, adult presentation

- The clinical presentation of NPC is highly variable. It may include systemic and neurological signs, and may present from birth to late adulthood [4].
- Systemic and neurological involvement may begin at different times and they follow an independent course, suggesting that the underlying pathophysiology may be different.
- Systemic features include hepatic involvement (cholestasis, hepatic insufficiency, hepatomegaly), splenomegaly, and, rarely, lung infiltration. Prolonged neonatal cholestatic jaundice is common. It usually resolves spontaneously and hepatic disease is not a significant feature after the neonatal period. Splenomegaly may be absent in 15 per cent of the patients and, when present, tends to regress with age. Neurological involvement starts after visceral involvement, but is progressive [4].
- Nearly all patients eventually develop neurological symptoms, including:
  - cognitive impairment
  - cerebellar ataxia
  - bulbar signs (dysarthria, dysphagia)
  - pyramidal signs
  - psychiatric symptoms
  - movement disorders
  - epilepsy.
- Characteristic neurological signs of this disease include the following.
  - Vertical supranuclear gaze palsy (see above).
  - Gelastic cataplexy: cataplexy is a sudden loss of muscular tone, not associated with loss of consciousness (different from syncope or seizures), which is often triggered by emotional stimuli. Patients with NPC may show cataplexy, often induced by laughter (gelastic cataplexy). This sign has been reported in 20 per cent of juvenile patients and can easily be confused with other symptoms, especially falls or seizures.
- According to the age of onset different forms of presentation are recognized, with overlapping symptoms [4]. Adult-onset forms show some peculiarities [4, 5].
  - Systemic features may be absent or mild in up to 50 per cent of patients. If the condition is suspected, abdominal ultrasound may allow detection of an otherwise non-apparent hepatosplenomegaly.
  - Psychiatric symptoms may be the presenting feature in up to 30 per cent of the cases [4, 6]. Most often these will include psychotic features (hallucinations, delusions, thought disorders), but other problems have also been reported (depression, bipolar disorder, obsessive-compulsive disorder, personality change). If carefully examined, most of these patients will show neurological signs (e.g. vertical supranuclear gaze palsy).
  - Altered vertical saccades and cerebellar, bulbar, and cognitive abnormalities are the most common neurologic signs. Cognitive impairment often involves executive function and verbal memory [7].
  - Movement disorders, including dystonia, myoclonus, parkinsonism, and chorea [6, 8], are more common than in patients with an earlier age of onset and may be present in up to 60 per cent of the cases. Occasionally they may be the presenting sign.
  - Epilepsy is less common than in younger patients.

Cholesterol esterification and filipin staining were assayed in cultured fibroblasts from the skin biopsy. Cholesterol esterification was undetectable and fibroblasts displayed an intense punctuate perinuclear fluorescence, confirming the diagnosis. Genetic testing showed that the patient was compound heterozygous for two previously described pathogenic mutations in the gene *NPC1*, which were later also identified in his brother.

Learning point Diagnostic tests for NPC

- The definitive diagnosis of an IEM requires at least one of the following:
  - biochemical demonstration of a defect in the relevant metabolic pathway
  - molecular confirmation of a pathogenic mutation(s) in the relevant gene.

  These tests are often complex, expensive, and not widely available. Abnormal metabolites may be detected in blood, urine, or CSF. Functional assays require cell or tissue samples (leucocytes, skin fibroblasts, muscle), are technically demanding, and require a high level of expertise for interpretation. It is important that the right samples are taken and that they are correctly processed before being sent to specialized laboratories.
- Sometimes secondary biochemical features can also be detected. These tests, which are less specific but more widely available, often involve determination of metabolites in body fluids (urine, plasma, CSF). In NPC these can include [4, 8]:
  - altered liver function tests
  - low platelet count
  - raised chitotriosidase activity (measured in plasma or leucocytes).
- The biochemistry of NPC is not well understood. It appears to be a disorder of intracellular lipid trafficking. Cholesterol and a number of other lipid species are stored, with different patterns of storage present in different tissues.
- Traditionally, diagnosis has relied on filipin staining of cultured fibroblasts. Fibroblasts obtained from a skin biopsy are incubated with low-density lipoprotein and then stained with the fluorescent dye filipin which binds to cholesterol. Fibroblasts from NPC patients show strong perinuclear staining in a vesicular pattern. In 15 per cent of patients, the test may show less strong staining, the so-called 'variant' phenotype. Mutation screening would still be advised to confirm the diagnosis [4, 8], and molecular genetic analysis is now becoming the diagnostic test of choice, with filipin staining reserved for those with previously unreported genetic variants of doubtful significance.
- The disease is caused by mutations of one of two genes *NPC1* (95 per cent of the cases) located in 18q11-q12, or *NPC2* (<5 per cent) located in 14q24.3. NPC1 is an integral membrane protein and NPC2 is a soluble lysosomal protein which may have enzymatic activity [4, 8]. The exact function of these proteins is not yet well understood.

Following diagnosis the patient was started on substrate reduction therapy with miglustat 200mg three times daily. He developed mild weight loss and mild diarrhoea. Reducing the dose to 100mg three times daily resolved these issues. At follow-up, a year after diagnosis, his symptoms remained stable.

Learning point Treatment strategies in LSDs

- LSDs are characterized by the accumulation of undegraded macromolecules within the endosomal–lysosomal system. Treatment strategies include the following.
  - Enzyme replacement therapy, aimed at restoring normal catabolism.
  - Substrate reduction therapy, aimed at reducing the substrate to a level where the residual enzymatic activity is enough to prevent accumulation.
  - Enzyme enhancement (chaperone) therapy, aimed at stabilizing mutant enzyme to allow it to reach its site of action in the lysosome and express its residual enzyme activity. This approach depends on the precise nature of the mutation.

(Continued)

- Enzyme replacement therapy (ERT) has been successfully used for the systemic manifestations of Gaucher disease, Fabry disease, Pompe disease, and some of the mucopolysaccharidoses. Unfortunately, because circulating enzymes cannot cross the blood–brain barrier this approach is not useful for conditions with involvement of the CNS [9].
- The iminosugar miglustat is an inhibitor of the ceramide-specific glucosyltransferase that catalyses the first step in the synthesis of glycosphingolipids. Unlike ERT, it is administered orally and can cross the blood–brain barrier. It has been trialled for substrate reduction therapy in a number of glycosphingolipid storage disorders, including neuronopathic forms of Gaucher disease, Tay–Sachs disease and NPC (where there is marked accumulation of gangliosides in neurons) [10, 11]. Clinical trials have shown slowing of the progression of the neurological manifestations of NPC with this treatment [11–13].

Evidence base Miglustat for NPC [11]

- A randomized controlled clinical trial comparing the effects of miglustat with standard symptomatic care in patients over 12 years of age with a biochemically confirmed diagnosis of NPC and neurological manifestations (n =29). An additional cohort of children (under 12 years of age; n =12) was included, all receiving miglustat.
- The study had two stages. During the first stage one group of patients (n = 20) was treated with oral miglustat 200mg three times daily and the second group (n = 9) received standard care (symptomatic treatment, rehabilitation, speech and occupational therapy). During the second stage all patients received miglustat.
- The primary outcome measure was horizontal saccadic velocity, which correlates with disease progression. Secondary outcome measures included swallowing assessment, ambulatory assessment (standard ambulation index), auditory acuity, and cognitive assessment (Mini-Mental State Examination).
- A significant improvement in horizontal saccadic velocity was seen in treated patients. Some improvements in swallowing and cognitive function, slowing of ambulatory deterioration, and stabilization of auditory function were also reported.
- The most commonly reported side effects were weight loss and gastrointestinal symptoms (diarrhoea, abdominal pain, flatulence, nausea).

Discussion

With an estimated prevalence ranging between 0.35 and 2.2 per 100,000 cases, NPC can be considered a rare disorder [4]. However, it is important for physicians to be aware of this condition, as specific treatment may prevent or slow further deterioration [13]. A high index of suspicion is necessary for diagnosis. This case also illustrates several important clinical points applicable to other LSDs and IEMs.

Metabolic disorders should be suspected in patients presenting with chronic progressive neurological or psychiatric symptoms or with a complex phenotype that involves several neurological systems, such as cerebellar, bulbar, cognition, pyramidal, or extrapyramidal. The most common neurological features of NPC are abnormal vertical saccades, cerebellar ataxia, bulbar signs, and cognitive impairment. The differential diagnosis should include a number of other conditions, including:

- other LSDs, such as Gaucher disease type 3 and GM2 gangliosidosis (Table 16.1) other IEMs, such as cerebrotendinous xanthomatosis
- heredodegenerative conditions, such as complicated spinocerebellar ataxias
- sporadic neurodegenerative disorders, such as multiple-system atrophy.

Expert comment

NPC, like most IEMs, is an autosomal recessive disorder. Siblings may be affected, but often the family history is non-contributory. A history of consanguinity makes a genetic condition much more likely. The phenotypic variability of NPC means that careful questioning for visceral (i.e. neonatal cholestasis, splenectomy) as well as neurological symptoms in siblings is important.

Table 16.1 Clinical features in adult forms of lysosomal storage disorders*

Disease	Neurological symptoms and signs	Characteristic clinical features	Characteristic imaging findings
Niemann-Pick type C	**Cerebellar ataxia**, dystonia, myoclonus, cognitive impairment, psychiatric features	Vertical supranuclear gaze palsy, gelastic cataplexy	-
Gaucher type 3	Dystonia, myoclonus, parkinsonism, **cognitive impairment**, epilepsy	Horizontal supranuclear gaze palsy, hepatosplenomegaly	-
GM1-Gangliosidosis	**Dystonia**, parkinsonism, cognitive impairment	Kyphoscoliosis, vertebral and hip dysplasia	Posterior putaminal lesions
GM2-Gangliosidosis	**Cerebellar ataxia**, dystonia, psychiatric features	Lower motor neuron disease, small-fibre peripheral neuropathy	Cerebellar atrophy
Krabbe disease	**Spastic paraparesis**, cerebellar ataxia, peripheral neuropathy	Demyelinating peripheral neuropathy	Leucoencephalopathy involving corticospinal tracts
Metachromatic leucodystrophy	**Cerebellar ataxia**, dystonia, spastic paraparesis, **cognitive impairment, psychiatric features**, peripheral neuropathy	Demyelinating peripheral neuropathy	Leucoencephalopathy sparing U-fibres
Fabry disease	Cerebrovascular events	Small-fibre peripheral neuropathy (acroparaesthesia), angiokeratomata, corneal dystrophy, renal impairment, heart disease	Posterior thalamic lesions

*Note the overlap of neurological signs and symptoms. Frequent presenting signs are shown in bold. Characteristic features are not necessarily frequent.

Expert comment

Always think of metabolic disorders in patients of all ages, especially if multiple neurological systems are involved. A progressive course and the presence of associated systemic signs raises the possibility of an IEM; careful evaluation of the eyes, skin, bones, and abdominal viscera is recommended. Bone dysplasia and hepatosplenomegaly suggest an LSD. If the history is of metabolic decompensation, with acute deterioration at a time of metabolic stress (e.g. fasting, intercurrent infection) a disorder of intermediate metabolism should be considered.

Characteristic neurological findings in NPC include abnormalities in vertical saccades, which are seen in at least 75 per cent of patients, and gelastic cataplexy. Type 3 Gaucher disease may also impair saccades, but usually horizontal gaze is affected first and most severely and there is prominent systemic involvement with hepatosplenomegaly and bone disease. Other conditions presenting with a chronic progressive neurological disorder and altered vertical saccades in a similar age range include, among others, Huntington disease [14] (particularly early-onset cases), Kufor–Rakeb syndrome [15], Whipple disease [16], neuronal brain iron accumulation syndromes [17, 18], and spinocerebellar ataxias [19].

Common diagnostic tests are of limited use. Imaging of the brain is often normal or shows non-specific abnormalities, such as cerebral or cerebellar atrophy [4].

Definitive diagnosis is difficult as NPC1 has no known enzymatic activity and hence its function cannot be assayed in leucocytes. Instead, it is necessary to demonstrate pathological cholesterol storage in cultured skin fibroblasts by filipin staining. Genetic testing is easier, but is not easy to interpret if novel mutations of uncertain clinical significance are detected [8]. Such tests are expensive, often difficult to interpret, and not widely available; thus referral to a specialist centre for assessment may be useful.

If the diagnosis is confirmed, substrate reduction therapy with miglustat should be considered, particularly in the early stages of disease, as it may lead to stabilization of the neurological symptoms [13].

Final word from the expert

Routine tests are often normal or non-specific, but may allow exclusion of other conditions. Diagnosis of an IEM relies on a combination of demonstration of abnormal metabolites, measurement of deficient activity of the relevant metabolic pathway, and molecular analysis of the associated gene. In most LSDs definitive diagnosis has involved measuring the activity of the deficient enzyme, often in white blood cells and/or plasma. This requires careful specimen handling and delays in getting specimens to the laboratory can invalidate the assays. Increasingly, tests on dried blood spots (like those used in newborn screening) are becoming available and have the advantage that the specimens are stable at room temperature for prolonged periods.

However, NPC is not caused by deficiency of a lysosomal enzyme and therefore diagnosis is more difficult. Molecular genetic analysis of the *NPC1* gene should be requested first. If this shows two mutations of known pathogenic significance, the diagnosis is secure. If there is a novel mutation, or only one mutated allele is identified, it is necessary to procede to analysis of cultured fibroblasts by filipin staining and cholesterol esterification studies. This can be a time-consuming process but, as treatment is available, it is important to make the diagnosis.

References

1. Jimenez-Sanchez G, Childs B, Valle D. Human disease genes. *Nature* 2001; 409(6822): 853-5.
2. Saudubray JM, Nassogne MC, de Lonlay P, Touati G. Clinical approach to inherited metabolic disorders in neonates: an overview. *Semin Neonatol* 2002; 7(1): 3–15.
3. Leigh RJ, Zee DS. *The Neurology of Eye Movements* (New York: Oxford University Press); 2006.
4. Vanier MT. Niemann–Pick disease type C. *Orphanet J Rare Dis* 2010; 5: 16.
5. Sévin, M., Lesca G, Baumann N, et al. The adult form of Niemann–Pick disease type C. *Brain* 2007; 130(Pt 1): 120–33.
6. Josephs KA, Van Gerpen MW, Van Gerpen JA. Adult onset Niemann–Pick disease type C presenting with psychosis. *J Neurol Neurosurg Psychiatry* 2003; 74(4): 528–9.
7. Klarner B, Klünemann HH, Lürding R, Aslanidis C, Rupprecht R. Neuropsychological profile of adult patients with Niemann–Pick C1 (*NPC1*) mutations. *J Inherit Metab Dis* 2007; 30(1): 60–7.
8. Patterson MC, Hendriksz CJ, Walterfang M, et al. Recommendations for the diagnosis and management of Niemann–Pick disease type C: an update. *Mol Genet Metab* 2012; 106(3): 330–44.

9. Lachmann RH. Enzyme replacement therapy for lysosomal storage diseases. *Curr Opin Pediatr* 2011; 23(6): 588–93.
10. Lachmann RH. Miglustat: substrate reduction therapy for glycosphingolipid lysosomal storage disorders. *Drugs Today (Barc)* 2006; 42(1): 29–38.
11. Patterson MC, Vecchio D, Prady H, et al. Miglustat for treatment of Niemann–Pick C disease: a randomised controlled study. *Lancet Neurol* 2007; 6(9): 765–72.
12. Patterson MC, Vecchio D, Jacklin E, et al. Long-term miglustat therapy in children with Niemann–Pick disease type C. *J Child Neurol* 2010; 25(3): 300–5.
13. Wraith JE, Vecchio D, Jacklin E, et al. Miglustat in adult and juvenile patients with Niemann–Pick disease type C: long-term data from a clinical trial. *Mol Genet Metab* 2010; 99(4): 351–7.
14. Rupp J, Dzemidzic M, Blekher T, et al. Comparison of vertical and horizontal saccade measures and their relation to gray matter changes in premanifest and manifest Huntington disease. *J Neurol* 2012; 259(2): 267–76.
15. Williams DR, Hadeed A, al-Din AS, et al. Kufor Rakeb disease: autosomal recessive, levodopa-responsive parkinsonism with pyramidal degeneration, supranuclear gaze palsy, and dementia. *Mov Disord* 2005; 20(10): 1264–71.
16. Averbuch-Heller L, Paulson GW, Daroff RB, Leigh RJ. Whipple's disease mimicking progressive supranuclear palsy: the diagnostic value of eye movement recording. *J Neurol Neurosurg Psychiatry* 1999; 66(4): 532–5.
17. Egan RA, Weleber RG, Hogarth P, et al. Neuro-ophthalmologic and electroretinographic findings in pantothenate kinase-associated neurodegeneration (formerly Hallervorden–Spatz syndrome). *Am J Ophthalmol* 2005; 140(2): 267–74.
18. Paisan-Ruiz C. Bhatia KP, Li A, et al. Characterization of PLA2G6 as a locus for dystonia–parkinsonism. *Ann Neurol* 2009; 65(1): 19–23.
19. Burk K, Abele M, Fetter M, et al. Autosomal dominant cerebellar ataxia type I clinical features and MRI in families with SCA1, SCA2 and SCA3. *Brain* 1996; 119 (Pt 5): 1497–1505.

CASE

17 A worsening acute psychosis

Umesh Vivekananda

Expert commentary: Dimitri M. Kullmann

Case history

A 20-year-old female student was admitted to hospital and detained under the Mental Health Act by the psychiatry team after being found wandering outside in a confused state. Four days earlier she had been complaining of headaches and her family had noticed changes in her behaviour. They reported that she had displayed odd ideas and had been suspicious of them. Two days before admission, the patient reported visual hallucinations and delusions ('I'm able to see inside people's bodies'), and her speech was nonsensical. While in hospital the patient was mute and noted by the duty psychiatrist to demonstrate abnormal posturing with 'dance-like movements with her arms'. On examination she was tachycardic with a heart rate of 150bpm and had an oxygen saturation of 88 per cent on pulse oximetry. She was reviewed by the medical team for an organic cause of her illness. Because of her unstable cardiovascular state and requirement for sedation, she was transferred to the neurocritical care unit.

On examination the patient was afebrile. Although consciousness was depressed and she did not obey commands, she had a preserved vestibular-ocular reflex, normal pupillary reaction, normal tone and reflexes in all four limbs, and bilateral flexor plantar response. Blood tests, including blood cultures, an autoimmune profile (ANA, ANCA, ENA, RhF), vitamin B12, thyroid screen, and porphyrin screen, were all normal. A CT scan of the head, performed under anaesthesia with intubation and ventilation because of severe agitation, revealed no abnormality. The results of a subsequent lumbar puncture and serum antibodies are shown in Table 17.1. An EEG showed excess rhythmic slow activity in keeping with an encephalopathy, but

Table 17.1 Results of initial cerebrospinal fluid and anti-neuronal antibody screen

Screen	Result (reference)
CSF	
Protein	0.2 (0.2–0.5)g/L
Glucose	4.6 (2.5–4.4)mmol/L
White blood cells	10 (0–5)/mm^3
Red blood cells	3 (0)mm^3
Culture	Negative
Virology	HSV1, HSV2, VZV, CMV, EBV negative
Serum antibodies	
Anti-Hu	Negative
Anti-Purkinje cell	Negative
Anti-myelin	Negative
Voltage-gated potassium channel	Negative

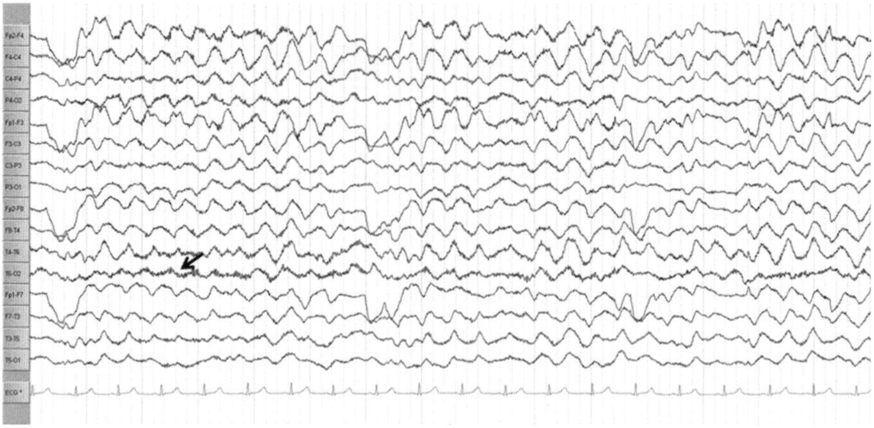

Figure 17.1 The EEG shows continuous generalized rhythmical delta slow activity that is evidence of a severe generalized encephalopathy. In addition there is evidence of 'extreme delta brush' (arrow), defined as beta activity overlying delta activity. This phenomenon has only recently been observed as a unique feature in patients with anti-NMDA-receptor encepahilitis [2]. There are no definite epileptiform abnormalities and no evidence to suggest non-convulsive status epilepticus.

no epileptiform activity (Figure 17.1). An MRI scan of the brain also showed normal brain appearance. An attempted extubation resulted in the patient having a generalized tonic-clonic seizure and so she was reintubated and given an intravenous loading dose of sodium valproate. With the sequence of events and investigations noted, an autoimmune encephalitis was suspected.

A transvaginal ultrasound revealed a right-sided ovarian teratoma and this was removed surgically five days later. Antibody tests to the *N*-methyl-D-aspartate receptor (NMDAR) were positive, further confirming the diagnosis.

Immunosuppressive therapy followed with two courses of plasma exchange, two courses of intravenous immunoglobulin (IVIG), and one course of high-dose steroids given over a period of five months. NMDAR antibodies remained detectable despite removal of the tumour and immunosuppressive therapy. The patient remained very agitated requiring intravenous sedation. She had continued dyskinesias, mainly orofacial, and episodes of hypotension and supraventricular tachycardias during this period. In addition, serial EEGs showed evidence of electrographic seizures, which were initially controlled with sodium valproate, and then with levetiracetam and clonazepam.

Two infusions of rituximab were given, and despite an episode of *Klebsiella* sepsis between courses the dyskinesias slowly started to abate over the following four months, which allowed the patient to be gradually weaned from sedation and ventilatory support. Mild cog-wheel rigidity was noted, but this was attributed to neuroleptic medication which was given in an attempt to manage the agitation. EEGs performed at this point did not demonstrate any further seizure activity, but showed a pattern in keeping with severe encephalopathy. She began making automated movements and at the end of four months was recognizing family and speaking a few words such as 'mum' and 'dad'. Even during this phase of improvement repeated NMDAR antibodies were positive. However, as the patient was being readied for transfer to a rehabilitation unit, she suffered a sudden cardiac arrest and, despite resuscitation, did not survive. Although unclear, it was thought that death was secondary to acute myocarditis. Table 17.2 gives a summary of the time course for the patient whilst in the ICU.

Expert comment

The progression of symptoms is typical of anti-NMDA-receptor encephalitis. There is an early phase of confusion, psychiatric disturbance, and/or seizures. About 10–20 days later, there is onset of movement disorders, followed by reduced consciousness and autonomic instability.

Fifty-eight per cent of cases are associated with a malignancy, notably ovarian teratoma.

Clinical tip Testing for anti-NMDA-receptor encephalitis

An immunofluorescence assay based on co-expression of GluN1 and GluN2 subunits of the NMDAR can detect antibodies in serum and CSF [1].

Clinical tip Intensive care unit management

As NMDAR encephalitis frequently affects consciousness, respiratory function (hypoventilation), cardiac function (arrhythmias), and autonomic function (labile blood pressure), the most appropriate place for treatment is an intensive care unit.

Table 17.2 Summary of the time course for the patient in theneurocriticalcare unit

Time in neurocritical care unit	Investigations/management
Day 1	Patient admitted for respiratory and cardiovascular support. Autoimmune encephalitis was suspected
Day 5	MRI head normal EEG demonstrated encephalopathy Ultrasound of ovaries revealed right-sided ovarian teratoma.
Day 10	Ovarian teratoma removed Anti-NMDA receptor antibodies return positive
Day 12	First course of plasma exchange
Day 45	Initiation of high-dose steroids
Day 71	Second course of plasma exchange
Day 104	First course of IVIG
Day 130	Second course of IVIG
Day 147	Patient still symptomatic Anti-NMDA receptor antibodies still positive
Day 176	First course of rituximab
Day 188	Episode of *Klebsiella* sepsis
Day 204	Second course of rituximab Patient gradually shows improvement
Day 250	Unexpected cardiac arrest and subsequent death

Discussion

Antibody-mediated encephalitis has been increasingly recognized in recent years. The discovery of antibodies to central nervous system (CNS) proteins was first reported from studies of limbic encephalitis (LE) in the 1960s. LE was initially considered a paraneoplastic disorder because of the detection of associated onconeuronal antibodies such as anti-Hu. It is now increasingly recognized that there are non-paraneoplastic forms of LE, and as a result the field of antibody-mediated CNS disorders has expanded to include encephalopathy, psychiatric disorders, epilepsy, and dementia.

Paraneoplastic limbic encephalitis (PLE)

The first three patients with suspected limbic encephalitis were reported in 1960 by Brierley and colleagues who described the features as 'subacute encephalitis of later adult life mainly affecting the limbic areas' [3]. At autopsy, two of their patients were shown to have probable bronchial carcinoma. The term 'limbic encephalitis' was coined by Corsellis and colleagues in 1968 [4] when commenting on more cases that had emerged. It was this association of malignancy and the CNS that supported the hypothesis of an immune-mediated pathogenesis.

The diagnosis of PLE remains difficult, as common presenting features are shared with a number of disorders including brain tumours and infective encephalitis. In a recent study of 50 patients with PLE [5] the main symptoms were loss of short-term memory (84 per cent); seizures (50 per cent) mainly emanating from the temporal lobes; psychiatric abnormalities (42 per cent) including behavioural changes and hallucinations, and hypothalamic dysfunction (22 per cent) including hyperthermia, hypersomnia, and endocrine abnormality. These features normally developed over days and weeks. Even more challenging, it appears that neurological symptoms usually predate the diagnosis of malignancy. The main associated malignancy is lung cancer, particularly small-cell lung cancer which accounts for 59 per cent of PLE cases reported in the literature. Other malignancies include testicular germ-cell tumours (6 per cent), breast cancer (3 per cent), and Hodgkin's disease (7 per cent) [5].

> **Learning point** Investigations in paraneoplastic limbic encephalitis
>
> - **MRI** The most common abnormality on T2-weighted MRI is mesial–temporal enhancement. Other affected areas are the brainstem and hypothalamus.
> - **CSF** The majority of PLE patients show pleocytosis, elevated proteins, presence of oligoclonal bands, and intrathecal IgG production on CSF.
> - **Paraneoplastic antibodies** can be found in serum, CSF, or both. They include anti-Hu, anti-Yo, anti-Ma, anti-Ta (also known as anti-Ma2), and anti-CV2, with new antibodies being found but not yet characterized. Anti-Hu is usually associated with small-cell lung cancer, whereas anti-Ma2 is associated with testicular tumours. The other antibodies are associated with a more heterogeneous list of malignancies, with anti-Yo relating more to paraneoplastic cerebellar degeneration.

Anti-neuronal antibodies were found in 60 per cent of cases, with anti-Hu being the most common and strongly associated with lung cancer, followed by anti-Ta, associated with testicular germ-cell tumours, and then anti-Ma. Indeed, the positive finding of an anti-neuronal antibody has commonly resulted in the diagnosis of an underlying malignancy. The most successful management of PLE is appropriate treatment of the underlying tumour. Other immunomodulatory options include steroids, cyclophosphamide, IVIG, and plasma exchange. In the series mentioned above, neurological status post treatment improved in fifteen cases, remained stable in eight, and worsened in eleven, six of which resulted in death.

Limbic encephalitis associated with voltage-gated potassium-channel antibodies

The presence of an LE associated with voltage-gated potassium-channel antibodies (VGKC-Abs) has recently been recognized in patients who have demonstrated LE-like clinical features, but had no evidence of malignancy and negative results for paraneoplastic antibodies [6]. In addition they show raised serum/CSF VGKC-Abs levels (i.e. >400μM). More recently it has been recognized that VGKC-Abs do not bind directly to subunits of VGKCs but to one or other of two associated proteins, LGI1 and CASPR2. CASPR2 antibodies also occur in acquired neuromyotonia and Morvan's fibrillary chorea.

Limbic encephalitis with VGKC-Abs can present with the symptoms described earlier for PLE, but the predominant feature is a pervasive and generalized impairment of memory. Interestingly, patients can also present with hyponatraemia in the form of SIADH, presumably a hypothalamic-related phenomenon. T2-weighted MRI again shows mesial–temporal enhancement but, unlike PLE, CSF cell count and protein level is either normal or marginally raised, usually with matched oligoclonal bands. Encouragingly, immunosuppressive treatment in this group does seem successful. Use of steroids, IVIG, and plasma exchange in varying combinations has been found to improve neuropsychological status when tested formally, convey a reduction in VGKC-Ab titre, and resolve SIADH-related hyponatraemia.

Other much less frequent anti-neuronal antibodies have been associated with LE. Patients with AMPA receptor antibodies (AMPAR-Abs) demonstrate a predominantly psychiatric phenotype, and patients with $GABA_B$ receptor antibodies ($GABA_BR$-Abs) tend to have seizures. Both are associated with malignancy, and it is thought that $GABA_BR$-Abs are responsible for the previously documented antibody-negative small-cell lung cancer cases. [7]

Anti-NMDA-receptor encephalitis

Anti-NMDA-receptor encephalitis (ANMDARE) was first discovered by Dalmau and coworkers in 2007 and since then has been found to be the second most common cause of immune mediated encephalitis after acute disseminated encephalomyelitis (ADEM) [8]. As in our case, the clinical syndrome appears to have a stereotypical progression starting with a prodrome of fever and headache. Within 48 hours patients can have seizures, and psychiatric symptoms begin to manifest such as anxiety, insomnia, and behavioural disturbances. This is followed by a characteristic movement disorder consisting of oro-facial dyskinesias, including grimacing and tongue protrusion, and axial and symmetric limb jerking. Other movements include choreoathetosis, oculogyric crisis, and dystonia. [9] Within days or weeks reduced consciousness develops with hypoventilation and autonomic imbalance manifesting as hyperthermia, tachycardia, hypersalivation, hypertension, bradycardia, hypotension, urinary incontinence, and erectile dysfunction. At this stage intensive care support is often required, as illustrated by our case who received ventilation for her hypoventilation and was monitored for tachycardia.

Evidence base

Dalmau J, Gleichman AJ, Hughes EG, et al. Anti-NMDA-receptor encephalitis: case series and analysis of the effects of antibodies [9]

A case series of 100 patients with anti-NMDAR encephalitis was reported.

- Median age of patients was 23 years (range 5–76 years); 91 were women.
- All patients presented with psychiatric symptoms or memory problems; 76 had seizures, 88 unresponsiveness (decreased consciousness), 86 dyskinesias, 69 autonomic instability, and 66 hypoventilation.
- Fifty-eight of 98 patients (59 per cent) for whom results of oncological assessments were available had tumours, most commonly ovarian teratoma. Patients who received early tumour treatment (usually with immunotherapy) had better outcome ($p = 0.004$) and fewer neurological relapses ($p = 0.009$) than the rest of the patients. Seventy-five patients recovered or had mild deficits, and 25 had severe deficits or died.
- Improvement was associated with a decrease of serum antibody titres.

Pathophysiology

Anti-NMDAR antibodies recognize an extracellular epitope and therefore are likely to be pathogenic. Studies on cultured rat hippocampal neurons show that antibodies from patients with anti-NMDAR encephalitis led to the rapid and reversible loss of surface NMDAR by antibody-mediated internalization, leading to impaired NMDAR-mediated synaptic transmission. How the decrease in NMDAR function leads to the clinical manifestations is unclear, but it has been suggested that pathways in multiple areas of the brain are disinhibited because of impaired recruitment of GABAergic interneurons that express NMDARs. This may be responsible for the neuropsychiatric (frontostriatal region), movement disorder (brainstem), and autonomic (dopaminergic, noradrenergic and cholinergic systems) symptoms seen in the disease. [10]

Learning point Investigations in anti-NMDA receptor encephalitis

- MRI can show increased FLAIR or T2-signal in one or several brain regions which do not appear to correlate with patient symptoms
- EEG normally shows generalized or predominantly fronto-temporal slow or disorganized activity (delta-theta) without epileptic discharges, in keeping with an encephalopathy. A 'delta brush' pattern (fast waves superimposed on the crests of delta waves) has been reported in some cases. (Figure 17.1)
- CSF demonstrates marked pleocytosis and the presence of oligoclonal bands. More specifically, it is now possible to test for intrathecal production of NR1 antibodies.

Unlike typical PLE, encephalidites with antibodies to cell surface antigens, such as ANMDARE, can respond to immunosuppressive therapy or improve spontaneously without identification of a possible tumour. However, it appears that tumour removal does accelerate improvement and reduces the number of relapses. One study suggested that 80 per cent of patients with a tumour (mostly teratomas) had substantial improvement after tumour removal and first-line immunotherapy, and only 48 per cent of those without a tumour had a similar degree of improvement after first-line immunotherapy and needed second-line immunotherapy more often. Overall, second-line immunotherapy resulted in substantial improvement in 65 per cent of patients [10]. Although randomized trial evidence is lacking, Figure 17.2 summarizes

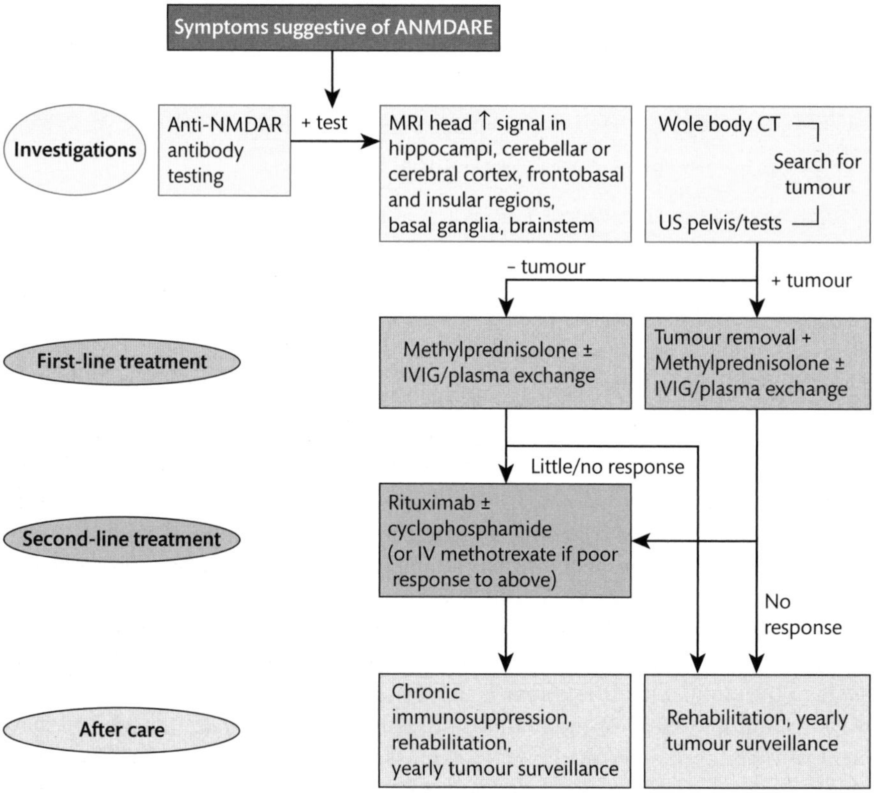

Figure 17.2 A suggested pathway for the diagnosis and treatment of ANMDARE.

Adapted from *Curr Opin Pediatr* 22(6), Florance-Ryan N, Dalmau J, Update on anti-*N*-methyl-D-aspartate receptor encephalitis in children and adolescents, pp. 739–44, © 2010, with permission from Wolters Kluwer Health.

a pathway for the diagnosis and treatment of patients suspected to have ANMDARE. There is a 25 per cent relapse rate, particularly in patients where no tumour was identified or who received suboptimal immunosuppression. [1]

ANMDARE cases we have seen in our unit usually have prolonged hospital admission with further months of physical and cognitive rehabilitation. It is recommended that these patients are screened for malignancy every two years, even if they have recovered neurologically. Relapses of ANMDARE do occur and may be associated with presence of an occult tumour, insufficient immunotherapy during the first episode, or withdrawal of the immunosuppression [1].

Stiff person syndrome (SPS)

SPS is characterized by fluctuating rigidity and stiffness of the axial and proximal lower limb muscles, with superimposed painful spasms and continuous motor unit activity on electromyography. It is believed the prevalence is 1–2 cases per million in the UK. Currently the Dalakas criteria can be used to potentially make a diagnosis of SPS [11].

Clinical tip Diagnosis of stiff person syndrome

- Stiffness in the axial muscles (predominantly in the abdominal and thoracolumbar paraspinal muscles leading to a fixed deformity or hyperlordosis).
- Superimposed painful spasms precipitated by unexpected noises, emotional stress, tactile stimuli.
- Confirmation of the continuous motor unit activity in agonist and antagonist muscles by electromyography.
- Absence of other neurological or cognitive impairments that could account for the stiffness.
- Positive serology for GAD65 (or amphiphysin) autoantibodies, assessed by immunocytochemistry, Western blot, or radio-immunoassay. About 60–80 per cent of cases have associated GAD antibodies.
- Response to diazepam.

Treatments for SPS are directed at the symptoms and the immune process. Benzodiazepines (GABA-A agonist), baclofen (GABA-B agonist), and anti-epileptics such as levetiracetam (GABAergic action) can be used for the symptoms[12]. IVIG, plasma exchange, or rituximab can be considered for modulating the immune process.

SPS variants

Progressive encephalomyelitis with rigidity (PERM)

PERM was initially described in 1976 [13] as a subacute disorder characterized by muscular rigidity, stimulus-sensitive spasms, brainstem dysfunction, and the pathological finding of perivascular lymphocyte cuffing and neuronal loss in the brainstem and spinal cord with relative sparing of the cortex. Further case reports have described stiffness associated with generalized myoclonus, hyperekplexia, cerebellar ataxia, and autonomic dysfunction. In 2008 glycine receptor antibodies were shown to be present in a typical PERM patient and since then ten further cases have been reported [14]. CSF analysis may show a pleocytosis. Management is similar to that for SPS.

Paraneoplastic SPS

Paraneoplastic variants comprise 5 per cent of SPS patients and manifest as stiffness mostly in the neck and arms, in contrast with the distribution of typical SPS [12]. It is associated with malignancies of the breast, colon, lung, and thymus, and Hodgkin's lymphoma, occasionally manifesting before the cancer does. Autoantibodies against amphiphysin and gephyrin may occur.

Final word from the expert

This case exhibits many typical features of NMDA receptor encephalitis. The patient was a young female with an ovarian teratoma, and presented with psychosis followed rapidly by seizures and autonomic instability, as well as a pathognomonic movement disorder. We have seen approximately a dozen patients with this disorder on the neurological intensive care unit at the National Hospital for Neurology and Neurosurgery, and management can be complicated by the need for long-term sedation and artificial ventilation. Although no randomized clinical trial data are available, our experience suggests that improvement is faster with early identification and removal of the teratoma if present, and aggressive immunosuppression. There is an argument for not delaying rituximab, because it is less effective once plasma cells are established.

References

1. Irani SR, Bera K, Waters P, et al. *N*-methyl-D-aspartate antibody encephalitis: temporal progression of clinical and paraclinical observations in a predominantly non-paraneoplastic disorder of both sexes. *Brain* 2010; 133: 1655–67.
2. Schmitt SE, Pargeon K, Frechette ES, et al. Extreme delta brush: a unique EEG pattern in adults with anti-NMDA receptor encephalitis. *Neurology* 2012; 79: 1094–1100.
3. Brierley JB, Corsellis JAN, Hierons R, Nevin S. Subacute encephalitis of later adult life mainly affecting the limbic areas. *Brain* 1960; 83: 357–69.
4. Corsellis JA, Goldberg GJ, Norton AR. 'Limbic encephalitis' and its association with carcinoma. *Brain* 1968; 91: 481–96.
5. Gultekin SH, Rosenfeld MR, Dalmau J. Paraneoplastic limbic encephalitis: neurological symptoms, immunological findings and tumour association in 50 patients. *Brain* 2000; 123: 1481–94.
6. Vincent A, Buckley C, Palace J. Potassium channel antibody-associated encephalopathy: a potentially immunotherapy-responsive form of limbic encephalitis. *Brain* 2004; 127: 701–12.
7. Zuliani L, Graus F, Vincent A. Central nervous system neuronal surface antibody associated syndromes: review and guidelines for recognition. *J Neurol Neurosurg Psychiatry* 2012; 83: 638–45.
8. Granerod J, Ambrose HE, Davie NW. Causes of encephalitis and differences in their clinical presentations in England: a multicentre, population-based prospective study. *Lancet Infect Dis* 2010; 10: 835–44.
9. Dalmau J, Gleichman AJ, Hughes EG, et al. Anti-NMDA-receptor encephalitis: case series and analysis of the effects of antibodies. *Lancet Neurol* 2008; 7: 1091–8.
10. Dalmau J, Lancaster E, Balice-Gordon R. Clinical experience and laboratory investigations in patients with anti-NMDAR encephalitis. *Lancet Neurol* 2011; 10: 63–74.
11. Dalakas MC, Fujii M, Li M, et al. The clinical spectrum of anti-GAD antibody-positive patients with stiff-person syndrome. *Neurology* 2000; 55: 1531–5.
12. Hadavi S, Noyce AJ, Leslie RD, Giovannoni G. Stiff person syndrome. *Pract Neurol* 2011; 11: 272–82.
13. Whiteley AM, Swash M, Urich H. Progressive encephalomyelitis with rigidity. *Brain* 1976; 99: 27–42.
14. Stern WM, Howard R, Chalmers RM, et al. Glycine receptor antibody mediated Progressive Encephalomyelitis with Rigidity and Myoclonus (PERM): a rare but treatable neurological syndrome. *Pract Neurol* 2014; 14: 123–7.

CASE

18 An unusual case of basilar stroke

Fiona Kennedy

Expert commentary: Martin M. Brown

Case history

A 54-year-old female accounts manager woke from sleep at 2a.m. with nausea and dizziness. She described the sensation as the 'world spinning'. On waking she also vomited. She had been feeling well the previous day and had gone to bed around 11p.m. with a mild headache. When she had woken up her partner noticed that her speech was different and she was slurring her words. She was also unable to move her left arm or leg and was noticeably unsteady. In addition, she described paraesthesia on the right side of her body.

She had a past medical history of treated hypertension and hypercholesterolaemia and was a smoker. She also suffered from bilateral carpal tunnel syndrome, and had had a nephrectomy for a staghorn calculus. Her medication included amlodipine 5mg and simvastatin 40mg. There was a family history of stroke; her mother had had a non-fatal stroke at the age of 68.

Learning point Risk factors for posterior circulation stroke

- Unmodifiable factors:
  - older age
  - male sex
  - ethnicity
  - family history of stroke or transient ischaemic attack (TIA).
- Modifiable factors:
  - hypertension
  - smoking
  - diabetes mellitus
  - high cholesterol
  - previous stroke or TIA
  - atrial fibrillation
  - atherosclerosis
  - structural cardiac abnormalities
  - alcohol
  - obesity
  - physical inactivity
  - thrombophilia
  - inflammation
  - infection
  - connective tissue disease.

Her partner called an ambulance and she arrived at her local hospital at 6a.m. On examination on admission her Glasgow coma scale (GCS) was 14/15. Examination of the cranial nerves revealed nystagmus on left lateral gaze, and she was dysarthric. She had left-sided weakness with hypotonia. Reflexes were all present and symmetrical. She had an extensor left plantar response. She was ataxic on the left and had a positive Romberg test. Sensory examination revealed reduced pinprick sensation on the right side of the body. Given these symptoms and signs, the patient was transferred to the emergency department at a tertiary hospital where she had been accepted for admission by the acute stroke team.

On arrival at the tertiary hospital, the patient's GCS was still 14. However, within minutes of arrival it dropped to 3. On examination at this point her pupils were dilated and unreactive, and she required intubation. A CT scan of her brain, including a CT angiogram (CTA), was performed under general anaesthetic. The CT showed an area of low density in the midbrain extending to the right, suggestive of an acute infarct. An acute intravascular thrombus, extending into the P1 segments of both posterior cerebral arteries (PCAs), was identified at the top of the basilar artery (Figure 18.1). As a result of this non-invasive imaging the patient was transferred urgently for angiography. Angiography demonstrated near occlusion at the basilar artery tip from a large filling defect, which extended into both the posterior cerebral and superior cerebellar arteries (Figure 18.2). The neurointerventional radiologist performing the procedure attempted clot extraction several times with a Solitaire™ stent and also attempted a loop snare that was unsuccessful. Successful suction thrombectomy was then performed with restoration of the normal artery lumen. Normal flow was re-established in the vessels (Figure 18.3). CT brain was repeated post-procedure to exclude haemorrhage, new infarction, or hydrocephalus.

Following the procedure the patient was extubated and improved rapidly, regaining a GCS of 15/15. She was transferred to the stroke unit for further investigation into the aetiology of the basilar artery thrombus and to commence rehabilitation. The investigations performed included normal urea and electrolytes, liver function, and thyroid function tests. The white cell count (WCC) was raised at 17.44×10^9/L, which is common after stroke but may also be a sign of concurrent infection. Glucose was 6.3mmol/L and total cholesterol was 3.6mmol/L. Antinuclear antibodies, thrombophilia screen, and antiphospholipid antibodies were all negative. An echocardiogram was performed to look for a cardiac source of embolus, and this was normal. Her electrocardiogram (ECG) showed sinus rhythm and a chest radiograph (CXR) revealed aspiration pneumonia, which was thought to account for the raised WCC. She was commenced on aspirin 75mg and clopidogrel 75mg, and continued on antihypertensive and lipid-lowering medications.

The patient was returned to her local stroke unit, and at this point she was mobilizing with the physiotherapists. On discharge she continued to have a mild left-sided weakness of MRC grade 4/5. She also had left-sided ataxia, intention tremor, and left fourth cranial nerve palsy causing diplopia on right lateral gaze. She did not require a lengthy stay at her local stroke unit and was discharged home on a community physiotherapy programme. MRI brain was performed following her discharge from hospital. The scan showed a small mature right-sided paramedian pontine infarct and further small regions of mature ischaemic damage within the right middle cerebral peduncle and left superior cerebellar artery territory. There were normal flow voids in the intradrual vertebral and basilar arteries.

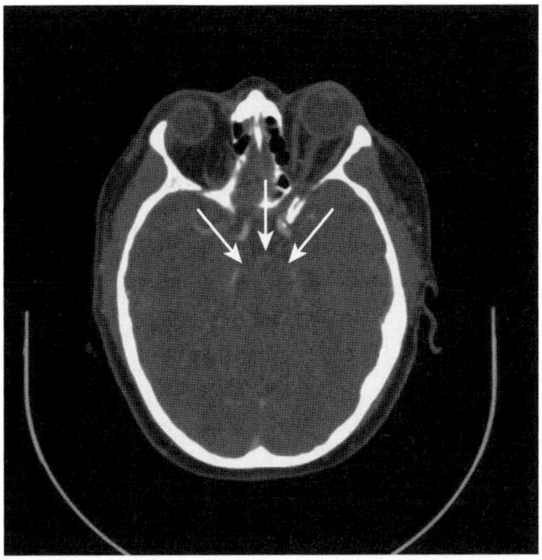

Figure 18.1 CTA performed approximately 8 hours after the patient woke up with symptoms. The white arrows demonstrate thrombus within the basilar artery and both P1 arteries, seen as absence of contrast. There is normal flow within the right P2.

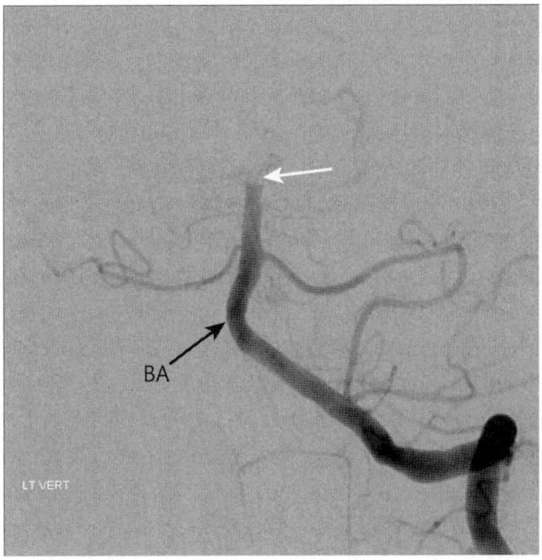

Figure 18.2 Angiogram prior to clot retrieval showing thrombus at the tip of the basilar artery (BA) (whitearrow).

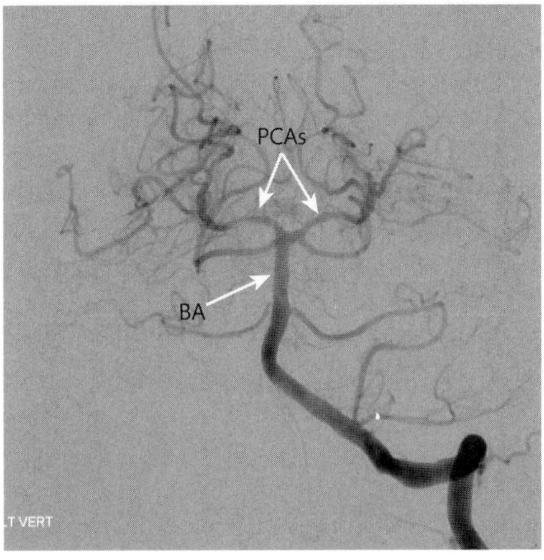

Figure 18.3 Angiogram following successful clot retrieval showing flow in the recanalized basilar artery (BA) and posterior cerebral arteries (PCAs).

As an outpatient she underwent a transoesophageal echocardiogram (TOE) but this did not show any evidence of patent foramen ovale (PFO) or significant valvular lesion. During stroke clinic follow-up, she was doing extremely well, mobilizing independently with a stick. She continued to attend physiotherapy and had been able to return to work on a part-time basis. Although independently mobile, she still had some problems with balance and therefore was cautious when she was outdoors in crowds. Blood pressure had been well maintained with the addition of bendroflumethiazide.

Discussion

The posterior circulation

The vertebrobasilar system and the posterior cerebral arteries supply the posterior part of the circle of Willis. The circle of Willis joins the anterior and posterior circulations of the brain. The vertebral artery arises from the subclavian artery and ascends through the foramina in the transverse processes of the cervical vertebrae and enters the skull through the foramen magnum. At the lower border of the pons it joins the contralateral vertebral artery to form the basilar artery. Branches of the vertebral artery supply the brainstem and cerebellum. The basilar artery and its branches supply the thalamus, pons, cerebellum, midbrain, occipital lobe, and temporal cortex. The vertebrobasilar system, like all blood vessels, can be affected by atherosclerosis, embolism, thrombosis, dissection, aneurysms, and inflammatory conditions [1]. The result of any of these disease processes is a patient presenting with a posterior circulation TIA or stroke. Vertebrobasilar disease accounts for approximately 20 per cent of all ischaemic strokes [2].

Clinical tip Decreased consciousness in posterior circulation strokes

Rapid deterioration in the GCS of a patient presenting with symptoms of posterior circulation stroke should alert the physician to considering basilar artery thrombosis as the mechanism of stroke.

Basilar artery thrombosis is an uncommon cause of stroke but it carries with it a very poor prognosis. The mortality rate associated with basilar artery thrombosis has been reported as high as 90 per cent [2, 3]. Patients who do survive rarely regain functional independence and are at risk of recurrent strokes [4, 5]. In the case reported here, the patient presented with a hemiparesis and sensory symptoms in the contralateral limbs. She also presented with a fourth cranial nerve palsy and involvement of the bulbar muscles, causing dysarthria. In this case, infarction extended to involve the middle cerebellar peduncle and superior cerebellar artery territory, which led to her clinical deterioration and reduced level of consciousness.

Learning point Presentation of basilar artery thrombosis

The symptoms and signs of basilar artery thrombosis are:

- drowsiness
- coma
- dizziness
- ataxia
- confusion
- headache
- hemiparesis
- hemisensory disturbance
- locked-in syndrome
- oculomotor palsies
- nystagmus
- facial palsy
- oropharyngeal palsy
- crossed signs in face and limbs
- homonymous hemianopia
- cortical blindness.

Atherothrombotic occlusions within the basilar system are common at areas of underlying narrowing, for example at the vertebrobasilar junction (proximal basilar) and the mid-basilar region. Atherothrombotic occlusion is rarely seen in the distal basilar artery. Intracranial large artery stenosis is more common in African American and Asian populations and is more prevalent in the older population [6, 7].

Embolism from cardiac, aortic, or proximal large-vessel sources accounts for 45–54 per cent of posterior circulation strokes [8]. Embolic rather than atherothrombotic occlusion is more commonly found in younger people [6]. Studies suggest that cardioembolic occlusions are more common in the distal portion of the basilar artery. Studies have also shown a poor prognosis in distal basilar artery occlusions (BAOs), especially when recanalization does not occur [9].

Basilar artery disease

The clinical presentation of basilar artery disease varies depending on the level of the stenosis or occlusion. More than 60 per cent of patients give a history of preceding symptoms of transient ischaemia in the vertebrobasilar territory [4, 10]. These symptoms include vertigo and nausea, headache, diplopia, dysarthria, homonymous hemianopia or cortical blindness, hemiparesis, and hemisensory disturbance. It can be difficult to time the onset of arterial occlusion in patients who describe this stuttering onset of posterior circulation symptoms. Patients with atherothrombotic occlusion of the posterior circulation can present with symptoms including hemiparesis, reduced level of consciousness, cranial nerve palsies, and locked-in syndrome. Locked-in syndrome manifests with quadriplegia, loss of horizontal eye movements, and relative preservation of consciousness. Communication with the patient can only be established through vertical eye movements and blinking. Locked-in syndrome occurs when there is occlusion of the proximal and middle segments of the basilar artery, causing infarction in the basis pontis.

Embolism to the basilar artery with temporary occlusion can present with transient ischaemic symptoms including acute transient loss of consciousness and brainstem symptoms. 'Top of the basilar' syndrome, described by Caplan [11], can present with an array of symptoms including reduced level of consciousness, motor and sensory abnormalities, visual and oculomotor abnormalities, somnolence, and hallucinations. Emboli can propagate to the posterior cerebral arteries and their branches, which supply the midbrain, thalamus, and temporal and occipital lobes. Infarction of the medial temporal lobe can present with memory impairment or amnesia in some patients.

Clinical tip Causes of basilar artery occlusion

Potential causes of BAO:

- vertebrobasilar atherothrombosis
- cardioembolism
- vertebral artery dissection.

Learning point Locked-in syndrome

The clinical picture of locked-in syndrome is:

- normal cognition
- quadriplegia
- loss of horizontal eye movements
- inability to speak.

Learning point Lateral medullary syndrome

Lateral medullary syndrome, also known as Wallenberg syndrome, is a consequence of dorsolateral medulla infarction.

- Aetiology: occlusion of posterior inferior cerebellar artery (PICA), vertebral artery, or perforating medullary arteries
- Classical symptoms:
  - ipsilateral Horner's syndrome
  - loss of pain and temperature sensation on the contralateral limbs and trunk and ipsilateral face
  - vertigo, nausea, vomiting
  - nystagmus
  - ipsilateral ataxia
  - dysarthria
  - dysphagia.

Imaging in posterior circulation stroke

CT is of limited value when imaging the posterior fossa of the brain. However, CT angiography (CTA) is an extremely useful tool for identifying large-vessel stenosis or occlusion in the posterior circulation. CTA has sensitivity and specificity of more than 90 per cent for identifying BAO and stenosis [12]. MRI is of greater value for identifying acute posterior circulation infarction. Magnetic resonance angiography (MRA) can also be employed to detect stenosis and occlusion in the posterior

> **Expert comment**
>
> MRI is more sensitive than CT at identifying posterior circulation infarction. CT angiography (CTA), time-of-flight magnetic resonance angiography (TOF MRA), and contrast-enhanced magnetic resonance angiography (CEMRA) are all valuable for detecting basilar stenosis/occlusion and the presence of thrombus. Digital subtraction angiography (DSA) remains the gold standard. Doppler ultrasound can also be used to diagnose basilar thrombosis/occlusion but is technically limited.

> **Clinical tip** Angiography in basilar artery disease
>
> Although conventional angiography is the gold standard for diagnosing basilar artery disease, it carries a risk of stroke of approximately 1 per cent.

circulation. Time-of-flight (TOF) techniques and contrast-enhanced MRA are able to produce high-resolution images. Extracranial and intracranial Doppler ultrasound can be used to identify BAO but is technically limited. In a study of 19 patients with BAO, Doppler ultrasound proved to be inconclusive in over 50 per cent of cases [12]. Conventional digital subtraction angiography (DSA) still remains the gold standard investigative tool. However, angiography is invasive, time-consuming, and limited to specialist centres, and has an associated risk of stroke of approximately 1 per cent. Non-invasive techniques are being used more widely for diagnostics, with DSA being reserved for patients with diagnostic uncertainty and those who require endovascular intervention.

Treatment

Most evidence to support the use of intravenous thrombolysis, intra-arterial thrombolysis, or endovascular clot retrieval in the context of BAO is based on small case series or single-case reports. There have been no completed randomized controlled trials (RCTs) in this area. Even RCTs of intravenous thrombolysis in acute stroke have not included many patients with posterior circulation ischaemia, and there have been no RCTs for acute posterior circulation stroke alone. Carotid endarterectomy, stenting, and angioplasty have been evaluated extensively and are shown to prevent recurrent stroke in patients with recently symptomatic carotid artery stenosis. However, such RCT evidence does not exist for stenosis or occlusion in the vertebrobasilar circulation.

An observational study from Helsinki of 50 consecutive patients with BAO treated by intravenous thrombolysis has been reported [13]. Recanalization was achieved in 60 per cent of cardioembolic and atherothrombotic BAOs, and in 71 per cent of dissection cases. At three months, 46 per cent of patients in whom recanalization was achieved were independent. None of those with failed recanalization were independent at three months. The complications reported in this observational study were intracerebral haemorrhage, multifocal haemorrhage, subarachnoid haemorrhage, intraparenchymal haemorrhage, and asymptomatic haemorrhagic transformation.

A study of 40 patients with acute BAO treated with intra-arterial thrombolysis showed that recanalization of the basilar artery was achieved in 80 per cent of the cohort [14]. Low baseline NIHSS and recanalization were predictors of favourable outcome, and there was a non-significant trend that patients treated within six hours did better than patients treated later. At three months 35 per cent of patients had a favourable outcome (modified Rankin score (MRS) ≤2), 23 per cent had a poor outcome (MRS 3–5), and 42 per cent had died. This study suggests that intra-arterial thrombolysis may be beneficial in selected patients with BAO.

A systematic analysis of published case series comparing treatment of basilar artery thrombosis with intravenous thrombolysis (IVT) or intra-arterial thrombolysis (IAT) [15] found that the rate of death or dependency was the same (78 per cent for IVT versus 76 per cent for IAT, $p=0.82$). Survival rates, percentages of good outcomes, and frequency of complications were also the same in the two groups. Recanalization was achieved more frequently with IAT than with IVT (65 per cent versus 58 per cent, $p=0.05$). In this analysis the likelihood of good outcome without recanalization was ‘close to nil’.

Several endovascular mechanical devices and techniques have been used to retrieve or lyse clots from the cerebral vasculature. These include the use of clot aspiration, laser, ultrasound, angioplasty, stenting, microwire clot manipulation, microsnares, and more recently the MERCI clot retriever device [16–20].

One small study adds further weight to the argument that recanalization improves outcome and provides evidence that mechanical clot extraction can be considered in certain patients with BAO [17].

Expert comment Summary of evidence from published case series

- Patients treated with IA thrombolysis within six hours of presentation did better than patients treated after six hours.
- Low baseline NIHSS, good collateral vessels, and evidence of recanalization were predictors of favourable outcome.
- Recanalization can be achieved with intravenous thrombolysis, intra-arterial thrombolysis, and clot extraction.
- Clot retrieval can be achieved using aspiration, laser, ultrasound, angiography, stenting, microwire clot manipulation, microsnares, and the MERCI clot retriever.
- The likelihood of a good outcome without recanalization is 'close to nil'.

Evidence base

The Basilar Artery International Cooperation Study (BASICS) was a prospective observational study of patients with radiologically confirmed BAO [21]. A total of 592 patients were analysed between 2002 and 2007. They were divided into three groups depending on the treatment they received: antithrombotic treatment only (AT), primary intravenous thrombolysis (IVT) including subsequent intra-arterial thrombolysis, or intra-arterial therapy (IAT) which included thrombolysis, mechanical clot retrieval, stenting, or a combination of these techniques. This observational study did not show any evidence to suggest significant superiority of any of the treatment groups. However, consistent with other published data, the authors showed that recanalization did protect against poorer outcome.

Bringing together the evidence from published studies, there is a non-significant trend for favourable outcome in patients who are treated within six hours, patients who have a low baseline NIHSS, patients with sufficient collaterals, and patients with little ischaemic damage on baseline imaging. Therefore, in the absence of clinical trial evidence, treating patients with BAO with either intravenous or intra-arterial therapy should be considered on a patient-to-patient basis at centres with the appropriate resources.

Conclusion

Without recanalization good recovery virtually never occurs. The PROACT II trial showed that survival in patients without recanalization ranged from zero to 20 per cent versus 40–80 per cent in those with recanalization [22]. Therefore the key to effective management of BAO is rapid diagnosis and early achievement of recanalization [23]. Although there is no randomized controlled evidence regarding the treatment of basilar artery thrombosis, studies that have been published have shown that a favourable outcome can be achievable with recanalization of the basilar artery. Therefore patients who were traditionally faced with a dismal prognosis may actually have the opportunity to achieve a favourable recovery. Until results from an RCT have been published, centres will continue to treat patients with BAO on an ad hoc basis, taking each individual's circumstances into consideration.

Final word from the expert

Basilar artery thrombosis carries a grave prognosis with a high untreated mortality rate. To improve outcome, the diagnosis needs to be considered and confirmed promptly with CTA or MRA in order to deliver treatment. There is no randomized controlled evidence to guide physicians towards optimal management, but published studies show an improved outcome with recanalization of the basilar artery. The key message here is that patients who do not undergo treatment to recanalize the artery have a poorer outcome than patients who are successfully recanalized. Recanalization treatment should be considered in all patients, but until the results of an RCT are available, decisions concerning optimal treatment will need to be made on an individual basis with multidisciplinary input.

References

1. Voetsch B, DeWitt D, Pessin MS, Caplan LR. Basilar artery occlusive disease in the New England Medical Centre Posterior Circulation Registry. *Arch Neurol* 2004; 61: 496–504.
2. Baird TA, Muir KW, Bone I. Basilar artery occlusion. *Neurocrit Care* 2004; 1: 319–30.
3. Wijdicks EFM, Scott JP. Outcome in patients with acute basilar artery occlusion requiring mechanical ventilation. Stroke 1996; 27: 1301-1303.
4. Hornig CR, Lammers C, Buttner T, et al. Long-term prognosis after infratentorial transient ischaemic attacks and minor stroke. *Stroke* 1992; 23: 199–204.
5. Archer CR, Horenstein S. Basilar artery occlusion: clinical and radiographic correlation. *Stroke* 1977; 8: 383–91.
6. Levy E, Firlik A, Wisniewski S, et al. Factors affecting survival rates for acute vertebrobasilar artery occlusions treated with intra-arterial thrombolytic therapy: a meta-analytical approach. *Neurosurgery* 1999; 45: 539–45.
7. Gorelick PB, Caplan LR, Hier DB, et al. Racial differences in the distribution of posterior circulation occlusive disease. *Stroke* 1985; 16: 785–90.
8. Caplan L. Vertebrobasilar disease and thrombolytic treatment. *Arch Neurol* 1998; 55: 450–1.
9. DeWitte TC, Moran CJ, Akins PT, et al. Relationship between clot location and outcome after basilar artery thrombolysis. *Am J Neuroradiol* 1997; 18: 1221–8.
10. Ferbert A, Bruckman H, Drunmen R. Clinical features of proven basilar artery occlusion. *Stroke* 1990; 21: 1135–42.
11. Caplan LR. 'Top of the basilar' syndrome. *Neurology* 1980; 30: 72–9.
12. Brandt T, Knauth M, Wildermuth S, et al. CT angiography and Doppler sonography for emergency assessment in acute basilar artery ischaemia. *Stroke* 1999; 30: 606–12.
13. Lindsberg PJ, Soinne L, Tatlisumak T, et al. Long-term outcome after intravenous thrombolysis of basilar artery occlusion. *JAMA* 2004; 292: 1862–6.
14. Arnold M, Nedeltchev K, Schroth G, et al. Clinical and radiological predictors of recanalization and outcome of 40 patients with acute basilar artery occlusion treated with intra-arterial thrombolysis. *J Neurol Neurosurg Psychiatry* 2004; 75: 857–62.
15. Lindsberg PJ, Mattle HP. Therapy of basilar artery occlusion: a systematic analysis comparing intra-arterial and intravenous thrombolysis. *Stroke* 2006; 37: 922–8.
16. Gobin YP, Starkman S, Duckweiler GR, et al. MERCI I: a phase 1 study of mechanical embolus removal in cerebral ischaemia. *Stroke* 2004; 35: 2848–54.
17. Mayer TE, Hamann GF, Brueckman HJ. Treatment of basilar artery embolism with a mechanical extraction device: necessity of flow reversal. *Stroke* 2002; 33: 2232–5.

18. Leary MC, Saver JL, Gobin YP, et al. Beyond tissue plasminogen activator: mechanical intervention in acute stroke. *Ann Emerg Med* 2003; 41: 838–46.
19. Kerber CW, Barr JD, Berger RM, Chopko BW. Snare retrieval of intracranial thrombus in patients with acute stroke. *J Vasc Interv Radiol* 2002; 13: 1269–74.
20. Nedeltchev K, Remonda L, Do DD, et al. Acute stenting and thromboaspiration in basilar artery occlusions due to embolism from the dominating vertebral artery. *Neuroradiology* 2004; 46: 686–91.
21. Schonewille WJ, Wijman CAC, Michel P, et al. Treatment and outcomes of acute basilar artery occlusion in the Basilar Artery International Cooperation Study (BASICS): a prospective registry study. *Lancet Neurol* 2009; 8: 724–30.
22. Furlan A, Higashida R, Wechsler L, et al. Intra-arterial prourokinase for acute ischaemic stroke. The PROACT II study: a randomized controlled trial. Prolyse in acute cerebral thromboembolism. *JAMA* 1999; 282: 2003–11.
23. Ford GA. Intra-arterial thrombolysis is the treatment of choice for basilar thrombosis. *Stroke* 2006; 37: 2438–9.

CASE

19 Will I walk again, doctor?

Sara Ajina

Expert commentary Angela Gall

Case history

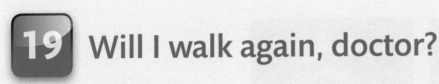

A 26-year-old woman was admitted to a tertiary neurology unit via her local hospital after falling from a first-floor balcony. She had been drinking with friends, when the railing she was leaning against suddenly gave way, causing her to fall 5 metres to the ground.

Paramedics who attended the scene recorded that her GCS was 15 and carried out the standard protocol of Advanced Trauma Life Support (ATLS). They administered high-flow oxygen, secured intravenous access, and started rapid fluid resuscitation. At all times the patient was assumed not only to have sustained a spinal cord injury (SCI), but also a potentially unstable spinal fracture. Paramedics carried out a basic examination, which included examination of the head, chest, abdomen, pelvis, and limbs for signs of multiple trauma. Diaphragmatic breathing and a flaccid paralysis of the lower limbs were noted. There was deformity of the upper thoracic spine, with the patient reporting severe back and neck pain.

As she was talking and able to maintain her airway, she was log-rolled to a supine position (optimal for spinal immobilization) and placed in a rigid collar with sandbags and a backboard for transport to hospital. It is during this initial stage that preventing extension of spinal cord injury is key, as well as maximizing oxygenation and circulation to optimize the chances of neurological recovery.

After the patient arrived at the hospital, monitoring showed a persistently low blood pressure and heart rate around 55bpm, which was attributed to neurogenic, rather than circulatory, shock. Management at this stage consisted of continued aggressive fluid resuscitation, whilst avoiding inotropic support which has been shown to be less effective at maintaining adequate spinal cord perfusion [1]. The patient was not given steroids, as per current recommendations [2].

Once the patient was medically stable, imaging was performed including an MRI scan of the whole spine (Figure 19.1a). This confirmed a fracture through the T9 vertebral body and an unstable T8/9 dislocation with significant compromise of the spinal canal and damage to the spinal cord below T6. A decision was made to perform spinal stabilization and the patient underwent posterior T6–T11 surgical fixation two days after injury. Figure 19.1b shows the post-operative imaging.

Clinical tip Immobilize the spine acutely

Because SCIs are likely to involve multiple levels, it is crucial to immobilize the entire spine during acute management. Ideally, log-rolling should be performed by five people as per MASCIP guidelines (<www.mascip.co.uk/guidelines>), with the head simultaneously moved through an arc, to minimize any movement to the spine.

Expert comment

Neurogenic shock is seen in approximately a fifth of patients admitted with cervical cord injury and a tenth of patients with thoracic SCI, with severity greatest in injuries above T1 because of complete interruption of sympathetic outflow [3, 4]. The situation in this case could be consistent with a high thoracic injury, causing at least partial interruption and thus impaired peripheral vascular tone and venous return.

Expert comment

There is no evidence to definitively recommend use of high-dose methylprednisolone in acute spinal cord injury, and it may have an adverse effect on early mortality and morbidity [5].

Weeks 1–4: early rehabilitation: *Assessment and rehabilitation planning*

Eighteen days after surgery, the patient was transferred to the spinal cord injuries centre (SCIC) for rehabilitation. Details of the injury and subsequent management were carefully reviewed, and a thorough assessment was carried out by all members of the rehabilitation team.

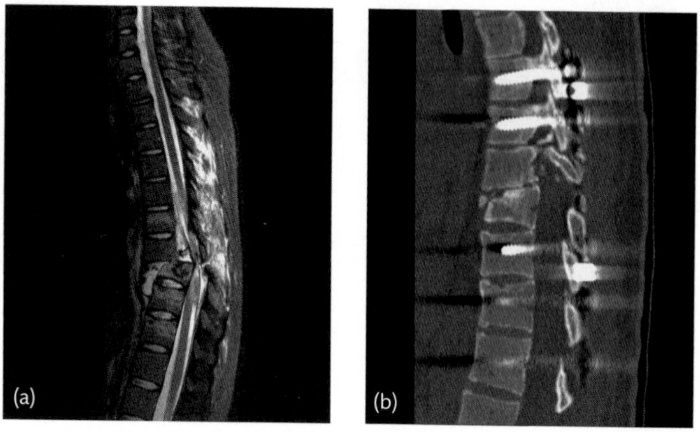

Figure 19.1 MRI and CT images taken before and after spinal fixation: (a) T2-weighted MRI showing the spinal cord injury, associated with a fracture dislocation at T8/9 with significant damage to the spinal canal; (b) CT scan demonstrating the posterior T6–T11 surgical fixation.

Apart from mild pain at the site of surgery, the patient was comfortable on a pressure-relieving mattress. Because the normal range for systolic blood pressure in SCI above T6 is often reduced to 90–110mmHg, it was necessary to adapt warning scores in her observation charts. Neurological assessment (Figures 19.2 and 19.3) demonstrated a neurological level at T5, AIS A (ASIA Impairment Scale A), with a zone of

ASIA Impairment Scale (AIS)

☐ **A = Complete.** No sensory or motor function is preserved in the sacral segments S4-S5.

☐ **B = Sensory Incomplete.** Sensory but not motor function is preserved below the neurological level and includes the sacral segments S4-S5 (light touch, pin prick at S4-S5: or deep anal pressure (DAP)), AND no motor function is preserved more than three levels below the motor level on either side of the body.

☐ **C = Motor Incomplete.** Motor function is preserved below the neurological level**, and more than half of key muscle functions below the single neurological level of injury (NLI) have a muscle grade less than 3 (Grades 0-2).

☐ **D = Motor Incomplete.** Motor function is preserved below the neurological level**, and at least half (half or more) of key muscle functions below the NLI have a muscle grade > 3.

☐ **E = Normal.** If sensation and motor function as tested with the ISNCSCI are graded as normal in all segments, and the patient had prior deficits, then the AIS grade is E. Someone without an initial SCI does not receive an AIS grade.

**For an individual to receive a grade of C or D, i.e. motor incomplete status, they must have either (1) voluntary anal sphincter contraction or (2) sacral sensory sparing with sparing of motor function more than three levels below the motor level for that side of the body. The Standards at this time allows even non- key muscle function more than 3 levels below the motor level to be used in determining motor incomplete status (AIS B versus C).

NOTE: When assessing the extent of motor sparing below the level for distinguishing between AIS B and C, the motor level on each side is used; whereas to differentiate between AIS C and D (based on proportion of key muscle functions with strength grade 3 or greater) the single neurological level is used.

Figure 19.2 The American Spinal Injuries Association (ASIA) Impairment Scale is used to classify SCI and can be useful in assessing prognosis.

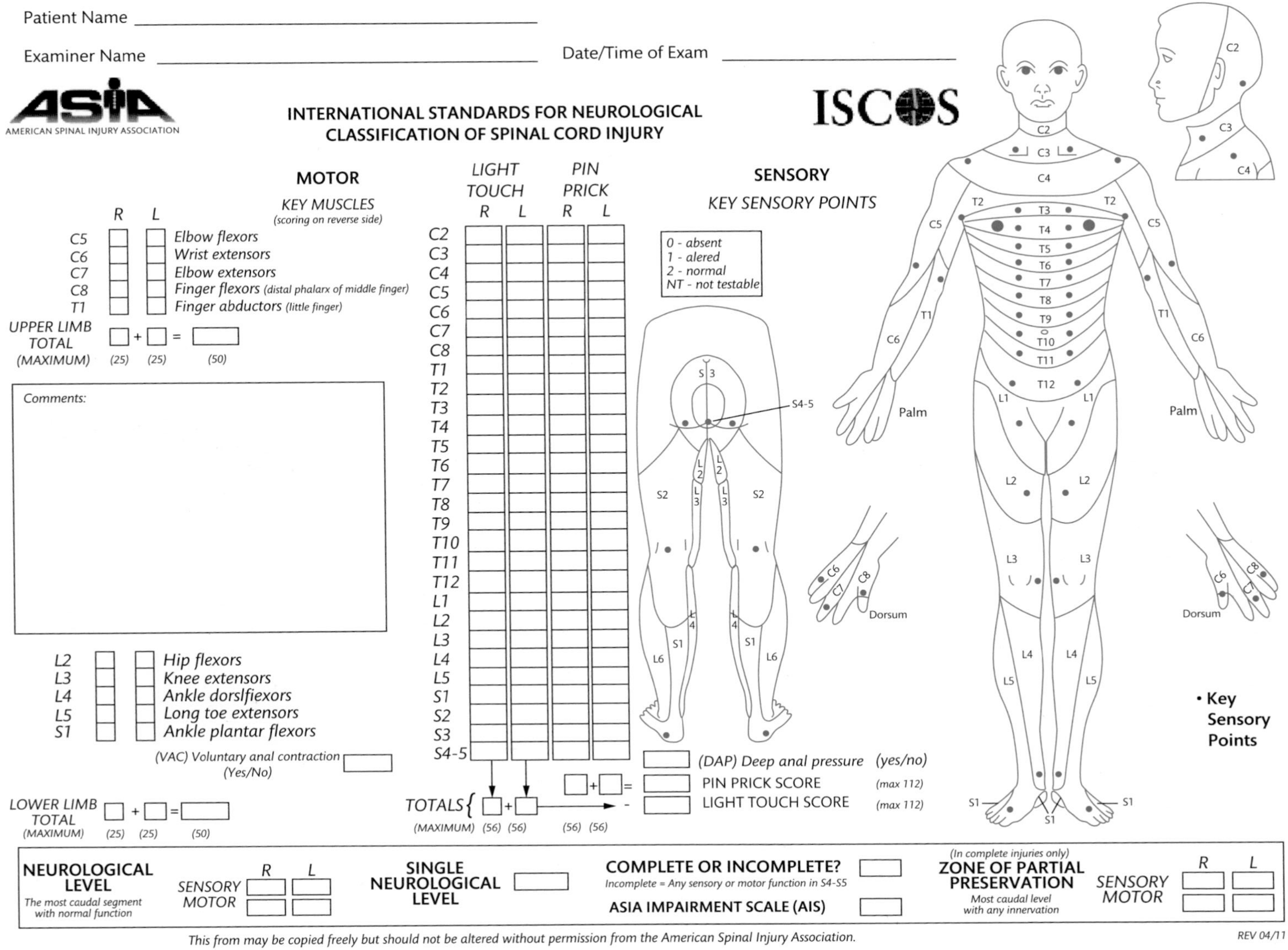

Figure 19.3 The ASIA score sheet allows the assessor to clearly demonstrate the sensory and motor levels of spinal cord injury, as well as its severity. This assessment should be carried out immediately on admission and repeated regularly, and if there are any signs of deterioration.

Reproduced with permission from the American Spinal Injury Association.

partial preservation spanning the caudal three levels (T6–T8). Muscle tone in the lower limbs was flaccid, with absent reflexes and unrestricted range of movement.

Clinical tip Carrying out the ASIA assessment

One of the most important tools for classifying and evaluating prognosis of SCI is based on the International Standards for Neurological Classification after Spinal Cord Injury (ISNCSCI), often termed the ASIA assessment. This determines the motor, sensory, and neurological levels of injury by giving a score for motor function (0–5) at ten index muscles bilaterally and for sensory function (0–2) at each spinal level below C1. Sensation is tested with light touch and sharp dull discrimination to pinprick, and it is useful to vary the stimulus a number of times for each level (i.e. when applying light touch versus no touch, or pinprick versus dull) to obtain as accurate an evaluation as possible. Sensation should be assessed on the front and back of the trunk and limbs. This must also include an assessment of voluntary anal contraction, deep anal pressure, and the sacral sensory dermatomes, which are essential to determine the overall impairment grade (see Figures 19.2 and 19.3) ranging from AIS A to E. If the injury is complete, it is necessary to determine the zone of partial preservation, representing an intermediate partially innervated zone caudal to the neurological level.

The routine management plan at this point is outlined in *Learning point: Critical points to consider at the start of rehabilitation*, with the addition of an up-to-date chest X-ray (Figure 19.4). The patient had been told what she considered a 'very basic' amount of information previously about her spinal injury and what it meant for the future, but was aware that she might not walk again (see Table 19.1 for prognosis in SCI). It was agreed that as soon as her scans and/or additional imaging had been obtained, a meeting would be held to discuss a number of issues: her diagnosis, what to expect for short- and longer-term prognosis, and what support was available to her. She was encouraged to attend with members of her family if she wished, and it would be an opportunity to show her images of the spinal injury, ideally with the meeting held in a consultation room, away from the ward. During her 12-week period of rehabilitation (Table 19.2), she would be issued with a weekly timetable incorporating additional time for a patient education programme about SCI, which is critical to achieving independence and self-management [6]. Fortnightly goal-planning sessions would be scheduled with an occupational therapist, a physiotherapist, a nurse, and a member of the medical team.

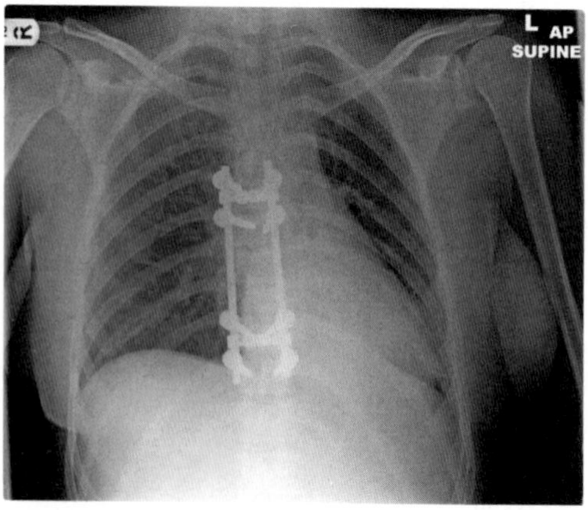

Figure 19.4 Chest X-ray on admission to the SCI unit confirms the absence of any significant chest injury and demonstrates the internal spinal fixation in-situ.

Table 19.1 Expected functional outcomes for complete spinal cord injuries

Level	Innervated muscles	Functional outcome
C1-C3	Sternocleidomastoid, cervical paraspinal, neck accessory muscles. Possible neck flexion, extension, and rotation.	Ventilator-assisted, with regular suctioning to clear secretions. Requires full-time personal care. Should have verbal independence. Power-assist wheelchair and environmental controls may be used with head or mouth controls.
C4	Upper trapezius, diaphragm, cervical paraspinal muscles. Possible neck flexion, extension, rotation, inspiration, shoulder shrug.	Able to breathe independently using diaphragm. Respiratory reserve may be low, secondary to paralysis of intercostal muscles. Dependency level and assisted devices as for C1-C3.
C5	Deltoid, biceps, brachialis, brachioradialis, rhomboids, serratus anterior (partial). Possible shoulder flexion and abduction, elbow flexion and supination.	Requires total assistance to sit up, but can be independent eating/drinking and basic grooming with adaptions and wrist splinting. May propel a manual wheelchair short distances, or power-chair via hand controls. Requires full-time care.
C6	Extensor carpi radialis longus and brevis, serratus anterior, latissimus dorsi. Possible forearm supination, wrist extension, and some horizontal adduction.	Can use a Tenodesis grip to provide basic but useful hand grasp function. Independent in eating and upper body care with adaptive devices. Needs some to total assistance in lower body personal care, bladder, and bowels, although most can perform ISC. May transfer independently on level surfaces. Independent propelling lightweight wheelchair. Able to drive an automatic car with hand controls. Requires part-time care.
C7-8	Latissimus dorsi, sternal pectoralis, triceps, pronator quadratus, extensor carpi ulnaris, flexor carpi radialis, flexor digitorum profundus and superficialis, flexor/extensor/abductor pollicis, lumbricals (partial). Possible elbow extension, ulnar/wrist extension, wrist flexion, finger flexion and extension, thumb flexion, extension, abduction.	Independent with all activities of daily living. Able to dress and undress independently, with intact overhead and broad reaching. Can transfer independently including split-level transfers, although may require assistance between wheelchair and floor. Can achieve advanced wheelchair skills.
T1-T9	Intrinsics of the hand, internal and external intercostals, erector spinae, lumbricals. Upper extremities fully intact, limited upper trunk stability.	Endurance and respiratory capacity may be increased secondary to innervation of intercostals. Independent with all aspects of care. Transferring independently with/without a sliding board. Independent standing with a standing frame. Below T6, not at risk of autonomic dysreflexia (although occurrence has been recorded with injuries as low as T8).
T10-L1	Fully intact intercostals, external obliques, rectus abdominis. Intact respiratory function, good trunk stability.	Some functional ambulation possible with forearm crutches or walker and caliper or KAFO to assist. May still require manual wheelchair for more functional mobility.
L2-S5	Fully intact abdominals and trunk muscles. Depending on level, some degree of hip flexors, extensors, abductors and adductors, knee flexors, extensors, ankle dorsiflexors and plantar flexors.	Excellent trunk stability. Partial to full control of lower limbs. May require frame or crutches (L3-5) and AFO to aid foot clearance on mobilizing (L3). Below S1 should have independent ambulation.

ISC, intermittent self-catheterization; AFO, ankle-foot orthosis; KAFO, knee-ankle-foot orthosis.

Table 19.2 Anticipated length of rehabilitation*

Ventilator-assisted tetra AIS A-C	20 weeks	Para AIS A–C	12 weeks
C3–C5 tetra AIS A–C	12 weeks	Incomplete UMN para AIS D	12 weeks
C6–C8 tetra AIS A–C	15 weeks	Ambulant cauda equina	6 weeks
Incomplete tetra AIS D	16 weeks		

*Example from a UK SCIC.

Learning point Critical points to consider at the start of rehabilitation

- Up-to-date ASIA within 24 hours of admission.
- Spasticity assessment: consider systemic and/or local antispasticity agents.
- Blood tests: FBC, U&E, LFT, Ca^{2+}, Gluc, PO^{4+}, Mg^{2+}, CRP, TFT, Vitamin B12, Fol, Ferritin, Vitamin D. Beware in particular of early hyponatraemia from excessive ADH secretion, and immobilization hypercalcaemia.
- MRI whole spine: check for multiple SCI levels, missed fractures/dislocations, post-traumatic syringomyelia.
- Definitive spinal management: ascertain spinal stability, any restrictions to spine movement, and orthosis requirements from spinal surgeons.
- Review all injuries if traumatic SCI, with optimal management plans.
- Head injury: review history for loss of consciousness, transient amnesia, and evidence of raised intracranial pressure. Assess cognition with six-item CIT and a more detailed tool if the CIT is abnormal. If at risk, must review or request CT head.
- Low-molecular weight heparin and TED hose: from 72 hours, for first 12 weeks of SCI unless contraindicated. High index of suspicion for thromboembolism.
- Anticholinergic: start 10mg oxybutinin XL early if suprasacral SCI.
- Proton pump inhibitor: prescribe acutely for 12 weeks in all patients. There is a 2–20 per cent risk of stress ulcer, with peak incidence at day 9.
- Ephedrine or/and fludrocortisone: prescribe prn if at risk of orthostatic hypotension with SCI, to use in addition to TED hose and abdominal binder.
- Nifedipine: prescribe 10mg prn in case of autonomic dysreflexia if SCI above T6
- Request urodynamic studies and renal tract US studies for 4–8 weeks post-SCI.
- Skin integrity assessment, provision of pressure-relieving mattress, and regular turning schedule as appropriate for current mobility level (high-risk, every 2–3 hours).
- Assess patient's understanding of current situation, expectations, and important cultural beliefs.

Learning point Prognosis of SCI

Table 19.1 describes the expected functional outcome for complete spinal cord injuries at every level, and normally provides a very accurate predictor of potential. However secondary complications or comorbidities may affect realization of the full functional potential. How patients progress in terms of recovery is difficult to predict, but may follow certain patterns with useful predictors from clinical examination. Data exists from observational studies and can be used as a guide in predicting prognosis, but it is important to acknowledge that it is not possible to provide an accurate prediction of outcome in an individual.

Complete SCI

Recovery and improvement is usually very limited in complete injuries. In tetraplegia, 70–80 per cent of patients will gain one level following a period of rehabilitation. Less than 1 per cent will gain functional lower limb power. In the upper limbs, if muscle groups show an initial strength of 1–2/5, one may expect an improvement to grade 3. In complete paraplegia, only 25 per cent of patients see an improvement in their neurological level, again with a possible improvement in muscle groups from 1–2/5 to 3/5. Generally speaking, cauda equina lesions have a better prognosis than lesions of the cord.

Incomplete SCI

In incomplete tetraplegia, more than 90 per cent of patients are expected to gain one neurological level. In particular, the patient's age and sensation to pinprick are useful prognostic indicators. If pinprick is preserved in the upper limbs, the majority of patients will gain power in the corresponding myotome to a score of over 3/5. If there is sacral and/or lower limb sparing of pinprick, patients are more likely to be ambulating at one year, and more than half will convert from ASIA C to ASIA D. In incomplete paraplegia, approximately 85 per cent of patients see an improvement of muscles graded at 1–2/5 to 3/5 by one year, and muscles graded 0/5 have a 26 per cent chance of improving to grade 3. Overall, 76 per cent of patients of all age-groups become community ambulators.

Expert comment

Weekly (or fortnightly) goal-planning meetings require the patient to work with the team to set specific long- and short-term targets to aim at during the admission. It also serves as an opportunity to record the current level of independence with the Spinal Cord Independence Measure (SCIM), providing an objective measure of progress similar to FIM-FAM used in non-specific neurological disorders [7].

Respiratory function

This is an important focus of therapy and nursing intervention in the early stages of rehabilitation. Patients with high thoracic and cervical lesions are particularly susceptible to respiratory complications, with an incidence of 67 per cent for SCI patients in the first month post-injury. With a T5 neurological level, volitional intercostal and abdominal muscle contraction is lost; the latter is normally important during the forceful expiration necessary to generate a cough. Therefore prophylactic chest treatment was started, including deep breathing exercises, percussion, and assisted coughing. This involves applying upward and inward pressure on either side of the lower ribs or upper abdomen as the patient attempts to cough, thus generating additional intrathoracic pressure.

Bladder

At this time the patient still had a urinary catheter on free drainage. This is useful early post-injury as a method of fluid balance monitoring, but is an obvious source of infection. Changes to the bladder after SCI can take several weeks or months to emerge in supra-sacral cord lesions, unlike the immediate acontractile bladder in conus medullaris and cauda equina lesions. Detrusor contractions can become associated with simultaneous contraction of the distal sphincter, causing obstruction of voiding—so-called 'dyssynergic distal sphincter' (DSD). This can cause high detrusor pressure, which can acutely trigger autonomic dysreflexia. If untreated over time, raised bladder pressures can lead to detrusor hypertrophy, vesico-ureteric reflux, and hydronephrosis, as well as incomplete bladder emptying causing recurrent urinary tract infections and pyelonephritis. Therefore a critical assessment of bladder structure, function, and pressures must be carried out; this is often done approximately six to eight weeks post-injury. This patient's results are displayed in Figure 19.5. Imaging of the renal tract with ultrasound should be repeated at least annually following discharge, and urodynamic studies should be performed every 12–18 months.

Clinical tip Neurogenic bladder management

Although the situation may still evolve, bladder management should be initiated early as achievable goals can be anticipated from the level and severity of SCI, predicted upper limb dexterity, and patient preference. Ultimately the aim is to maintain continence and prevent complications, and one of the best methods of long-term management in this case would be for intermittent self-catheterization (ISC) together with anticholinergic medication [8]; therefore oxybutynin XL 10mg was started on admission to the rehabilitation unit. This reduces contractility and increases bladder capacity, helping to lower detrusor pressures in a neurogenic bladder and prevent incontinence between catheterizations. With both techniques patients should be able to avoid the need to wear incontinence pads or urinary drainage apparatus, which was very important to this young patient. To learn ISC, the patient must be able to sit up, with nursing staff initially carrying out the procedure until the patient can confidently take over. The aim is to keep bladder volumes around 400ml, with catheterization initially performed every 4–6 hours on a timetable, changing on urge, if the patient has sensation, or to suit their daily routine as they become able to predict the times that their bladder will be full.

Clinical tip Autonomic dysreflexia

Incidence

Autonomic dysreflexia (AD) is a potentially life-threatening complication affecting 48–85 per cent of SCI patients injured at T6 and above, with onset after spinal shock has abated. It is most prevalent in individuals with complete lesions, although it does also occur in incomplete SCI.

(Continued)

Pathogenesis

AD develops due to interruption of the spinal sympathetic pathways linking supraspinal cardiovascular centres with the peripheral sympathetic outflow at the level of injury. The result is that sensory triggers below the lesion cause a massive imbalanced reflex sympathetic discharge, whose precise mechanism is uncertain. Hypotheses include disinhibition of sensory pathways or sympathetic systems, altered reflex responses in sympathetic preganglionic neurons, re-innervation of neurons by spinal interneurons, and denervation hypersensitivity.

Trigger factors

Common triggers include distension of hollow organs (commonly bladder and bowels), catheterization, UTI, urodynamics, activation of nociceptors, sexual activity, increased spasticity, functional electrical stimulation (FES), and heterotopic bone and skeletal fractures.

Signs and symptoms

Patients may develop a pounding headache associated with a sudden rise in systolic blood pressure (>20 per cent). Flushing and sweating of the skin above the lesion level, nasal congestion, and nausea can occur, reflecting attempted homeostatic parasympathetic activity above the injury level. If severe hypertension is sustained it can lead to retinal/cerebral haemorrhage, myocardial infarction, and seizures.

Management

Sit the patient up, remove any potential triggers, and if necessary administer an antihypertensive with rapid onset and short duration of action, such as 10mg nifedipine (bitten and held sublingually for rapid onset) or glyceryl trinitrate.

Bowels

As would be expected, sensation of the urge to defecate and voluntary control of the anal sphincter was absent in this patient. She was generally unaware when her bowels had opened, with frequent soiling of the bed sheets after being turned in bed. This was extremely distressing for her, exacerbated by a lack of understanding of why this was happening. As soon as possible after injury, a bowel regime should be instigated. Sadly, this is often not undertaken until the patient is admitted to the SCIC.

Together with a detailed education plan, the principle of this patient's bowel care was a pre-emptive strategy to routinely trigger defecation before reflex-mediated incontinence occurred. In the hyper-reflexic bowel, although voluntary control is impaired, connections between the spinal cord and colon as well as the myenteric plexus remain intact; therefore stool can be expelled via reflex activity. This can be further encouraged via the gastrocolic reflex where colonic activity is stimulated in the first 15–30 minutes after a meal or warm drink. Initially, this patient required a short period of laxative treatment as constipation (probably contributed to by post-operative analgesics, which were reduced on SCIC admission) had been causing rectal distension and incontinence. She was then started on a daily routine of glycerin suppositories with or without bisacodyl suppositories (more stimulating than glycerin), waiting 5–15 minutes before attempting digital rectal stimulation to encourage adequate stool passage. Typically, digital stimulation is continued for 30 seconds to 1 minute at a time, after which peristaltic activity and stool delivery occurs within seconds to a few minutes. This was initially carried out by nursing staff, although ultimately she would learn to perform this routine herself.

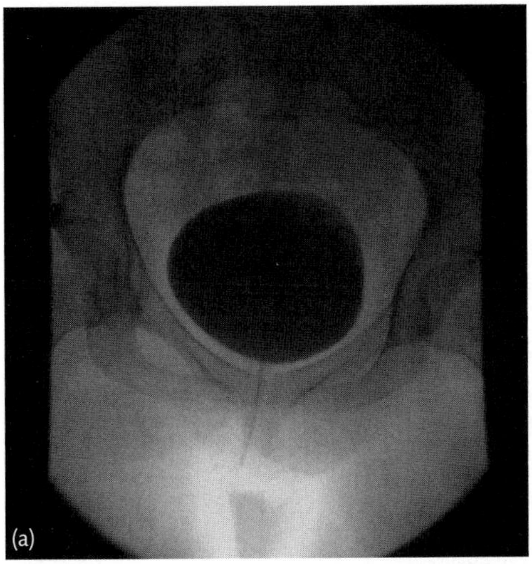

Cystometry

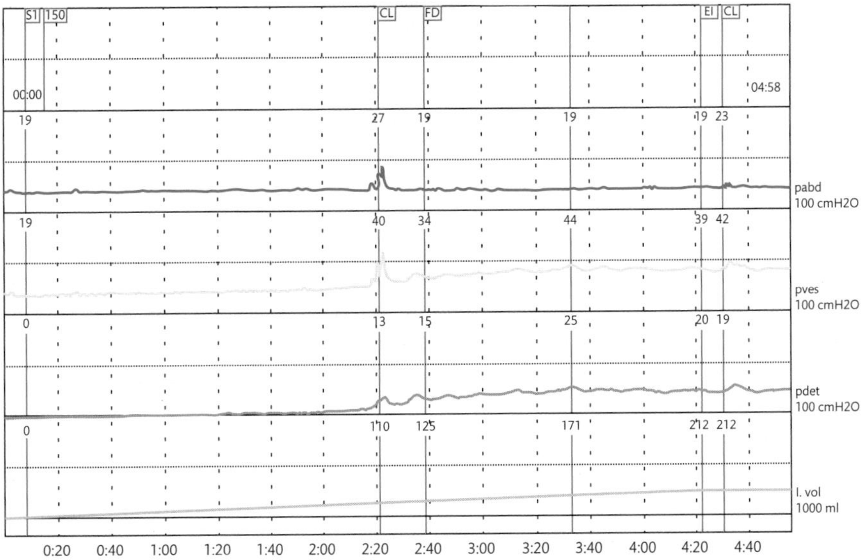

	First Desire	Normal Desire	Strong Desire	Urgency	pmax	@	Infused Vol
Vesical Pressure:	34 cmH2O	- - cmH2O	- - cmH2O	- - cmH2O	59		112
Abdominal Pressure:	19 cmH2O	- - cmH2O	- - cmH2O	- - cmH2O	43		112
Detrusor Pressure:	15 cmH2O	- - cmH2O	- - cmH2O	- - cmH2O	26		212
Urethral Pressure:	- - cmH2O	- - cmH2O	- - cmH2O	- - cmH2O	--		--
Ure. Closure Prs.:	- - cmH2O	- - cmH2O	- - cmH2O	- - cmH2O	--		--
Infused Volume:	125 ml	- - ml	- - ml	- - ml			
Compliance:	8 ml/cmH2O	- - ml/cmH2O	- - ml/cmH2O	- - ml/cmH2O			

Infusion Medium:	contrast	Max. Cysto Capacity:	- - ml	Max. Infused Capacity:	212 ml
Infusion rate:	50 ml/min	Min. Valsalva Leak Prs:	cmH2O	Min. Vesical Leak Prs.:	cmH2O
Position:	supine	EMG Coordination:		EMG Activity:	
Sensation:	normal	Compliance:		Detrusor:	hyper-reflexive
Unih Ura Relax:		Contraction inhibited:			
Catheter Type:		Provocation:			
EMG Electrode Type:		EMG Electrode Position:			

Comment:

nil fired off residual 450mls

(b)

Figure 19.5 Bladder investigations at eight weeks show reasonable filling volumes, with no early signs of vesico-ureteric reflux or detrusor muscle hypertrophy. Cystometry shows a mild reduction in bladder compliance associated with an increased detrusor muscle pressure (red line) for the volume of fluid infused (bottomline, abnormal if <10ml/cm), with no episodes of firing-off.

Posture management and physiotherapy

The patient had not yet sat out of bed and in view of her high thoracic level would be at risk of orthostatic hypotension. Furthermore, patients with tetraplegia or high paraplegia have paradoxically improved vital capacity when lying supine rather than sitting up. This is primarily due to gravity's effect on abdominal contents, causing a reduction in tidal volume when upright. To minimize this, staff were directed to apply an abdominal binder whenever she was to be positioned upright. This increases intra-abdominal pressure and places the diaphragm in a more efficient resting posture.

Trunk control was initially very poor, although the ability to balance would play a key role in learning to transfer independently. She would also need to work on the strength of her non-paralysed upper limb/shoulder girdle muscles that would be important in providing support. Once able, she was trialled on a generic stable self-propelling wheelchair before a custom-measured lightweight frame could be ordered through her local wheelchair service. She could then self-propel through the ward, which quickly increased her independence. Whilst still requiring assistance to transfer into the chair, she could attend gym sessions or the dining room on her own. Although, see clinical tip for the implications of increased wheelchair use on skin integrity.

Clinical tip Skin breakdown and pressure relief measures

Sitting in a wheelchair for prolonged periods of time can cause the skin to break down, with particular vulnerability over the ischia. Therefore it is advisable to build up time sitting in the chair over a number of days. It is also important to provide the correct cushion (in this case, a Jay 2 cushion for a high risk of skin breakdown) and to teach patients how to relieve pressure by leaning forward. This is ultimately their responsibility, and therefore should be emphasized at every opportunity. Most guidelines recommend two consecutive minutes of pressure relief for every 60 minutes sitting in a wheelchair.

She also started a supported standing programme. As well as significant psychological benefit, regular periods of standing can help prevent contractures, reduce spasticity, and aid bowel function. As the patient had already encountered problems with postural hypotension, she was given ephedrine 15–30mg prophylactically before each session. She was then able to lie on a tilt-table for 15 minutes at a time, with the vertical angle increased with each session as tolerated. By the fifth week, she could stand in an Oswestry standing frame for 30 minutes at a time.

Weeks 5–8: intermediate rehabilitation

Approximately mid-way through the admission, a meeting was scheduled between the patient, her family, and the rehabilitation team. Staff from her local area were invited to attend so that they would understand her likely health and social needs following discharge. This case conference was an opportunity for everyone to be updated on progress, what outstanding areas were left to focus on, and the expected destination and date of discharge. It was also an opportunity for the patient to voice any particular concerns or questions for the team, such as her interest in 'research' organizations offering patients the chance to walk again.

Expert comment Ethical approach to 'research' organizations:

The patient in this case started to express a strong interest in exploring electrically assisted walking devices and research into 'reactivation' of the nervous system, after one of her relatives had noticed a clinic online claiming to cure her spinal injury. This is a common scenario as patients, families, and

(Continued)

friends try and find solutions, with the internet and significant progress in biomedical engineering leading to a number of commercially available applications claiming to restore function. A useful approach would be to arrange a meeting for an open discussion of the current standards for treatment and issues around the absence of a cure. The importance of rigorous research should be explained, as well as the potential for harm and the absence of evidence from many of the centres worldwide offering so-called cures. If your own unit is engaged in research in any capacity, it may be helpful to provide a summary of current projects, with leaflets if available, and offer to pass on the patient's details in case relevant projects arise. It is also worth referring patients to the <http://www.escif.org> and <http://www.closerlookatstemcells.org> websites, which have details of the current state of science and information on unproven treatment clinics.

Spasticity

To date the patient had been progressing well with therapy. However, at around the fifth and sixthweeks, therapists had noticed increasing lower limb spasms and clonus that were starting to interfere with her transfer-board transfers, as well as her posture in the wheelchair. At this point, no obvious triggers to the onset of spasticity could be found, and its presence was felt to reflect the natural offset of spinal shock (see Table 19.3 for spasticity grading). Physical interventions had already been attempted; therefore it was necessary to consider additional approaches to work synergistically with stretching regimes. The patient was started on baclofen 5mg three times daily, to be uptitrated every few days if indicated and if side effects allowed, and she also trialled functional electrical stimulation.

Table 19.3 The modified Ashworth Scale*

0	No increase in muscle tone
1	Slight increase in muscle tone, manifested by a catch and release or by minimal resistance at the end of the range of motion when the affected part (s) is moved in flexion or extension
1+	Slight increase in muscle tone, manifested by a catch, followed by minimal resistance throughout the remainder (less than half) of the range of movement
2	More marked increase in muscle tone through most of the range of movement, but affected part (s) easily moved
3	Considerable increase in muscle tone, passive movement s difficult
4	Affected part (s) rigid in flexion or extension

*May be useful for grading spasticity to monitor progress over time and when assessing the efficacy of treatments such as botulinum toxin injection. It is also as an objective and universally recognized measure.

Learning point Spasticity

Definition

Spasticity is characterized by a velocity-dependent increase in tonic stretch reflexes and increased alpha-motor neuron excitability. **Spasms** can occur due to disinhibited polysynaptic reflexes and can be precipitated by stretch or other peripheral, noxious, or visceral afferents. In contrast, **increased tone** is the enhanced and prolonged response to muscle stretch at rest, via Ia and IIa afferents, which can be associated with connective tissue changes and abnormal co-contraction over time.

Assessment

This is a multidisciplinary approach, evaluating the pattern of spasticity, its severity (Table 19.3), obvious precipitants, and what effect its reduction would have, particularly on muscle power. Common or

(Continued)

important triggers include pain, constipation, infection, skin irritation, heterotopic ossification, and development of a syrinx within the spinal cord. Therefore it is useful to consider the assessment as a way of identifying underlying problems whose treatment may correct spasticity without the need for systemic agents.

Management

This can be divided into physical and medical therapies, involving systemic, regional, and local treatments.

1. **Systemic treatments** These can target centrally acting GABA receptors through baclofen, gabapentin, and benzodiazepines. Alternatively, centrally acting alpha-noradrenergic agonists, such as tizanidine and clonidine, can be targeted to inhibit release of glutamate and aspartate. Peripherally acting medications include dantrolene, which inhibits intracellular calcium release, and cannabinoids. Whilst there is no agreed protocol on choice of medication, all can be advantageous in generalized patterns of spasticity, and their actions are easily reversed. Disadvantages include a range of side effects such as drowsiness (most agents), postural hypotension and hepatotoxicity (tizanidine), and weakness that may worsen previous levels of function.
2. **Regional treatments** These can target afferent or efferent pathways. Afferent target options include topical anaesthetics, FES, epidural spinal cord stimulation, and surgical deafferentation. Efferent target options include intrathecal baclofen or, in extreme cases, intrathecal phenol which causes rapid protein denaturation. Whilst rarely considered at this stage in rehabilitation, intrathecal baclofen delivers doses of approximately a hundredth of the oral dose, resulting in marked potency to a targeted region but minimal systemic side effects. There is considerable evidence for its efficacy and functional benefits, although it requires surgical implantation, is expensive, and demands careful maintenance and monitoring for complications. Patients are evaluated beforehand by lumbar puncture, and test doses of 25–100μg baclofen are administered via slow injection. Muscle tone and function is then evaluated over a number of hours, using spasticity measures such as the modified Ashworth Scale (Table 19.3) [9].
3. **Local treatments** These include quick-acting peripheral nerve blockade to achieve focused relaxation of entire muscle groups, or botulinum toxin injection whose effect peaks at four weeks and lasts for up to 3 months. Botulinum toxin can be extremely effective by targeting individual muscles with a pure motor effect, although the dose can be limited, particularly in lower limb treatment (maximum 400 units of Botox® or 1000 units of Dysport®), and patients may develop resistance over time due to antibody formation.

Learning point Functional electric stimulation (FES)

FES works by applying safe levels of electric current to the distal ends of innervating nerves to cause muscle contraction. FES can be used by physiotherapists to aid muscle strengthening, improve range of motion, provide transient inhibition of spasticity, and facilitate voluntary motor function in incomplete SCI. For individuals with tetraplegia, FES can also be used to restore hand grasp and release. In paraplegic patients such as in the present case, FES can be useful for cardiac conditioning, improving venous return from the lower limbs, and possible prevention of osteoporosis although evidence for this is variable. This patient found particular psychological and cardiovascular benefit from using the FES-assisted bike for 30 minutes twice a week. This works via a series of surface electrodes to sequentially stimulate quadriceps, hamstrings, and glutei bilaterally through a computer-controlled device. The effect is to enable a patient with complete lower limb paralysis to experience coordinated and controlled movement of their legs in a way that would otherwise be impossible.

Whilst clearly beneficial, there are some issues to consider. First, patients with lesions above T5 may lose some cardiovascular benefit because of impaired sympathetic control, thus limiting the body's ability to increase their heart rate, stroke volume, and cardiac output. Secondly, the use of FES to restore **functional** movement lost due to neurological impairment is a relatively uncommon and expensive application that would not routinely be available.

Neuropathic bladder and recurrent urinary tract infection

By this stage, rehabilitation assistants were helping the patient perform intermittent catheterization every six hours, with volumes of 200–300ml, although she was experiencing increasing occasions of incontinence ('firing-off'), which in her case represented involuntary reflexive emptying between catheters, sometimes several times a day. She had now completed her urological assessment (see Figure 19.5), which confirmed that her detrusor pressures were raised with mild DSD. A urine sample showed no significant growth that would account for an increase in bladder symptoms. As she was only on a starting dose of anticholinergic medication (oxybutynin XL), this was increased to 20mg. It was also felt that commencing baclofen for her generalized spasticity might facilitate the bladder symptoms by action on striated pelvic floor muscles. If this was insufficient, a second anticholinergic agent [10] could be used before considering local therapies such as intravesical botulinum toxin.

The medication adjustments proved beneficial, but a couple of weeks later she started to complain of increased fatigue and a further exacerbation of lower limb spasms and urinary incontinence. She showed signs of UTI and therefore was treated with oral nitrofurantoin and increased oral fluids. However, by the end of the day, she had notably deteriorated with frequent distressing rigors, a heart rate of 130bpm, blood pressure of 85/60mmHg, and a temperature of 39.5°C. She was given high-flow oxygen and fluid resuscitated before being transferred to an acute bay for monitoring. Antibiotics were switched to intravenous piperacillin/tazobactam, according to local recommendations, and an indwelling urethral catheter inserted. Although she responded quickly to treatment, she developed two further UTIs and one further episode of sepsis during her rehabilitation.

Clinical tip Urinary tract infection

Individuals with neuropathic bladder are prone to bacterial colonization of the urinary tract. This risk is particularly high with indwelling catheters (98 per cent likelihood of bactiuria), although there is still a 70 per cent chance of bactiuria with intermittent catheterization, and these individuals are more susceptible to symptomatic UTIs. The vast majority of episodes of UTI in patients with SCI are caused by commensal bowel flora, primarily Gram-negative bacilli and enterococci. This puts patients at a significant risk of Gram-negative sepsis that can progress very rapidly, as in this case. Indeed, sepsis remains a common cause of morbidity and mortality in SCI [11]. Interestingly, colonizing micro-organisms often vary with gender or level of SCI; for example, *Escherichia coli* and *Enterococcus* account for over two-thirds of cases of UTI in female patients undergoing ISC [12]. Because of this high chance of colonization, clinicians must be guided by symptoms or signs of systemic infection when making a decision to treat. This is particularly difficult in instances of multiple bacterial growth, where it can be hard to ascertain which organism has been pathogenic in causing the infection. In such situations, where the patient is systemically unwell, it would not be unreasonable to treat all organisms grown.

Weeks 8-12: late rehabilitation

By this stage, the patient had decided to be discharged to her parents' home in the short-term, and move to her own flat when it was ready at a later date. The focus of therapy now was to maximize her independence prior to discharge. This included being able to self-medicate correctly, perform ISC and bowel management independently, perform split-level transfers, and check her own skin on a daily basis in case of early pressure sores or tears. At this stage it is also important to consider successful community reintegration, such as advanced wheelchair skills, facilitating a return to work, driving an adapted vehicle, encouraging hobbies or sports that were previously enjoyed, giving opportunities to socialize with other patients, family, and friends, and offering counselling on sexual function, body image, and relationships.

Learning point Trans-anal irrigation

Trans-anal irrigation systems, such as Peristeen®, can offer a reasonable alternative to conservative bowel management, and have been shown to offer some benefit in constipation, faecal incontinence, and symptom-related quality of life in SCI [13], as well as other causes of neurogenic bowel dysfunction. The principle behind it is effectively emptying the descending colon, so that the patient will be less likely to experience faecal incontinence, and the period between planned evacuations can also be extended. Although rare, there is an associated risk of bowel perforation, and incontinence may worsen in the short term. Therefore it is important to consider contraindications such as active inflammatory bowel disease before considering this option.

Reproduction and sexual function

As this patient was in her mid-twenties, it was necessary to approach the topic of conception and pregnancy proactively to avoid anxiety through misunderstanding and to provide a basic idea of what to expect. Most women of child-bearing age with SCI can successfully conceive, carry, and deliver a baby, although potential complications make it important for the process to be overseen by an SCI specialist.

Expert comment Sexual and reproductive function following SCI

Ovarian function in female SCI patients is less affected than testicular function in males, who invariably show a decreased number and motility of spermatozoa and abnormal morphology after SCI. This means that men may require vibro-ejaculation, electro-ejaculation, or direct aspiration of sperm from the testicle to retrieve viable sperm for artificial insemination, although care must be taken in SCI above T6, as autonomic dysreflexia usually occurs near or at ejaculation requiring nifedipine to be available. In women, reproductive function itself is generally unaffected, although care is needed to maintain good physical health and safe wheelchair positioning during pregnancy; for example, there is increased rate of complicated UTI, thromboembolism, and skin breakdown. In labour, because afferent innervation of the uterus comes from T10–L1, 25 per cent of women are unable to detect its onset. Uterine contractions also arise from T10–T12, and so women (including this patient) with SCI above T10 should have effective uterine contractions enabling normal progression of labour, although lack of voluntary abdominal contractions leads to a slightly higher incidence of assisted delivery with forceps or vacuum. However, one would expect abdominal muscle spasms to shorten labour duration. Most women with SCI above T6 are at risk of autonomic dysreflexia with uterine contractions, which can be life-threatening for both mother and baby. Spinal or epidural anesthesia extending to T10 at the start of labour can prevent this, but if this is insufficient they must be treated with antihypertensives or magnesium sulphate, or by expediting delivery [14].

Neurogenic heterotopic ossification

During the two weeks before discharge the patient developed a warm swollen right thigh, associated with pyrexia of 38°C. Blood tests revealed raised inflammatory markers with CRP 234 and CK 2700, but normal full blood count, liver, and renal function. Because of the high risk of thromboembolism in this patient group, urgent Doppler ultrasound was requested but was normal. Her symptoms continued to worsen, exacerbating lower limb spasms and stiffness. An MRI scan was performed see (Figure 19.6) which confirmed marked muscle oedema around the right buttock and thigh with features consistent with developing heterotopic ossification (HO).

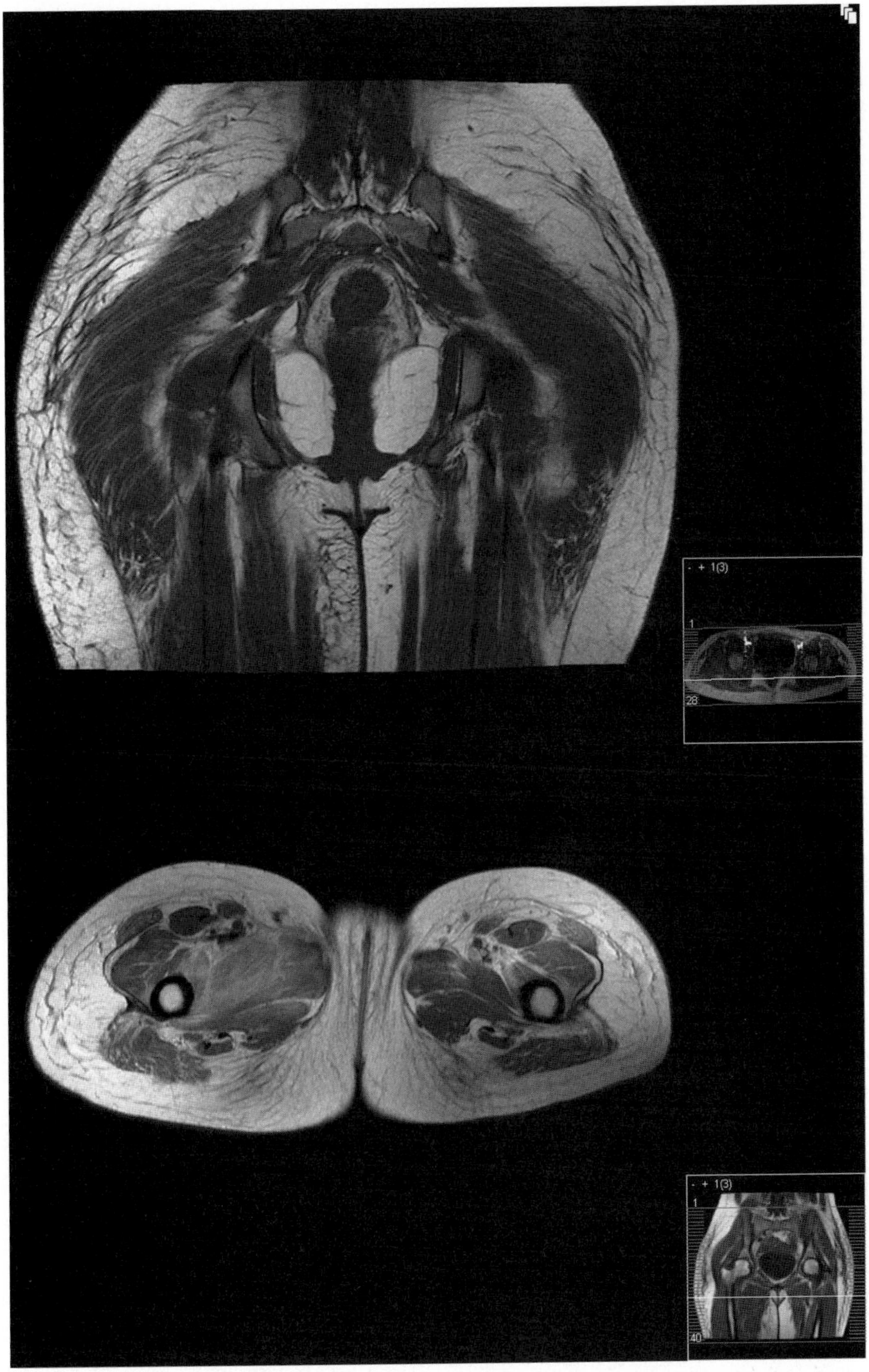

Figure 19.6 MRI T1-weighted coronal and axial images demonstrating early neurogenic heterotopic ossification. There is clear evidence of muscle oedema around the right buttock and proximal thigh region, involving predominantly the gluteus medius and minimus, the iliacus, and the adductor muscle groups. Perifascial fluid is also seen on both sides, with mild oedema within the distal aspect of the left gluteus maximus and around the left psoas insertion into the proximal femur.

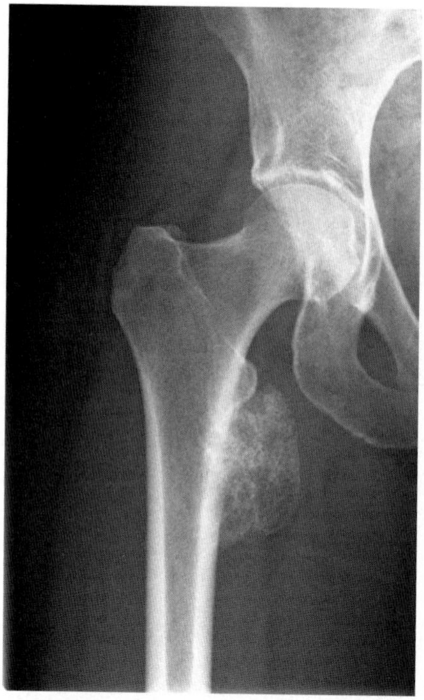

Figure 19.7 Late radiographic changes in neurogenic HO demonstrate calcification around the lesser trochanter of the right femur. When severe, this can progress to ankylosis of the joint with a restricted range of movement affecting transfers and spasticity, and causing marked discomfort.

HO diagnosis requires a combination of clinical, haematological, and radiological findings, with X-ray signs of calcification often absent early on. As in this case, inflammatory markers are elevated acutely, particularly with an increase in alkaline phosphatase (see the learning point on neurogenic HO for the underlying pathophysiology). Ultrasound can be useful early, although its value will depend on the experience of the radiologist; it is most useful for excluding important differentials such as deep vein thrombosis, haematoma, or tumour. The gold standard for early diagnosis was a three-phase technetium-99m bone scan, which can also be useful in monitoring maturation. However, MRI is increasingly the investigation of choice, demonstrating an increased signal from oedema in muscles, fascia, and subcutaneous tissue during acute onset [15]. Two to six weeks after the bone scan, one would start to see soft tissue calcification on a plain film (Figure 19.7) which can be highly specific for HO.

Learning point Neurogenic heterotopic ossification

Neurogenic HO is the formation of new lamellar bone in the soft tissue around a joint and is a major complication of brain injury and SCI, where it is seen in 16–53 per cent of patients. It typically develops 1–4 months post-injury, and presents with swelling, erythema, and warmth in the soft tissue close to a joint affected by neurological disease, with associated reduced range of movement and a low-grade fever. Pathophysiologically, there is inappropriate differentiation of mesenchymal cells to bone precursor cells, causing inappropriate osteoblastic activity which is associated in its early stages with increased blood flow, oedema, and formation of osteoid. The osteoid calcifies over a number of weeks, before more gradually remodelling and maturing into trabecular bone by approximately 18 months. The aetiology of HO is not precisely understood, although local tissue trauma is probably important, and starting all SCI patients with early gentle passive range-of-motion exercises seems to be preventative. Consequences can be problematic, including pain (if sensation is preserved), increased spasticity, peripheral nerve entrapment, and reduced range of movement leading to limitations in function, difficulty with posture and seating, and increased risk of pressure sores.

There are no specific pharmacological guidelines for management of HO, but in the acute phase vigorous movement of the joint should be avoided as this may exacerbate bone formation. The mainstays of drug treatment in most centres are non-steroidal anti-inflammatory drugs (NSAIDs) and sometimes bisphosphonates, although both lack supportive RCTs and NSAIDs may only minimize progression rather than reverse pathology. Bisphosphonates suppress mineralization of osteoid tissue and have been shown to reverse up to half of early lesions [16]. This patient was started on high-dose etidronate (20mg/kg/day) for two weeks, followed by half-dose for a further 10 weeks. She was also prescribed indometacin with stomach protection (a proton pump inhibitor) whilst her inflammatory markers remained elevated. This only affected a few days of rehabilitation and she was able to resume normal activities after a week, although she did not use the FES-bike until all signs of inflammation had resolved.

By the time of discharge, this patient had achieved an expected level of independence and education about SCI and its complications. She had spent a couple of successful weekends at home and knew that after discharge she could access the community liaison team, and would attend a follow-up at three months.

Final word from the expert

In the long-term management of SCI, it is essential for clinicians to remain alert to a number of complications associated with increased morbidity and mortality. These include late spinal instability and post-traumatic syringomyelia causing ascending myelopathy (in trauma cases), increased and early-onset cardiovascular disease, osteoporosis, respiratory complications, and the ongoing risk of pressure sores causing osteomyelitis. Therefore it is important to address these issues at regular intervals, as well as optimizing and maintaining function over time, monitoring psychosocial well-being, using the patient support network, and checking for any ongoing symptoms as presented in this case. Ultimately the goal of rehabilitation is to optimize health, to prevent and minimize disability resulting from this condition, and to achieve an optimal community participation and sustained quality of life.

References

1. Gilbert J. Critical care management of the patient with acute spinal cord injury. *Crit Care Clin* 1987; 3: 549–67.
2. Consortium for Spinal Cord Medicine. Early acute management in adults with spinal cord injury: a clinical practice guideline for health-care professionals. *J Spinal Cord Med* 2008; 31(4): 403–79.
3. Gulya HR, Bouamrab O, Leckyc FE. The incidence of neurogenic shock in patients with isolated spinal cord injury in the emergency department. *Resuscitation* 2008; 76: 57–62.
4. Nacimiento W, Noth J. What, if anything, is spinal shock? *Arch Neurol* 1999; **56**: 1033–5.
5. Short DJ, El Masry WS, Jones PW. High dose methylprednisolone in the management of acute spinal cord injury: a systematic review from a clinical perspective. *Spinal Cord* 2000; 38(5): 273–86.
6. Williams S. The role of patient education in the rehabilitation of people with spinal cord injuries. *Int J Ther Rehabil* 2008; 15(4): 174–9.
7. Catz A, Itzkovich M, Agranov E, et al. SCIM—spinal cord independence measure: a new disability scale for patients with spinal cord lesions. *Spinal Cord* 1997; 35: 850–6.

8. Nosseir M, Hinkel A, Pannek J. (2007) Clinical usefulness of urodynamic assessment for maintenance of bladder function in patients with spinal cord injury. *Neurourol Urodyn* 2007; 26(2): 228–33.
9. Bohannon RW, Smith MB. Interrater reliability of a modified Ashworth scale of muscle spasticity. *Phys Ther* 1987; 67(2): 206–7.
10. Kennelly MJ, Devoe WB. Overactive bladder: pharmacologic treatments in the neurogenic population. *Rev Urol* 2008; 10(3): 182–91.
11. Thietje R, Pouw MH, Schulz AP, et al. Mortality in patients with traumatic spinal cord injury: descriptive analysis of 62 deceased subjects. *J Spinal Cord Med* 2011; 34(5): 482–7.
12. Bennett CJ, Young MN, Darrington H. Differences in urinary tract infection in male and female spinal cord injury patients on intermittent catheterization. *Paraplegia* 1995; 33: 69–72.
13. Christensen P, Bazzocchi G, Coggrave M, et al. A randomized, controlled trial of transanal irrigation versus conservative bowel management in spinal cord-injured patients. *Gastroenterology* 2006; 131(3): 738–47.
14. Ghidini A, Simonson MR. Pregnancy after spinal cord injury: a review of the literature. *Top Spinal Cord Inj Rehabil* 2011; 16(3): 93–103.
15. Wick L, Berger M, Knecht H, et al. Magnetic resonance signal alterations in the acute onset of heterotopic ossification in patients with spinal cord injury. *EurRadiol* 2005; 15(9): 1867–75.
16. Banovac K. The effect of etidronate on late development of heterotopic ossification after spinal cord injury. *J Spinal Cord Med* 2000; 23(1): 40–4.

CASE

20 Parkinsonism with little response to levodopa

Karen M. Doherty

Expert commentary: Henry Houlden

Case history

A 57-year-old woman developed a tremor, stiffness, and weakness in her left hand and arm. She described difficulty stirring cake mixes and brushing her hair. There was no sensory disturbance or pain. The symptoms had developed gradually over a few months and there was no clear precipitating event or injury. She was otherwise in good health; her only medication was an ACE inhibitor for mild hypertension. There was no family history of neurological disease. When she attended her GP, examination revealed an intermittent rest tremor of the left hand, cogwheeling rigidity, and asymmetrically brisk reflexes of the left arm. She was referred to a neurologist for assessment and management of suspected Parkinson's disease.

At the neurology appointment she described a feeling of inner tremulousness and an occasional shake of her left hand. She was right-handed but had noticed difficulty doing kitchen chores which required her to use both hands. On occasion she had dropped items from her left hand. She also described vivid dreams, and her husband reported that she often moaned in her sleep. On examination she was hypomimic, had reduced arm swing during walking and her gait was slow. There was moderate cogwheeling rigidity of the left arm and subtle rigidity of the right. Speed and amplitude of rapid alternating movements (finger taps, pronation–supination of the hands, heel taps) were reduced bilaterally but were worse on the left. She had slightly increased axial tone on neck flexion–extension. Limb reflexes were generally brisk and slightly asymmetrical (left > right) but plantar responses were flexor. A diagnosis of probable Parkinson's disease was made and she was started on levodopa therapy.

A few months later she returned to clinic and complained that her condition had deteriorated. She denied any significant improvement in her symptoms on a levodopa dose of 250mg/day. She reported general slowing down, and her husband reported a slowness and quietness of her speech. She described feelings of loss of balance and a tendency to fall, especially when she was turning. On examination her facial expression was flat, she was hypophonic, and her speech was mildly dysarthric. There was moderate cogwheeling rigidity and bradykinesia in both upper limbs. On the pull test she took six steps back to stop herself from falling. It was suggested that she increase her daily dose of levodopa to at least 600mg.

Six months later she was taking 800mg of levodopa daily but still felt that there was little improvement. She described no 'on' or 'off' fluctuations and had no limb dyskinesias. She described a 'giddy' feeling after walking up the stairs and after rising from a deep chair. Her GP had recently stopped her antihypertensive medication. Examination was relatively unchanged except that she was noted to have grimacing movements around her lower face involving her mouth and lips. Her blood pressure fell from 120/80mmHg lying to 90/65mmHg after standing for two minutes, and it was considered that she might have an atypical parkinsonian condition, possibly multiple system atrophy (MSA).

At review three years from onset she complained of worsening balance and tending to fall to the left. She described her handwriting as miniscule and illegible. She had begun to have difficulty swallowing and had developed neck stiffness and urinary incontinence. She continued to take levodopa as she felt that perhaps it reduced her stiffness, but when 'on' levodopa she continued to have pouting and grimacing movements of her face. The dose had been reduced to 500mg/day because of the orofacial dystonia and orthostatic hypotension. She felt that her tremor had become more jerky and intermittent. On examination she was hypophonic and dysarthric, and her tongue movements were slow. She was slow to respond to questions but there was no evidence of cognitive impairment. Eye movements and saccades were of normal speed and range, but pursuit eye movements were broken (saccadic). There was no nystagmus or cerebellar signs on limb examination. There was no resting tremor but she had tiny side-to-side movement of her outstretched fingers (polyminimyoclonus) and occasional jerks of her arms (myoclonus); tone was moderately increased in her limbs but was worse axially. She had slow and small amplitude finger taps and hand movements and tended to hold her hands in a flexed posture. Her head position was dropped forward but neck muscles were hypertrophic, rigid, and strong, typical of antecollis. Reflexes remained brisk and she now had bilateral extensor plantar responses. She walked with a stoop and leant to the left, with no arm swing. A 40mmHg drop in her systolic blood pressure was present on standing from the supine position. Her diagnosis was felt to be probable MSA, and an MRI brain scan was requested to look for specific features supportive of this. She was started on domperidone for orthostatic hypotension (OH) and solifenacin for bladder instability.

Learning point Criteria for diagnosis of MSA [1, 2]

Definite MSA

Extensive glial cytoplasmic inclusions staining positively with α-synuclein accompanied by striatonigral and/or olivopontocerebellar degeneration on neuropathological examination.

Probable MSA

Sporadic progressive disease beginning at >30 years of age with autonomic failure (urinary incontinence plus erectile dysfunction in males) or orthostatic hypotension and at least one of the following:

- poorly levodopa-responsive parkinsonism
- cerebellar syndrome

Possible MSA

Sporadic progressive disease beginning at >30 years of age with parkinsonism or a cerebellar syndrome and

- at least one feature of dysautonomia
- at least one of the following:
    - upgoing plantar response with hyperreflexia
    - stridor

(Continued)

- o rapid progression of parkinsonism
- o poor levodopa response
- o postural instability within three years
- o gait/limb ataxia, cerebellar dysarthria, or oculomotor dysfunction
- o dysphagia within five years
- o atrophy on MRI of putamen, middle cerebellar peduncle (MCP), pons, or cerebellum
- o hypometabolism on FDG-PET in putamen, brainstem, or cerebellum
- o parkinsonism
- o presynaptic nigrostriatal dopaminergic denervation on SPECT/PET (abnormal DaT scan).

Brain MRI was significant for the 'hot cross bun' sign in the mid pons (Figures 20.1a and 20.1b). More superiorly there was also evidence of T2 hypointensity in the putamina bilaterally, with a rim of high signal at the lateral putamina ('slit-like void' sign) (Figure 20.1c). There was mild generalized atrophy of the cerebral hemispheres and cerebellum, and the pons also appeared a little reduced in volume on sagittal view (Figure 10.1d). These findings, together with the clinical history, were supportive of the diagnosis of MSA.

Learning point MRI findings to look for in suspected MSA [3–6]

- The 'hot-cross bun' sign (Figures 20.1a and 20.1b)—a cruciform hyperintensity on T2-weighted MRI in mid pons (thought to reflect loss of the pontine neurons and myelinated transverse cerebellar fibres but sparing the corticospinal tracts).
- Cerebellar atrophy (especially of the vermis and MCPs).
- The 'middle cerebellar peduncle sign'—MCP hyperintensities on T2-weighted MRI.
- Pontine atrophy.
- Putaminal atrophy or the 'slit-like void' sign (Figure 20.1c)—hypointense signal on T2-weighted MRI with a hyperintense rim in the external putamen (due to gliosis), highly specific for MSA but less commonly found than the features above.

At the age of 62, five years from disease onset, the patient attended clinic in a wheelchair. She was still able to walk very slowly with assistance. She complained of headaches radiating to the back of her neck which improved when she was lying supine, suggestive of 'coat-hanger pain'. Urinary frequency, nocturia, and incontinence had become more problematic despite antimuscarinic treatment. Her husband reported snoring and disrupted noisy breathing at night. On standing she was noted to have 'bobbing legs'—a jerky up-and-down motion which is a manifestation of negative myoclonus. Polyminimyoclonus was widespread in the fingers of both outstretched hands and generalized myoclonus was observed around her shoulders, legs, and trunk. She communicated mainly via light writer. Speech, swallowing, and salivation were complicated by 'jaw-opening' and occasional 'tongue-protrusion' dystonia which necessitated further reduction in her levodopa treatment to 300mg/day and focused botulinum toxin injections. Postural hypotension was again present and provoked feelings of dizziness. She was started on fludrocortisone 100μg/day for OH and clonazepam 0.5mg bd for the generalized myoclonus. Formal autonomic function testing and ENT review were requested.

Urodynamic studies revealed poor bladder emptying with a post-void residual volume of 70ml and features of mixed stress urge incontinence. Orthostatic hypotension was present on head-up tilt; hypotension also occurred during mental arithmetic. Respiratory sinus arrhythmia was absent during deep breathing and there was

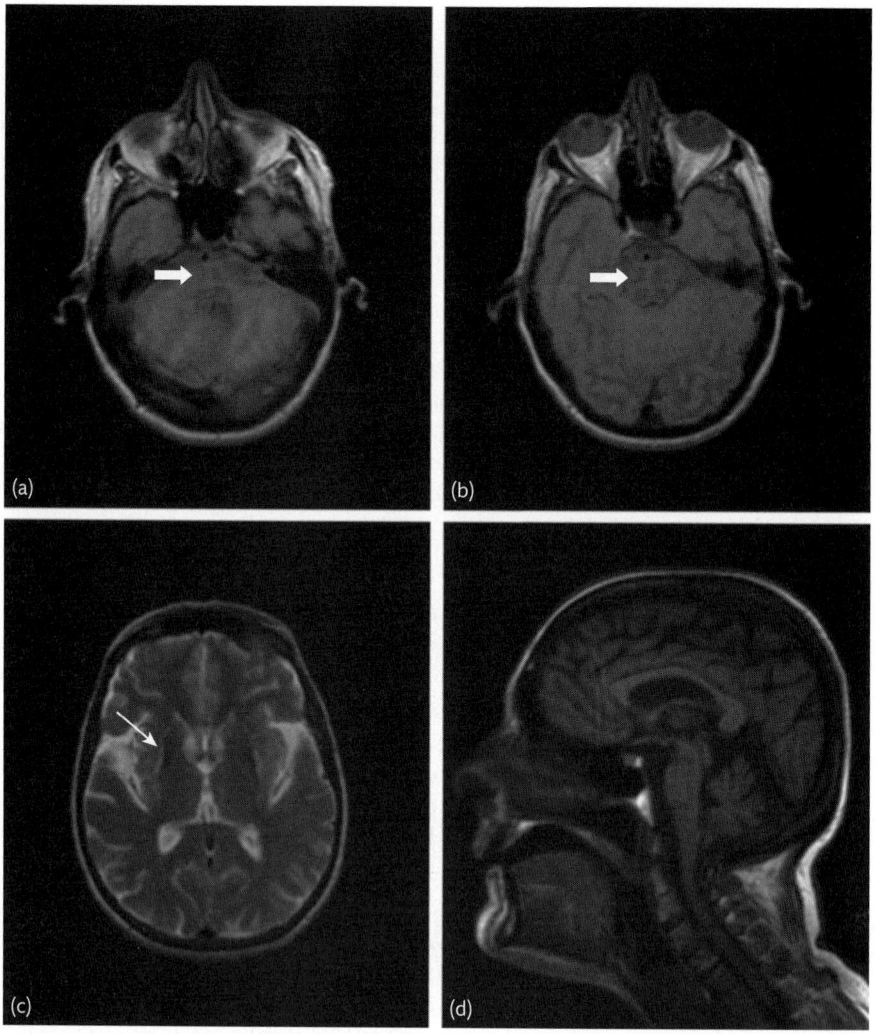

Figure 20.1 (a, b) The 'hot-cross bun' sign at the level of the mid pons (arrowed); (c) the 'slit-like void' sign (arrowed at right putamen); (d) mild cerebellar, cerebral, and pontine atrophy. (a)–(c) T2-weighted axial views; (d) T1-weighted sagittal view.

no increase in heart rate during hyperventilation. The Valsalva manoeuvre appeared to be blocked. In conclusion there was evidence of widespread cardiovascular autonomic failure. ENT review confirmed paradoxical movements of the vocal cords and poor abduction, probably giving rise to her inspiratory sighs. Arrangements were made for suprapubic catheter placement.

Clinical tip Autonomic testing in MSA [7, 8]

Autonomic function tests can be supportive of a diagnosis of MSA over Parkinson's disease (PD) when there is evidence of widespread severe cardiovascular autonomic dysfunction (abnormal cardiovascular reflex responses to deep breathing, Valsalva manoeuvre, and upright tilt) and

(Continued)

sudomotor dysfunction (thermoregulatory sweat test). However, cardiovascular autonomic dysfunction in a parkinsonian patient without other red flags suggestive of MSA is as likely to be caused by PD with dysautonomia as it is by MSA.

Cardiac MIBG scintigraphy, which identifies the noradrenaline-containing nerve terminals in the myocardium using $[^{123}I]$meta-iodobenzylguanidine, was previously advocated as reliably distinguishing PD (reduction in post-ganglionic sympathetic cardiac innervation) from MSA (normal uptake). It has recently been found to be a less robust discriminator, as reduced uptake has been reported in MSA patients in several studies. Therefore cardiac MIBG scintigraphy is no longer promoted as the key diagnostic test for differentiating between the disorders. The use of sphincter EMG in the diagnosis of MSA is a matter for debate and is no longer frequently performed.

At the age of 64 the patient was mainly bedbound, unable to use her light writer, and mute. She required a purée diet and had frequent chest infections, but she declined placement of an enteral feeding tube. She was doubly incontinent. Events suggestive of anoxic seizures—jerking when in an upright position following a report of dizziness—occurred on occasion. Midodrine 7.5mg three times daily was added to fludrocortisone and domperidone for management of OH. Because of reports by her husband of persistent disrupted breathing at night, she underwent polysomnography which showed frequent central sleep apnoeas of the Cheyne–Stokes pattern. Nocturnal oxygen was advised, as CPAP was deemed too difficult for her to manage.

At her last clinical examination she was noted to have bilateral flexion contractures of both hands and anterocollis, as well as pout and snout reflexes. Her cognition appeared intact, but she had become very depressed. The following year she died of aspiration pneumonia after eight years of symptomatic MSA. Her final clinical diagnosis had been refined to MSA-P, and post-mortem examination revealed widespread glial cytoplasmic inclusions in the putamen, substantia nigra, and pontine base, and to a lesser extent in the cerebellar white matter. Neuronal loss and gliosis was evident and predominated in the striatonigral regions with milder involvement of the cerebellar cortex, leading to a pathological diagnosis of MSA–striatonigral degeneration (SND) predominant.

Clinical tip Features of MSA

- Symptoms to enquire about in suspected MSA:
  - urinary frequency, urgency, incontinence
  - erectile dysfunction
  - dizziness on rising from bed, seat, climbing stairs
  - fainting
  - cold hands and feet with discoloration
  - coat-hanger pain (pain in the back of the head, neck, and shoulders relieved by lying flat)
  - vivid dreams, restless legs, thrashing out during sleep (suggestive of REM sleep behaviour disorder)
  - heavy snoring, stridor, or apnoeic episodes during sleep.
- Signs to look for in suspected MSA:
  - parkinsonism—rest tremor, bradykinesia, rigidity (often more symmetrical than PD)
  - early postural instability - positive pull test (retropulsion)
  - minimyoclonus (polyminimyoclonus in fingers, generalized limb or trunk myoclonus 'lightning jerks', negative myoclonus 'bobbing legs')
  - postural deformity such as antecollis, torticollis, lateral flexion or kyphoscoliosis (mixed lateral flexion and forward stoop)
  - cerebellar signs (nystagmus, saccadic pursuit eye movements, dysmetria/finger–nose ataxia/heel–shin ataxia)
  - pyramidal signs—hyper-reflexia, pathological reflexes, Babinski signs

(Continued)

  - primitive reflexes—pout, snout, grasp, palmomental
  - dysphonic, dysarthric speech of low volume
  - postural hypotension (fall of at least 30/15mmHg at two minutes from supine to standing)
  - Orofacial dyskinesias/dystonia in response to levodopa therapy.
- Likely to be absent in MSA:
  - significantly impaired cognition/dementia
  - impaired sense of smell
  - hallucinations
  - gaze palsy.

Clinical tip Management of MSA [9–12]

Approximately a third of MSA patients will have a degree of response to levodopa, so it is always advised to trial levodopa therapy in any patient suspected of having MSA. The development of severe orthostatic hypotension and/or orofacial dystonia may limit levodopa therapy, and most patients do not manage to take any more than 600mg/day. Other anti-parkinsonian therapies which are sometimes tried include dopamine agonists, MAO-B inhibitors, and amantadine. Conservative measures, such as increasing fluid and salt intake, head-up tilt during the night, and compression stockings, should be used initially in the management of OH. Pharmacological agents used to treat OH include fludrocortisone which supports sodium retention, ephedrine (a sympathomimetic) which might be limited because it causes increased tremor, midodrine, and droxidopa. Bladder dysfunction may be helped by antimuscarinic agents or intermittent self-catheterization; erectile dysfunction may be helped in the early stages with sildenafil which is simpler to manage than intracavernosal papaverine. Clonazepam can be useful for generalized myoclonus. Botulinum toxin therapy may be indicated for hypersalivation, blepharospasm, dyspraxia of eyelid opening, and limb and peri-oral dystonia, and to prevent contractures from chronic severe hand or foot dystonic posturing. Many patients will have depression and may be helped by antidepressant medication and cognitive behavioural therapy. CPAP or nocturnal oxygen may be necessary if sleep apnoea and/or stridorous respiration are causing breathing difficulty at night. Long-term management of MSA patients will also demand discussion regarding the use of suprapubic catheters, a PEG tube for feeding, and decisions about long-term care and DNAR orders.

Final word from the expert

MSA is a difficult diagnosis where patients often present with suggestive signs of MSA and rapidly progress with time. Always consider MSA in any patient with parkinsonism that responds poorly to drug therapy and patients with late-onset rapidly progressive ataxia. Early bladder involvement is a key feature.

The management of MSA is complex and multisystem, and requires support from several services and coordination through a specialist clinic with a clinical nurse specialist. Patients should be followed up closely to identify and best treat the manifestations of MSA as the disease progresses.

References

1. Gilman S, Wenning GK, Low PA, et al. Second consensus statement on the diagnosis of multiple system atrophy. *Neurology* 2008; 71(9): 670–6.
2. Trojanowski JQ, Revesz T. Proposed neuropathological criteria for the post mortem diagnosis of multiple system atrophy. *Neuropathol Appl Neurobiol* 2007; 33(6): 615–20.

3. Massey LA, Micallef C, Paviour DC, et al. Conventional magnetic resonance imaging in confirmed progressive supranuclear palsy and multiple system atrophy. *Mov Disord* 2012; 27(14): 1754–62.
4. Kraft E, Schwarz J, Trenkwalder C, et al. The combination of hypointense and hyperintense signal changes on T2-weighted magnetic resonance imaging sequences: a specific marker of multiple system atrophy? *Arch Neurol* 1999; 56(2): 225–8.
5. Ling H, Lees AJ. How can neuroimaging help in the diagnosis of movement disorders. *Neuroimaging Clin N Am* 2010; 20: 111–23.
6. Lang AE, Curran T, Provias J, Bergeron C. Striatonigral degeneration: iron deposition in putamen correlates with the slit-like void signal of magnetic resonance imaging. *Can J Neurol Sci* 1994; **21**(4): 311–18.
7. Kimpinski K, Iodice V, Burton DD, et al. The role of autonomic testing in the differentiation of Parkinson's disease from multiple system atrophy. *J Neurol Sci* 2012; 317(1-2): 92–6.
8. Riley DE, Chelimsky TC. Autonomic nervous system testing may not distinguish multiple system atrophy from Parkinson's disease. *J Neurol Neurosurg Psychiatry* 2003; 74(1): 56–60.
9. Kollensperger M, Geser F, Ndayisaba JP, et al. Presentation, diagnosis, and management of multiple system atrophy in Europe: final analysis of the European multiple system atrophy registry. *Mov Disord* 2010; **25**(15): 2604–12.
10. Mathias CJ, Kimber JR. Postural hypotension: causes, clinical features, investigation, and management. *Annu Rev Med* 1999; 50: 317–36.
11. Rajrut AH, Uitti RJ, Fenton ME, George D. Amantadine effectiveness in multiple system atrophy and progressive supranuclear palsy. *Parkinsonism Relat Disord* 1997; 3(4): 211–14.
12. Colosimo C, Tiple D, Wenning GK. Management of multiple system atrophy: state of the art. *J Neural Transm* 2005; 112: 1695–1704.

CASE

21 Non-convulsive status epilepticus

Jan Novy and Krishna Chinthapalli

Expert commentary: Marco Mula

Case history

A 70-year-old woman was admitted because of stupor [1]. She was a heavy tobacco smoker (over 100 pack-years total exposure) and three years earlier had suffered from a urinary bladder cancer without metastases which had been treated by complete cystectomy with an ileal conduit.

Five months before admission her family noticed that her behaviour progressively changed as she became aggressive and had episodes of singular behaviour. She also suffered, for the first time, from two unprovoked generalized convulsive seizures, but refused to see a doctor. There was no known past medical history or family history of epilepsy.

While on holiday abroad, she developed progressive difficulties in oral and written comprehension. She was admitted to a local hospital after a new generalized convulsive seizure, which resulted in rib fractures. A CT scan of her brain revealed a left temporal hypodense lesion, thought to be subacute, which did not correspond to any vascular territory. Clonazepam was started at a dose of 1mg daily. A lumbar puncture was performed and revealed a lymphocytic pleocytosis (10 cells/μl), slightly increased protein (50.1mg/dl, range 15–46mg/dl), and normal glucose. A real-time qualitative PCR test for herpes simplex virus (HSV) was negative for HSV-1 but positive for HSV-2. HIV serology was negative. An MRI scan of her brain showed T2 hyperintensity in the lateral temporal regions, predominantly on the left. Otherwise, there was no metabolic or electrolyte disturbance on blood tests. Intravenous aciclovir (30mg/kg daily) was started for three weeks. During this treatment the patient progressively worsened, becoming somnolent. She had several episodes of forced deviation of the head and eyes to the right. Clonazepam was increased and then phenytoin was added (450mg daily). The patient was transferred to a tertiary centre with suspected non-convulsive status epilepticus several months after the beginning of the symptoms.

Learning point: Classifying status epilepticus

From the electroclinical point of view, status epilepticus (SE) can be classified as focal or generalized and as convulsive or non-convulsive. The generalized convulsive form (where motor convulsive movements are bilateral) is the worst subtype because it quickly leads to a general metabolic disturbance and permanent brain damage, and so should be treated very aggressively. If not treated rapidly, it evolves into a 'subtle' status epilepticus where clinical manifestations are minimal (subtle jerking, twitching, or blinking) but the EEG continues to show generalized epileptic activity. This eventually evolves to a complete electromechanical dissociation where the patient is comatose

(Continued)

without any clinical suggestive signs while he/she continues to be in status. Focal convulsive status (epilepsia partialis continua) consists of localized clonic (often irregular) muscular jerks. Generalized non-convulsive status epilepticus encompasses mostly absence status and its variants. In absence status the patient shows a variable degree of cognitive impairment ranging from mild slowing to stupor; this is associated with generalized (sub-)continuous 3Hz spike and wave discharges. Focal non-convulsive status can manifest with a wide range of symptoms and a variable degree of cognitive impairment according to the location of the epileptic focus. Focal temporal non-convulsive status is the most common form of non-convulsive status epilepticus. Motor and orofacial automatisms as well as autonomic changes are frequently present and consciousness can be variably affected. Extra-temporal forms may manifest with variable disturbances and a different spectrum of cognitive impairment (e.g. dysexecutive symptoms or speech problems are present in frontal dominant non-convulsive status). These symptoms are typically fluctuating.

On admission, the patient was stuporous, scoring 9/15 on the Glasgow coma scale, and had transient episodes of forced gaze and head version to the right and intermittent right peribuccal myoclonic jerks. Her neurological examination did not disclose any other focal signs. The EEG confirmed focal non-convulsive status epilepticus with waxing and waning multifocal bilateral seizures (Figure 21.1). Levetiracetam and then topiramate were introduced and rapidly titrated upwards to 2000mg daily and 200mg daily, respectively, over several days without success.

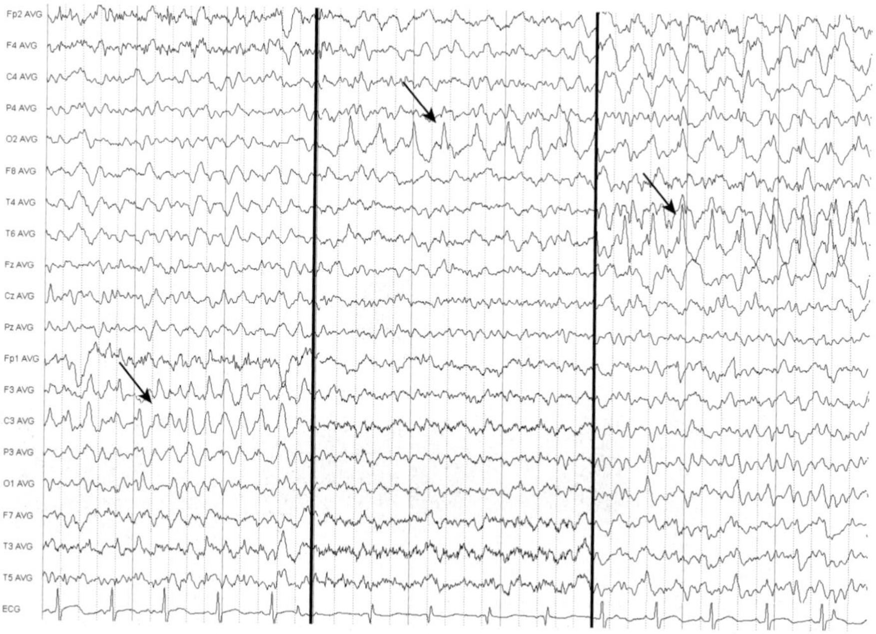

Figure 21.1 Three sequential EEG recordings (30mm/sec; 70μV/cm; HFF 70 Hz; LFF 0.5 Hz) in average referential montage showing left fronto-central (left panel), right occipital (middle panel), and right temporal (right panel) ongoing epileptic discharges (arrows).

Reproduced from *BMJ Case Rep*, Novy J, Carota A, Eggimann P, et al., Encephalitis with herpes simplex-2 in the cerebrospinal fluid and anti-RI (ANNA-2) antibodies: an infectious or a paraneoplastic syndrome? © 2009, with permission from BMJ Publishing Group Ltd.

> **Clinical tip** EEG interpretation in non-convulsive status epilepticus
>
> Diagnosis of non-convulsive status epilepticus always requires EEG for confirmation. EEG interpretation may not always be straightforward, and a treatment trial can be useful to ascertain the diagnosis. This test is performed by administering IV benzodiazepine, often at a lower dose than in normal first-line treatment (see Treatment section), under EEG monitoring. A significant clinical and electrophysiological improvement (disappearance of seizures or rhythmic discharges) is strongly supportive of the diagnosis of non-convulsive SE. However, improvement of the EEG is not necessarily supportive of a SE diagnosis: triphasic waves found in encephalopathies can disappear after administration of benzodiazepines, giving a false impression of improvement, but the patient may become more somnolent due to sedation. In unclear situations, a longer treatment trial with non-sedating anti-epileptic drugs (AEDs), such as phenytoin, valproate, levetiracetam, or lacosamide, may be needed with regular repeated EEG recordings.

In the meantime, investigations were repeated with a further lumbar puncture disclosing a slight lymphocytic pleocytosis (6 cells/μl), increased protein content (69.8mg/dl) and normal glucose. There was intrathecal IgG synthesis, and viral PCR for HSV-1 and HSV-2, human herpes virus type 6 (HHV6), varicella-zoster virus (VZV), Epstein—Barr virus (EBV), and enteroviruses was negative. Blood serology revealed signs of immunity to HSV, cytomegalovirus (CMV), EBV, and VZV, without signs of reactivation. HIV serology was repeated and was negative. General medical investigations including thyroid tests were unremarkable. Anti-nuclear antibodies were elevated (positive at a titre of 1:1280), but antinucleoprotein double-stranded DNA and anti-neutrophil cytoplasm antibodies were all negative. A second MRI scan of the brain confirmed the bilateral temporolateral T2 hyperintensities with extension into the left parietal region, and no enhancement with contrast (Figure 21.2). These abnormalities extensively involved the lateral aspect of the hemispheres, but spared the mesial temporal lobes. Diffusion-weighted sequences and an MR angiogram were unremarkable. Further analysis of the initial positive PCR for HSV-2 revealed that the PCR (qualitative) only became positive after 35–37 cycles, suggesting a low viral DNA load.

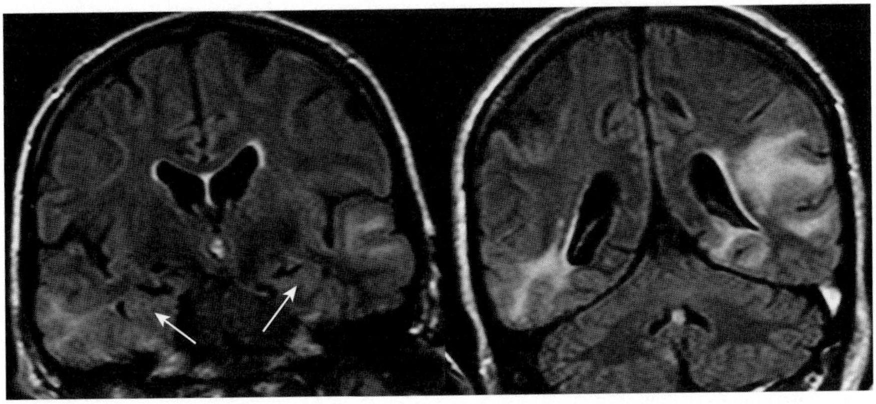

Figure 21.2 FLAIR MRI showing bilateral temporolateral lesions sparing the medial aspect of the temporal lobes (arrows).

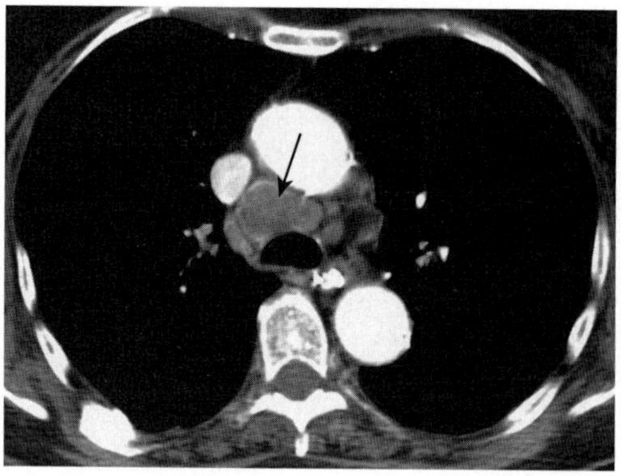

Figure 21.3 Contrast-enhanced thoracic CT scan showing a 3cm diameter pre-tracheal mass (arrow).

Reproduced from *BMJ Case Rep*, Novy J, Carota A, Eggimann P, et al., Encephalitis with herpes simplex-2 in the cerebrospinal fluid and anti-RI (ANNA-2) antibodies: an infectious or a paraneoplastic syndrome? © 2009, with permission from BMJ Publishing Group Ltd.

As the status epilepticus was refractory to a combination of four medications, a pharmacological coma was initiated after intubation. Thiopental was used, aiming for a burst-suppression pattern, and was started with a bolus of 5mg/kg and subsequently 5mg/kg/hour with EEG monitoring. This was done concomitantly with pulsed steroids (methylprednisolone 125mg/day). During the period of pharmacological coma, the dosages of levetiracetam and topiramate were increased (3000mg/day and 400mg/day, respectively). A thoraco-abdominal CT scan showed a pretracheal mass (Figure 21.3), and upon biopsy during mediastinoscopy a diagnosis of infiltrative small-cell lung carcinoma was made. After 48 hours of pharmacological coma, thiopental was progressively weaned. After four days, the EEG showed a relapse with continuous multifocal seizures. The hospital stay was then complicated by fever, and a chest radiograph showed bilateral pneumonia for which the patient was started on IV antibiotics.

Learning point Underlying causes of status epilepticus

Identifying the underlying cause of status epilepticus is crucial for management. The underlying cause was shown to be a major determinant of drug resistance [2] and of overall outcome [3] in status. People with de novo status epilepticus without a clear aetiology should undergo an extensive work-up, including full electrolyte/metabolic screening, imaging (a CT scan in an emergency followed by an MRI scan if the CT scan is inconclusive) with and without contrast. Vascular investigations should be carried out in cases where a stroke precedes the onset of status epilepticus or there is a persistent new neurological deficit during the episode of status epilepticus. In the absence of a clear aetiology a lumbar puncture should be performed to look for infectious, inflammatory, or neoplastic processes. This may require sedation and intubation. A slight pleocytosis is not uncommon in the context of status epilepticus, but a count of 10 cells/μl or higher should be considered abnormal. According to the results, the work-up should also include a search for auto-antibodies such as anti-VGKC, anti-NMDA, anti-GABA, anti-AMPA, anti-GAD, and other paraneoplastic (onconeural) antibodies. The search for an underlying cancer should be performed with appropriate imaging. Finally, depending on the clinical picture, investigations for mitochondrial diseases, genetic/chromosomal abnormalities, degenerative diseases (particularly dementias), and inborn errors of metabolism should be considered. Treatment of the underlying cause should be started promptly whenever possible. In this particular case, the investigations were complicated by the presence of a previously-treated infection which may have been due to reactivation or contamination. The investigations were repeated as the condition of the patient worsened despite treatment and finally showed the probable cause.

In this context, given the unresectable lung cancer and the frailty of the patient, who was not judged to be able to tolerate more aggressive immunosuppression or

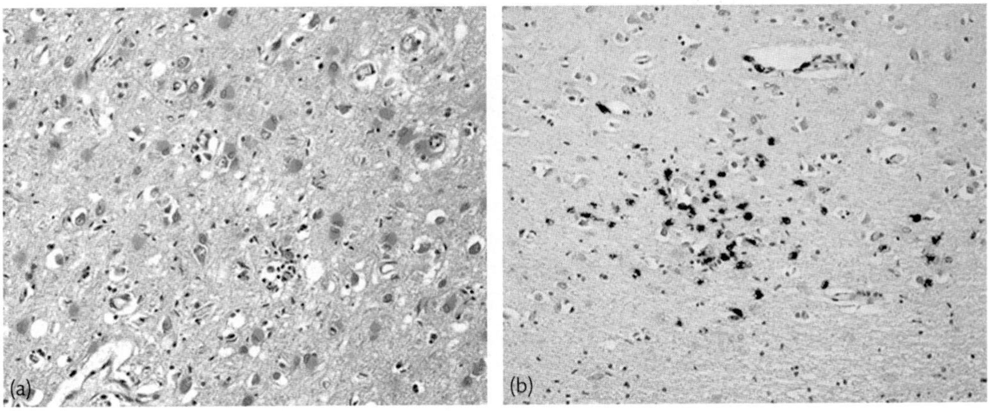

Figure 21.4 (a) Histology of the cerebral cortex (cingulate gyrus) showing neuronal loss, reactive gliosis, and lymphocytic infiltrate (H&E, 200x); (b) immunohistochemistry showing that the lymphocytic infiltrates are composed mostly of CD8 T cells (CD8, 100x). Please see colour plate section.

chemotherapy, it was decided, in agreement with her family's wishes, not to initiate any further treatment. She died a few days later.

After her death, the search for paraneoplastic auto-antibodies was completed and revealed positive anti-Ri (ANNA-2), whereas anti-Hu (ANNA-1), Anti Ma2 (Ta), anti-amphyphysin, and anti-CV2 (CRMP-5) were not present. The post-mortem examination confirmed the presence of small-cell lung carcinoma with local infiltration. Brain examination showed widespread foci of inflammation compatible with a paraneoplastic encephalitis. Lesions were predominantly in the fronto-parieto-temporal cortex, insula, cingulate gyrus, and brainstem, and consisted of neuronal loss, reactive gliosis, and multiple widespread lymphocytic infiltrates (Figure 21.4a) comprised mostly of CD8 T-cells (Figure 21.4b). There was no morphological or immunohistochemical evidence of HSV infection.

Discussion

Status epilepticus is a condition where an epileptic seizure(s) does not stop spontaneously and in the majority of the cases requires emergency intervention. It is classically defined as the continuous occurrence of seizures for at least 30 minutes (or recurrence of seizures without full recovery between them), mostly because this duration was historically shown to be associated with systemic metabolic disturbances [4] and with neuronal loss in animal models [5]. In practice, however, this duration should not be used to decide when to start treatment: an 'operational' definition of 5 minutes has been suggested [6], as seizures lasting longer than 5 minutes stop spontaneously within the first 30 minutes in only 40 per cent of cases. This operational definition is mostly relevant in generalised convulsive SE.

The diagnosis of non-convulsive status epilepticus can be difficult because it is dependent on an EEG. Patients with a previous diagnosis of epilepsy, prolonged personality changes, a recent-onset psychosis, or post-ictal confusion greater than 20 minutes should be investigated with EEG in order to rule out non-convulsive status.

Epidemiology and classification

Although 39–50 per cent of people presenting with SE are previously known to have epilepsy, it frequently represents a de novo neurological presentation. In Europe and North America its annual incidence varies between 6 and 41 per 100,000 and its overall mortality is in the range 7–39 per cent [7].

Cerebrovascular disease (acute or chronic), infectious encephalitis, brain tumours, head trauma, drugs (drug withdrawal, substance abuse, low anti-epileptic drug blood level), metabolic disturbances, and anoxia are the major causes of both convulsive and non-convulsive SE. More rarely, SE can be part of genetic, mitochondrial, metabolic, autoimmune, or paraneoplastic conditions [8]. In particular, autoimmune disorders causing SE with auto-antibodies against neuronal receptors (e.g. NMDA, AMPA, and GABA(b) receptors), ion channels (e.g. voltage-gated potassium channels (VGKC)), or enzymes (e.g. glutamic acid decarboxylase (GAD)) are increasingly reported, and may account for a considerable proportion of 'cryptogenic' SE (up to 10 per cent of SE) [2]. In a general intensive care unit, up to 9 per cent of critically ill comatose patients may be in non-convulsive SE; this percentage may be considerably higher in patients with acute and severe brain injury, such as cerebral anoxia.

Expert comment

Typical clinical scenarios for non-convulsive status epilepticus are:

- neonatal and infantile epileptic encephalopathies
- electroclinical status during sleep
- aftermath of convulsive status epilepticus
- critical illness.

The first two settings are rarely encountered by general neurologists (especially registrars) because they represent typical epileptological problems. Registrars have to be aware that specific epileptic syndromes are characterized by different risks of status epilepticus and some of them are characterized by recurrent episodes of non-convulsive status epilepticus, in some cases typically occurring during sleep (e.g. Lafora disease, Unverricht–Lundborg disease, Rett syndrome, Dravet syndrome, Landau–Kleffner syndrome).

As well as from non-convulsive status epilepticus, in intensive care it is often possible to encounter myoclonic status epilepticus. This term has been used to describe a wide variety of clinicoelectrographic presentations. It is a subtype of generalized convulsive status, and in patients with no history of epilepsy it is often symptomatic of severe brain damage (i.e. anoxic brain injury, paraneoplastic and metabolic encephalopathies including renal failure, sepsis, hypocalcaemia, drug or heavy metal intoxication). It is always associated with coma and the prognosis is poor. This entity should not be confused with Lance–Adams syndrome or chronic post-anoxic myoclonus. In fact, the treatment and prognosis are different.

Diagnosis

The diagnosis of SE relies on four main criteria: duration of the episode, clinical manifestations, EEG findings, and response to treatment (with a treatment trial if needed).

Non-epileptic psychogenic status due to prolonged non-epileptic attacks is probably the most frequent imitator of SE [9]. Useful clinical signs are resistance of eye opening in an apparently unconscious patient and ongoing breathing during prolonged convulsive movements. Absence of elevation of creatine kinase (CK) and lactate in an apparently generalized convulsive SE should also raise suspicion of a non-epileptic aetiology; although these may be elevated in very severe and prolonged non-epileptic attacks.

There is no unified consensus on EEG features in non-convulsive SE. In general terms, in patients with known epileptic encephalopathy the main EEG characteristic is the increase in prominence or frequency of the usual epileptic activity and improvement with IV benzodiazepines or AEDs.

Expert comment

The first approach is to differentiate patients with and without stupor or coma [10]. In patients without coma, it is possible to identify three major groups: typical absence status (3Hz spike-wave epileptic discharges), atypical absence status (2.5Hz), and focal non-convulsive status (<2.5Hz with or without rhythmic delta activity; >2.5Hz).

In patients without known epileptic encephalopathies, continuous epileptic discharges have to be differentiated from periodic discharges. At present, there is still uncertainty about the relevance of periodic lateralized epileptiform discharges (PLEDs). In general terms, they suggest severe focal parenchymal damage or brain injury. Some authors have argued that such discharges represent ongoing seizure activity and should be treated as such. However, given the multitude of aetiologies underling PLEDs, it seems reasonable to treat them as epileptic only if there is other evidence of ictal epileptic activity.

Pathophysiology

As a general framework, we have extensive information about generalized convulsive SE and several stages are recognized [4, 11]. Initial recurrent discrete seizures (<30 minutes) progressively merge (30–60 minutes). Generalized convulsions are progressively replaced by myoclonic jerks which then fade away ('subtle status'). In parallel, the EEG recording shows initially discrete seizures merging into continuous ictal discharges progressively intermixed with flat period, and evolving towards an electromechanical dissociation with periodic discharges over a flat background activity. This evolution carries a bad outcome. In the early stages (<30 minutes) compensatory mechanisms are effective, whereas later they progressively fail, leading to a mismatch between metabolic demands and delivery, leading to brain damage. Systemic factors such as convulsive movements and compromised breathing only partly account for the damage. The mechanisms underpinning SE self-sustainment are probably multiple and parallel. Recurrent seizures can decrease the response to GABA, the major inhibitory neurotransmitter in the brain, mostly by internalization of GABA(a) receptors. This internalization is thought to be the major cause of resistance to benzodiazepines, but it is unclear why SE becomes resistant to other treatments. Dysfunction of the other endogenous anti-convulsant pathways (adenosinergic, cannabinoid, and peptidergic) could also play an aggravating role. Excitatory NMDA receptors are also increasingly externalized to synapses after 60 minutes of SE. Inflammatory mediators are thought to be important in the pathophysiology too.

In generalized convulsive SE, brain damage occurs early; imaging shows hippocampal oedema and subsequent atrophy, with neuronal loss in both hippocampi as well as in the cerebellum at post-mortem examination. Neuronal death is probably the end result of overwhelming neuronal excitation (excitotoxicity). It is far less clear how much the brain is damaged by non-convulsive SE itself, as this is confounded by the inherent damage induced by the underlying cause. Animal models show that limbic SE causes milder neuronal loss in hippocampi than generalized SE, but these findings may not apply in humans. Clinically, there is conflicting evidence regarding

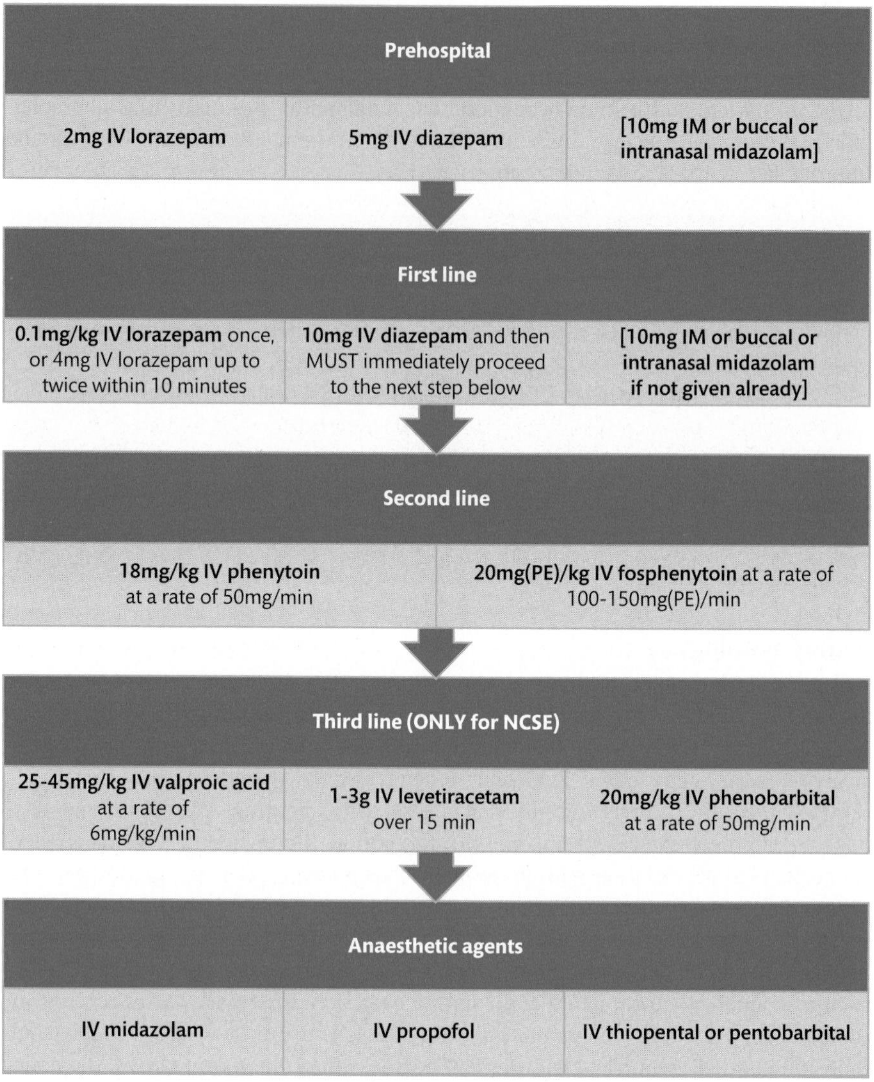

Figure 21.5 A treatment algorithm for status epilepticus based on the European Federation of Neurological Societies guideline [12] (IM, intramuscular; IV, intravenous; NCSE, non-convulsive status epilepticus). Intramuscular midazolam was not included as a first-line therapy in the guideline, but is mentioned here following evidence of efficacy in the RAMPART trial [15]. There are few data for buccal or intranasal midazolam, although they are widely used.

brain damage related to focal SE independent of the underlying cause. Absence status is widely regarded as harmless, with no convincing evidence of neuronal damage.

Treatment

Treatment should be carried out alongside investigations. SE in general is a medical emergency; along with its mortality and morbidity, it becomes less responsive to treatment as duration increases. Emergency cardiopulmonary resuscitation should be carried out first as needed. Up-to-date treatment guidelines are available for generalized convulsive status epilepticus (Figure 21.5) [12].

General management includes control of the airways and ventilation, arterial gas monitoring to see if there is metabolic acidosis or hypoxia requiring immediate treatment, an ECG, and blood pressure monitoring. Other preliminary measures may include IV glucose and thiamine, urea, creatinine, serum electrolyte and magnesium levels, full blood count, and liver function tests. In people with an established diagnosis of epilepsy who are already on a chronic regime with anti-epileptic drugs, serum drug levels should always be determined to assess compliance.

Current European guidance for first-line treatment is 0.1mg/kg IV lorazepam, a single dose of which proved to be effective in 80 per cent of patients [12]. If lorazepam is unavailable, diazepam 10 mg IV or rectal followed by phenytoin 18mg/kg IV may be given. Intramuscular midazolam at 10mg in adults may have the same efficacy as lorazepam, as shown in a pre-hospital study with paramedic administration of medication [15]. Phenytoin should be loaded rapidly at a rate of 50mg/min (20mg/min in the elderly). IV phenytoin loading should always be performed under cardiac monitoring and is contraindicated in people with arrhythmias. Phenytoin solution is very irritant at the injection site; in extreme cases this can result in purple glove syndrome (extensive cutaneous inflammation and venous thrombosis). Phenytoin has non-linear pharmacokinetics and liver-enzyme-inducing properties.

In this regard it is important to emphasize that IV infusion of diazepam and phenytoin takes 40 minutes compared with only 5 minutes for lorazepam. This approach should also be used for epilepsia partialis continua and non-convulsive status, although it is generally agreed that the therapeutic approach can be less aggressive than that adopted in generalized convulsive status.

Expert comment

Atypical absence status (continuous or frequent slow waves <2.5Hz), as seen in patients with Lennox–Gastaut syndrome, is usually refractory to benzodiazepines, which should be avoided in these patients anyway as they can induce a tonic status epilepticus.

Evidence base

Three important studies in the USA have demonstrated the efficacy of benzodiazepines as first-line treatment in generalized convulsive SE. In 1998, the Veterans Affairs Status Epilepticus Cooperative Study Group published the results of a double-blind RCT in adults presenting with status epilepticus in 22 hospitals [13]. Four IV drugs were compared: diazepam, lorazepam, phenytoin, and phenobarbital. In 384 adults with overt generalized convulsive SE, IV lorazepam terminated status in 64.9 per cent of patients, IV phenobarbital in 58.2 per cent, IV diazepam with subsequent IV phenytoin in 55.8 per cent, and IV phenytoin alone in 43.6 per cent. Lorazepam was significantly better than phenytoin but not the other two treatments.

Two double-blind RCTs have looked at pre-hospital administration of benzodiazepines. Alldredge et al. [14] enrolled 205 adults in a study of pre-hospital administration by paramedics of diazepam 5mg IV, lorazepam 2mg IV, or placebo. Lorazepam was successful in 59.1 per cent and diazepam was successful in 42.6 per cent, which was not significantly different statistically. Placebo terminated SE in 21.1 per cent. Benzodiazepines appeared to be safe in a pre-hospital setting, as the occurrence of cardiorespiratory complications (hypotension, cardiac arrhythmia, or respiratory dysfunction) was significantly lower than in the placebo group (10 per cent versus 22 per cent). In 2012, the Rapid Anticonvulsant Medication Prior to Arrival Trial (RAMPART) study showed that in 893 children and adults, intramuscular midazolam (10mg in adults) given by paramedics terminated SE in 73.4 per cent of patients by the time of arrival to hospital, compared with 63.4 per cent for IV lorazepam (4mg in adults) [15].

There have been no double-blind RCTs of other anticonvulsants in intravenous preparations (i.e. valproic acid, levetiracetam, lacosamide). A Cochrane systematic review in 2014 showed that there is limited evidence, usually from one or two underpowered open studies comparing levetiracetam with lorazepam and valproic acid with phenytoin [16]. Therefore new studies are urgently needed [17].

Nevertheless, US guidelines from the Neurocritical Care Society in 2012 state that phenytoin, phenobarbital, valproic acid, or levetiracetam may be used as second-line treatment after benzodiazepines [18].

Generalized convulsive status epilepticus refractory to phenytoin first-line treatment should be treated on an intensive care unit.

In non-convulsive status epilepticus, treatment with AEDs is usually recommended because of the lack of generally accepted guidelines, the lack of any head-to-head comparison studies, and the possible severe complications of general anaesthesia.

Valproic acid may be given as an IV bolus dose of 25-45mg/kg at an infusion rate of up to 6mg/kg. It has no arrhythmogenic properties and is the drug of choice in absence and myoclonic status. It is contraindicated in mitochondrial diseases. It is usually well tolerated, but can induce a hepatic encephalopathy often, but not invariably, associated with elevated serum ammonia. It is an inhibitor of liver enzymes.

Phenobarbital is usually given as a dose of 20mg/kg at a rate of 50mg/min. Its half-life is very long (up to 100 hours). Side effects include sedation, respiratory depression, and hypotension, and its extensive redistribution can delay their occurrence. Phenobarbital is less frequently used nowadays in SE. It is a potent liver enzyme inducer.

There is less experience with levetiracetam and lacosamide. The IV bolus dose of levetiracetam is usually 20mg/kg and its administration is well tolerated. The lacosamide IV bolus dose is usually 400mg. The major contraindication to its use is first-degree AV block. Neither drugs has any major interactions.

In the intensive care setting, the rate of complication is usually high: 50–66 per cent for infection requiring antibiotics and 50 per cent for significant hypotension. Midazolam seems to be the safest option, as it rarely induces a prolonged complete suppression of cerebral activity (in comparison with barbiturates), but it often needs to be combined with propofol to achieve seizure control. Pharmacological coma is usually maintained for 24–36 hours under EEG monitoring aiming for a burst-suppression pattern, which is easily recognizable with the absence of distinct seizures. The anaesthetic agent is then weaned off to assess for recovery. A potentially serious complication of propofol is propofol infusion syndrome (PRIS) characterized by circulatory collapse, lactic acidosis, hypertriglyceridaemia, and rhabdomyolysis. It has mostly been described in patients with infectious complications receiving catecholamines and/or steroids. Protracted use of propofol should be avoided, and careful monitoring of serum lactate, CK, and triglycerides is recommended for early detection of PRIS.

Several anaesthetic agents or pharmacological treatments (isoflurane, ketamine, etomidate, verapamil, lidocaine, magnesium) as well as procedures (hypothermia, ketogenic diet, respective surgery, vagus nerve stimulation, electroconvulsive therapy, transcranial magnetic stimulation) have been reported anecdotally in refractory SE. They are mostly described in small selected case series with mixed outcomes. These have been tried after failure of all conventional treatments.

Prognosis

SE has a significant mortality (6–39 per cent) and morbidity, either from the underlying condition or from SE itself. Major independent predictors of mortality are the underlying cause, patient age, the extent of impairment of consciousness (reflecting underlying brain dysfunction) [2], and the duration of the episode in generalized SE. This is particularly evident in non-convulsive status where the mortality rate is usually related to the underlying brain disorder.

Final word from the expert

Status epilepticus is a neurological emergency. Among the different subtypes, non-convulsive status is still under-diagnosed and under-treated. It can frequently be encountered by the general neurologist as it represents a complication of stroke, infectious diseases, metabolic encephalopathies, and in the critically ill patient. In these cases, EEG should be always part of the routine assessment. Treatment has to be tailored on the specific needs of the individual patient, taking into account generally accepted treatment guidelines for convulsive status epilepticus.

In patients with an already established diagnosis of epilepsy, rescue medications for the acute management of epileptic seizures are becoming increasingly popular. This is due to the increased awareness of clinicians, patients, families, and carers about the importance of a rapid and effective treatment of convulsions. Moreover, rapid changes in the organization of the health system and delivery of care are pointing to implementation in the pre-hospital setting, especially in chronic disorders such as epilepsy. Benzodiazepines still represent first-line agents for the acute treatment of convulsive seizures, with diazepam and lorazepam being the most widely used drugs in both adults and children. Diazepam is usually administered intravenously or rectally, while lorazapam is mainly administered via the IV, intramuscular, and transmucosal routes. Outside hospital, the IV route may be complex or almost impossible, making transmucosal routes quite popular. The intranasal or buccal delivery of midazolam, via the nasal or buccal mucosa, offers an attractive and cost-effective alternative, especially for the out-of-hospital setting. In this context, clinicians (and registrars in particular) must always be aware of any pre-hospital treatment in order to avoid overdoses of benzodiazepines in these patients.

References

1. Novy J, Carota A, Eggimann P, et al. Encephalitis with herpes simplex-2 in the cerebrospinal fluid and anti-RI (ANNA-2) antibodies: an infectious or a paraneoplastic syndrome? *BMJ Case Rep* 2009; 2009.
2. Novy J, Logroscino G, Rossetti AO. Refractory status epilepticus: a prospective observational study. *Epilepsia* 2010; 51(2): 251–6.
3. Rossetti AO, Hurwitz S, Logroscino G, Bromfield EB. Prognosis of status epilepticus: role of aetiology, age, and consciousness impairment at presentation. *J Neurol Neurosurg Psychiatry* 2006; 77(5): 611–15.
4. Lothman E. The biochemical basis and pathophysiology of status epilepticus. *Neurology* 1990; 40(5 Suppl 2): 13–23.
5. Meldrum BS, Horton RW. Physiology of status epilepticus in primates. *Arch Neurol* 1973; 28(1): 1–9.
6. Lowenstein DH, Bleck T, Macdonald RL. It's time to revise the definition of status epilepticus. *Epilepsia* 1999; 40(1): 120–2.
7. Neligan A, Shorvon SD. Frequency and prognosis of convulsive status epilepticus of different causes: a systematic review. *Arch Neurol* 2010; 67(8): 931–40.
8. Tan RYL, Neligan A, Shorvon SD. The uncommon causes of status epilepticus: a systematic review. *Epile Psy Res* 2010; 91(2–3): 111–22.

9. Dworetzky BA, Bubrick EJ, Szaflarski J P, et al. Nonepileptic psychogenic status: markedly prolonged psychogenic nonepileptic seizures. *Epile Psy Behav* 2010; 19(1): 65–8.
10. Bauer G, Trinka E. Nonconvulsive status epilepticus and coma. *Epilepsia* 2010; 51(2): 177–90.
11. Treiman DM, Walton NY, Kendrick C. A progressive sequence of electroencephalographic changes during generalized convulsive status epilepticus. *Epile Psy Res* 1990; 5(1): 49–60.
12. Meierkord H, Boon P, Engelsen B, et al. EFNS guideline on the management of status epilepticus in adults. *Eur J Neurol* 2010; 17(3): 348–55.
13. Treiman DM, Meyers PD, Walton NY, et al. A comparison of four treatments for generalized convulsive status epilepticus. *N Engl J Med* 1998; 339(12): 792–8.
14. Alldredge BK, Gelb AM, Isaacs SM, et al. A comparison of lorazepam, diazepam, and placebo for the treatment of out-of-hospital status epilepticus. *N Engl J Med* 2001; 345(9): 631–7.
15. Silbergleit R, Durkalski V, Lowenstein D, et al. Intramuscular versus intravenous therapy for prehospital status epilepticus. *N Engl J Med* 2012; 366(7): 591–600.
16. Prasad M, Krishnan PR, Sequeira R, Al-Roomi K. Anticonvulsant therapy for status epilepticus. *Cochrane Database Syst Rev* 2014; 9: CD003723.
17. Cock HR, ESETT Group. Established status epilepticus treatment trial (ESETT). *Epilepsia* 2011; 52 (Suppl 8): 50–2.
18. Brophy GM, Bell R, Claassen J, et al. Guidelines for the evaluation and management of status epilepticus. *Neurocrit Care* 2012; 17(1): 3–23.

CASE

22 A life-threatening drug reaction

Suchitra Chinthapalli

Expert commentary: Edel O'Toole

Case history

A 64-year-old South Asian woman was admitted to hospital with painful blisters, widespread skin peeling, and tiredness. She had noticed non-tense fluid-filled bullae, as large as 5cm in diameter, developing on her trunk and limbs over the preceding two days. She had been feverish and non-specifically unwell for one week. She had no past medical or family history of skin disease or of previous similar episodes.

She had been discharged from her local hospital two weeks earlier, following two generalized tonic-clonic seizures of unknown aetiology. A CT scan of the head was normal. She had received a loading dose of IV phenytoin in the emergency department and had subsequently commenced carbamazepine 200mg twice daily.

Past medical history included diabetes and hypertension. Her regular medications were metformin 500mg twice daily, aspirin 75mg once daily, simvastatin 40mg once daily, and ramipril 5mg once daily. She had been taking these medications for over five years. She had no known history of adverse reactions or allergies to drugs. She lived with her two children and was independent in her activities of daily living.

On examination she appeared unwell. Large areas of skin on her trunk and limbs had begun to detach, leaving exposed eroded areas (Figure 22.1). There were several large flaccid blisters on an erythematous base on her trunk and limbs. Approximately 50 per cent of her skin was involved. Nikolsky's sign was positive. Her oral and vulval mucous membranes were tender on palpation. Her lips were swollen and skin was beginning to slough off (Figure 22.2). No abnormalities were noted on cardiovascular, respiratory, abdominal, or neurological examination. Clinical observations, including temperature, heart rate, blood pressure, oxygen saturation, and respiratory rate, were within normal limits. Urine dipstick was negative.

A clinical diagnosis of toxic epidermal necrolysis (TEN) secondary to phenytoin and/or carbamazepine was made. She was admitted to a single room in the intensive care unit for supportive management and a skin biopsy was performed. The neurology team was informed and carbamazepine was stopped. If further seizures occurred during admission, their recommendation was to start levetiracetam 250mg twice daily.

The management of TEN is supportive: protection of the cutaneous and mucous membranes, adequate analgesia, and monitoring and treatment of complications (Table 22.1).

The patient's skin was treated with 50 per cent white soft paraffin plus 50 per cent liquid paraffin, which acts as a waterproof barrier reducing fluid loss and infection risk, and helps with pain and temperature regulation. There is significant transcutaneous fluid loss and also reduced oral intake, so the fluid balance was monitored carefully. Denuded areas were then covered with non-adhesive dressings

Learning point Nikolsky's sign

In 1896, Pyotr Nikolsky, a Russian dermatologist, reported that application of lateral pressure to affected skin in patients with pemphigus, usually using the thumb, led to blistering or denudation of the surrounding epidermis. This was later found to be associated with a range of bullous disorders.

Clinical tip Intensive care unit management

TEN is a serious life-threatening condition and referral to an intensive care unit should not be delayed whilst waiting for histological confirmation of the diagnosis. An urgent dermatology opinion should be sought for any blistering skin rash.

Clinical tip Stop any potentially causative drugs

Identifying and withholding the culprit drug immediately is very important and is associated with reduced mortality. Over 80 per cent of cases of TEN are due to the following medications: allopurinol, carbamazepine, lamotrigine, phenytoin, phenobarbital, nevirapine, oxicam NSAIDs (eg. piroxicam), and sulphonamides. Carbamazepine is the most common cause of TEN in some studies, but this depends on local prescribing patterns.

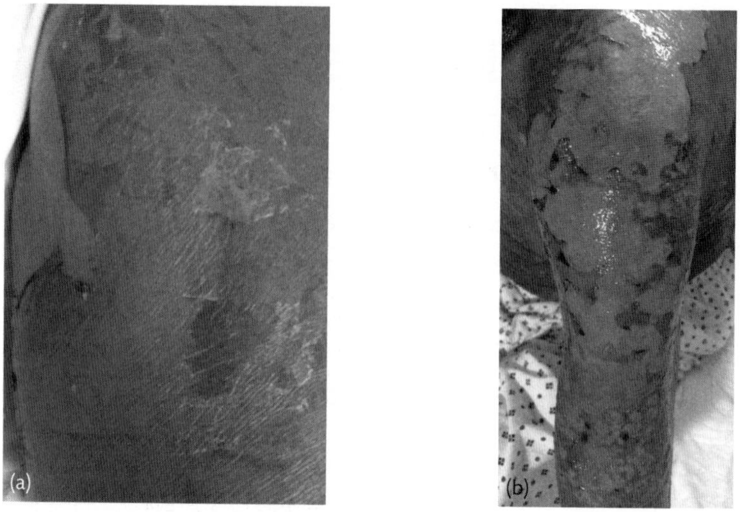

Figure 22.1 Clinical features of toxic epidermal necrolysis: (a) peeling skin; (b) denuded areas of skin. Please see colour plate section.

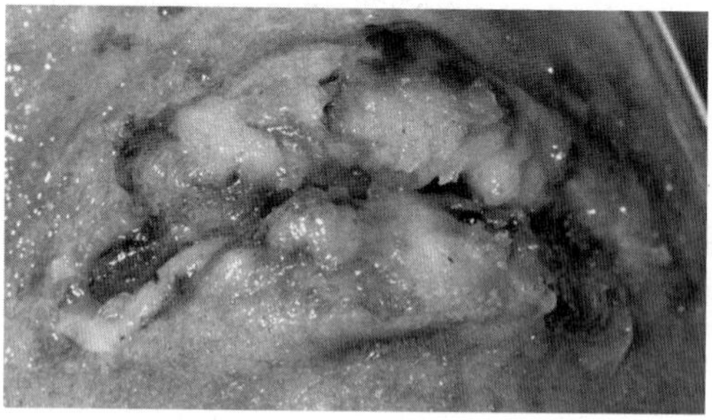

Figure 22.2 Clinical features of toxic epidermal necrolysis: oral mucosal involvement with sloughing and crusting of the lips. Please see colour plate section.

Image courtesy of Professor Rino Cerio, Queen Mary University of London.

and either bandaged or covered with high-density polyethylene wound dressing suits. Analgesia comprised paracetamol and short-acting morphine sulphate, although once the skin was covered the pain reduced significantly. Venous thromboprophylaxis was given. The ophthalmology team reviewed the patient to exclude ocular complications. Intravenous immunoglobulin (IVIG) was administered over three days.

Learning point Ocular symptoms

Ocular involvement occurs in 74 per cent of patients with TEN or Stevens–Johnson syndrome (SJS) in the acute phase and is one of the most serious long term sequelae of the disease [1]. It is important to seek ophthalmology review early. Symptoms can include dryness, pain, visual disturbance, and photophobia. Epithelial sloughing of the conjunctiva, cornea, and eyelids occurs, and there is an abnormal tear film. This leads to inflammation and increased risk of corneal scarring and infection, with the risk of blindness. Management includes topical lubricants, steroids, and antibacterial agents; more recently, clinical trials have used amniotic membrane transplants to cover the eyelids during the acute phase [2]. Up to 50 per cent of patients develop long-term complications, such as dry eyes, and the risk of this is unrelated to the degree of severity of the acute phase.

Table 22.1 Supportive management of skin loss in TEN

Skin function	Risk in TEN	Management
Prevent loss of moisture	Dehydration	Oral intake if possible IV access (peripheral or central) Urinary catheter
Temperature regulation	Hypothermia	Warming blankets Keep room warm
Protection against pathogens	Sepsis	Barrier nursing in a side room Frequently screen for infection and have low threshold for antibiotics (e.g. clinical examination, skin swabs, urine culture, blood cultures, chest radiograph) Antiseptic oral mouth washes
Sensation	Pain Trauma	Use a validated pain scoring system Provide adequate analgesia Avoid NSAIDs due to risk of gastric and renal injury
Nutrition (mucous membranes)	Malnutrition	Assess suitability for oral intake Consider nasogastric (NG) or total parental nutrition (TPN) Increased metabolic rate requiring increased calorie intake

Expert comment

There is currently no consensus on the use of systemic therapies to improve prognosis in TEN. Drugs used include steroids, ciclosporin, and immunoglobulins. There is conflicting evidence on the benefit of oral steroids early in the disease. Steroids may shorten the disease process, but may be associated with increased infection. Immunoglobulins are thought to inhibit Fas–Fas ligand binding which reduces keratinocyte apoptosis, and cohort studies have found improved survival with its use. However, in 2012 a systematic review and meta-analysis found no definite therapeutic benefit [3]. The decision to give systemic therapies is made by local dermatologists in conjunction with other clinicians involved in the patient's care.

Although this patient did not have complications at the time of presentation, she was at high risk when severity was assessed on admission using SCORTEN, an internationally recognized prognostic scoring system developed in 2000 [4, 5] (see Tables 22.2 and 22.3). The patient scored 4 for her age, degree of epidermal detachment, urea (16mmol/L) and glucose levels (22mmol/L), putting her at a 58 per cent risk of death.

Blisters continued to form and skin peeled off for a further 48 hours before subsiding. In the interim, new re-epithelialized skin had begun to form in some areas. At this time, the skin biopsy findings were discussed and were consistent with TEN (Figure 22.3).

By day 12 she was recovering well after a lower respiratory tract infection. Over 80 per cent of her denuded skin had re-epithelialized. She spent a further two weeks in hospital for rehabilitation. On discharge, she was advised that she should never take phenytoin or carbamazepine again, and this adverse drug reaction was documented in the clinical record. Her primary care physician was also informed that a further challenge with these medications or other aromatic AED compounds would be likely to lead to an even more serious reaction. She started levetiracetam on discharge, with no further seizures. At follow-up six months later the patient was well and had no lasting sequelae.

Clinical tip Adverse drug reactions

There is limited data on the epidemiology of drug adverse reactions because of under-reporting. Patients with serious adverse drug reactions should be reported to the relevant agency. In the UK the Yellow Card Scheme, run by the Medicines and Healthcare Products Regulatory Agency (MHRA) collects this data. Reporting can be done by physicians or patients and does not include patient-identifiable data. Patients should be advised to consider carrying bracelets, cards, or other methods of alerting health professionals to adverse reactions.

Table 22.2 A severity of illness score for toxic epidermal necrolysis (SCORTEN) for prognosis (valid when calculated within 24 hours of admission)

Parameter	Threshold	Score
Age	>40 years	1
Malignancy	Present	1
Epidermal detachment at time of admission	>10% of skin surface	1
Heart rate	>120bpm	1
Bicarbonate	<20mmol/L	1
Urea	>10mmol/L	1
Glucose	>14mmol/L	1

Adapted from *J Invest Dermatol.*, 115, Bastuji-Garin S et al., SCORTEN: A Severity-of-Illness Score for Toxic Epidermal Necrolysis, p. 149–153, Copyright (2000), with permission from Nature Publishing Group

Table 22.3 Predicted mortality based on total SCORTEN score.

SCORTEN score	Probability of death (%)
0–1	3
2	12
3	35
4	58
>5	90

Adapted from *J Invest Dermatol.*, 115, Bastuji-Garin S et al., SCORTEN: A Severity-of-Illness Score for Toxic Epidermal Necrolysis, p. 149–153, Copyright (2000), with permission from Nature Publishing Group

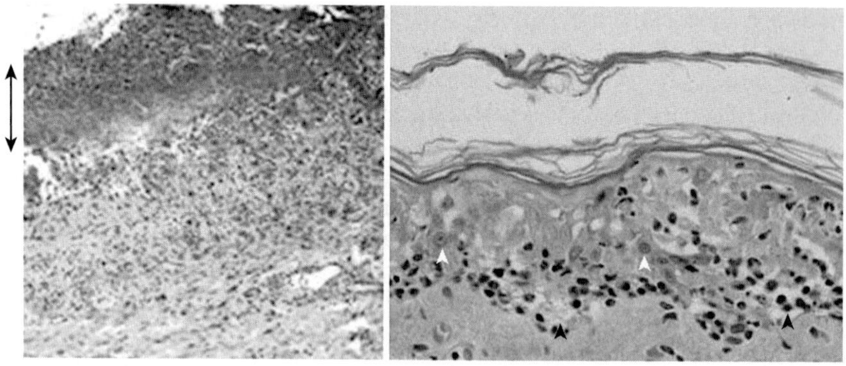

Figure 22.3 Histology of toxic epidermal necrolysis. Left panel: low-power view of skin biopsy with H&E staining showing full-thickness epidermal necrosis (double-headed arrow) with separation of epidermis and in some areas complete loss of epidermis. There is oedema in the underlying dermis with an inflammatory infiltrate. Right panel: medium-power view of early TEN lesional skin. There are scattered apoptotic keratinocytes (black arrowheads) and basal layer clefting (white arrowheads) with an inflammatory infiltrate in the upper dermis. Immunofluorescence was negative. Please see colour plate section.

Images courtesy of Professor Rino Cerio, Queen Mary University of London.

Discussion

Anti-epileptic drugs (AEDs) are frequently prescribed by neurologists and are widely recognized to be associated with a variety of adverse reactions, particularly skin eruptions which occur in approximately 15 per cent of users. Therefore it is important to understand and minimize the risk of skin eruptions with AEDs and to inform patients of this risk.

Risk factors for serious cutaneous adverse reactions (SCAR) with AEDs

In 2007, Arif et al. [6] published a retrospective study of 1890 patients exposed to 15 different anti-epileptic medications to compare and predict any rashes that occurred. The drugs most likely to cause a rash were phenytoin (5.9 per cent risk of rash), lamotrigine (4.8 per cent) and carbamazepine (3.7 per cent) [6]. This is in agreement with other published studies. The risk of developing a cutaneous reaction with an AED is five times greater if there has already been a previous reaction to another AED [6].

The highest risk of developing cutaneous reactions is within the first two months of commencing AEDs, as in this case [7, 8]. High initial serum concentrations of the drug may also be a risk factor [9]. Higher AED starting doses and quicker upward titration of doses are known to be associated with a higher risk of cutaneous reactions. For example, lamotrigine caused SJS in up to 1 in 100 children with high initial doses, but appears to cause it in less than 1 in 1000 users when titrated slowly [10]. The risk of lamotrigine causing cutaneous reactions is higher with concomitant administration of sodium valproate and is probably related to impaired lamotrigine metabolism. Lamotrigine should be started at a lower dose than usual in people taking sodium valproate. A suitable starting regimen for lamotrigine monotherapy would be 25mg daily for 14 days, followed by an increase in the daily dose in steps of no more than 50mg every 14 days. If it is used with sodium valproate, lamotrigine should be started at 25mg on alternate days for 14 days, then 25mg daily for at least 14 days, and then increased in steps of no more than 50mg every 14 days. Check national guidelines for up-to-date guidance on dosing. Patients should be told to seek medical attention urgently if they develop a rash.

Aromatic AEDs

Carbamazepine and phenytoin are aromatic AEDs, which means that their chemical structures contain an aromatic ring (Table 22.4). Symptoms of hypersensitivity are twice as common with aromatic AEDs as with non-aromatic AEDs [11, 12]. They are also more commonly associated with immunoglobulin E type 1 hypersensitivity and T-cell-mediated type 4 hypersensitivity reactions [12]. Studies have also shown there is cross-reactivity between the aromatic AEDs of the order of 40–58 per cent

Table 22.4 Aromatic AEDs

Carbamazepine	Oxcarbazepine
Eslicarbazepine	Phenobarbital
Felbamate	Phenytoin
Fosphenytoin	Primidone
Lamotrigine	Zonisamide

and 80 per cent in in vitro studies [13]. Therefore when a reaction as severe as TEN has occurred, it is best to avoid using other aromatic AEDs if possible.

Evidence base

In recent years there has been an increasing interest in the role of genetics in cutaneous drug eruptions. Genetic studies have begun to identify HLA alleles implicated in the development of severe cutaneous reactions. In 2004, Chung et al. [8] published findings of an association between HLA-B*1502 and SJS and TEN occurrence in 44 patients of Han Chinese origin in Taiwan taking carbamazepine. These researchers published further data including 91 patients in total with cutaneous reactions to carbamazepine and a control group of 144 patients. They found that 98.5 per cent (59/60) of patients with SJS or TEN had the HLA-B*1502 allele compared with 4.2 per cent (6/144) of the controls (odds ratio, 1357; 95% CI = 193.4–8838.3) [14]. Since then other studies have corroborated these findings and also demonstrated similar findings in other populations [15, 16].

The HLA-B*1502 allele is found in at least 10 per cent of Asians (including people from China, Thailand, Malaysia, Indonesia, the Philippines, and Taiwan) compared with 2–4 per cent of South Asians, 1–2 per cent of Caucasians, and less than 1 per cent of Japanese and Koreans [8, 14–16]. The MHRA in the UK and the Food and Drug Administration (FDA) in the USA currently advise that people of Asian ethnic origin should be offered screening prior to starting carbamazepine [17]. If they test positive for the allele then the drug should only be prescribed if the benefits outweigh the risks. The allele does not predict the risk of other skin reactions. A weaker association between the HLA-B*1502 allele and phenytoin-related severe cutaneous reactions has been identified, and there may also be a role for screening prior to phenytoin and fosphenytoin use.

A genome-wide association study published in 2011 identified HLA-A*3101, present in 2–5 per cent of Caucasians, as a predictor of hypersensitivity reactions with carbamazepine in those of Northern European ancestry [18]. This association has also been found in other populations. HLA-A*3101 presence is expected to be as high as 15 per cent in Japanese, South Indian, and Native American populations. Some experts are now also recommending genetic testing for HLA-A*3101 before initiation of carbamazepine in all carbamazepine-naive patients [19].

Stevens–Johnson syndrome (SJS) and toxic epidermal necrolysis (TEN)

SJS and TEN constitute a rare spectrum of diseases characterized by epidermal necrolysis. Approximately two cases per million population occur per year. Risk estimates based on the number of prescriptions or daily doses ranged from 1 to 10 per 10,000 new users for carbamazepine, lamotrigine, phenobarbital, and phenytoin, and were lower for valproic acid [20]. Although rare, SJS and TEN are acute in onset and life-threatening, with TEN mortality rates exceeding 30 per cent [4]. Incidence and mortality are higher with increasing age. Non-drug-related risk factors for SJS and TEN include the presence of HIV infection, malignancy, systemic lupus erythematosus (SLE), and female sex.

Patients usually present with a prodrome of non-specific symptoms including fever, malaise, and arthralgia. Within 72 hours, this progresses into mucocutaneous involvement such as burning eyes and difficulty swallowing. Erythematous macules develop, often beginning on the trunk and face, and rapidly coalesce. At the same time, the mucous membranes (eyes, mouth, and genitals) develop erythematous macules and erosions (Figure 22.2). Patients report severe pain out of proportion to the skin changes. Ocular involvement is frequently present and can vary from acute conjunctivitis to corneal ulceration. Subsequently, vesicles and blisters can form before large areas of epidermis begin to detach from the body (Figure 22.1). Nikolsky's sign is often positive but is not specific. The distinguishing feature between SJS and TEN is the degree of skin detachment present (see Table 22.5).

Table 22.5 Differentiation between SJS, TEN, and overlap syndrome

Factor	SJS	SJS-TEN overlap	TEN
BSA involved	<10%	10–30%	>30%
Medications implicated	>50%	50–95%	95%
Mortality	10%	30%	50%

BSA, body surface area.

The most common cause of TEN is prescribed medication and a culprit drug is identified in over 85 per cent of cases [21]. Diagnosis is based on clinical history and examination, supported by histological findings on skin biopsy (see Figure 22.3). Histology with immunofluorescence can be helpful in excluding other causes such as bullous pemphigoid, pemphigus vulgaris, acute generalized exanthematous pustulosis (AGEP), disseminated fixed bullous drug eruption, or staphylococcal scalded skin syndrome.

Expert comment

Studies have investigated the use of patch testing or lymphocyte drug-induced interferon-gamma (IFN-γ) assays to determine the culprit drug, but they are of uncertain diagnostic value and therefore are not currently recommended to be routinely performed. An algorithm of drug causality in epidermal necrolysis (ALDEN) was developed in 2010 and shown to be useful as a reference tool to exclude the causality of specific drugs [21]. It considers (1) the timing of when the drug was given in relation to onset of reaction, (2) whether the drug was present at the onset of the reaction, (3) whether there has been a previous similar reaction with the drug or a related drug, (4) whether the reaction process continues if the drug is continued, (5) whether studies have demonstrated the drug to be high risk for causing epidermal necrosis, and finally (6) whether another drug cause is more likely [21].

There are numerous theories regarding the disease mechanisms involved in drug-induced epidermal necrosis (Figure 22.4).

Epidermal loss disrupts all functions of skin including thermal and immune regulation as well as providing a barrier against physical injury (see Table 22.1). These patients require prompt assessment in collaboration with dermatologists and early recognition of the need for intensive supportive therapy in a suitable environment—often in an intensive care unit or burns unit. There may be a role for systemic therapies.

Erythema multiforme

This condition used to be considered as part of the same spectrum of diseases as SJS and TEN but is now recognized as a separate clinical entity. It is characterized by itchy erythematous targetoid lesions with a concentric variation in colour, with or without mucous membrane, usually oral, involvement (Figure 22.5). Lesions can occur anywhere, but are often on acral sites and extensor surfaces. Over 90 per cent of cases are attributed to infections, mainly herpes simplex virus (HSV). Drugs, including AEDs, account for less than 10 per cent of cases.

DRESS (drug rash with eosinophilia and systemic symptoms) syndrome (includes anticonvulsant hypersensitivity syndrome)

The most common causes of this serious idiosyncratic drug reaction are aromatic AEDs, in particular carbamazepine. Incidence is between 1 in 1000 to 1 in 10,000 exposures. It can also occur on reintroduction of a previously tolerated medication. It is characterized by a variety of clinical features (Table 22.6). Symptoms begin two

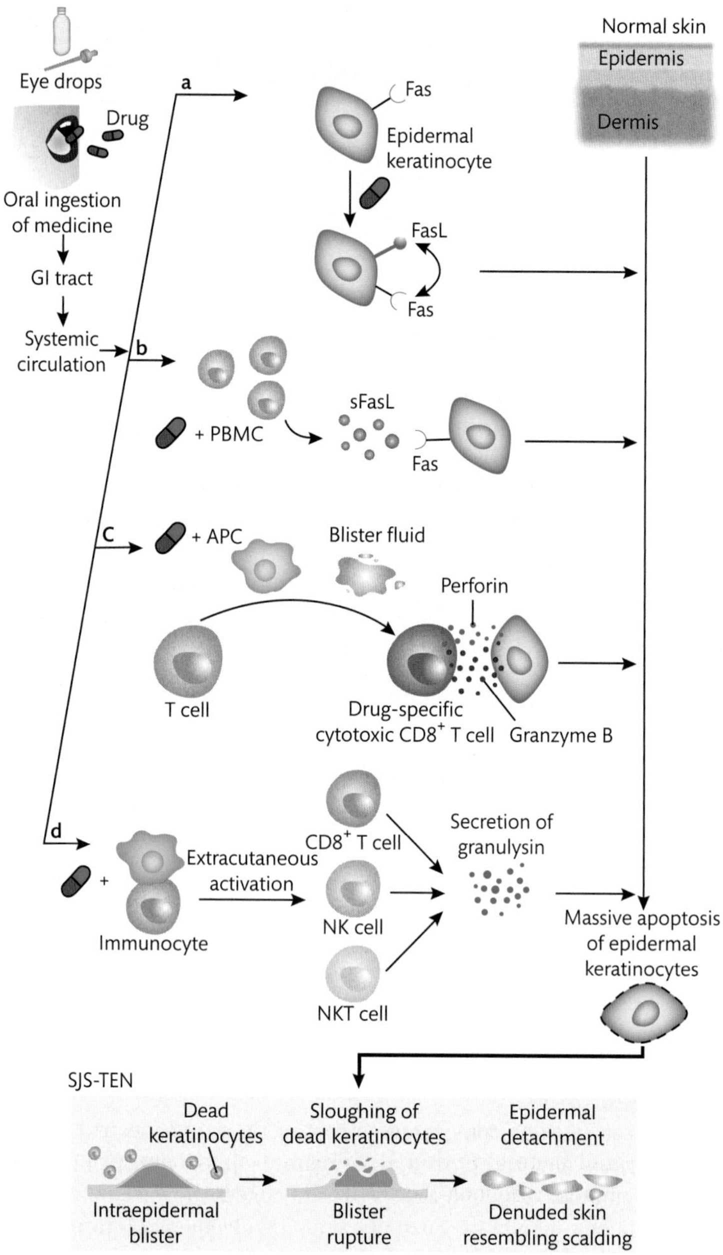

Figure 22.4 Mechanisms implicated in drug-induced keratinocyte death in SJS and TEN. Keratinocytes express Fas receptors which bind to Fas ligands (FasL) to form a death-complex that induces signalling for cell apoptosis. It is thought medications, such as aromatic AEDs, may induce keratinocytes and peripheral blood mononuclear cells (PBMCs) to upregulate FasL and increase production of soluble FasL, respectively, which then bind to keratinocyte Fas receptors leading to apoptosis (pathways A and B). Research has also suggested that the offending drugs interact with MHC Class I expressing cells, leading to activation and accumulation of cytotoxic CD8+ T cells in skin blisters. These T cells then release perforin and granzyme B which kill keratinocytes (pathway C). Alternatively, secretion of granulysin, which induces cell apoptosis, may occur due to drug-induced activation of cytotoxic CD8+ T cell, natural killer (NK) cells and NK T cells (pathway D).

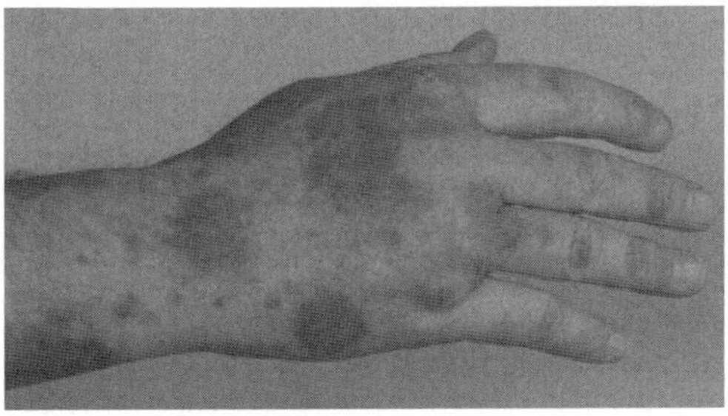

Figure 22.5 Erythema multiforme. Please see colour plate section.

to six weeks after the initiation of the medication, starting with fever and a macular rash beginning on the face, trunk, and upper limbs. The rash then becomes papular and spreads to the lower limbs. The face is often swollen. The rash may progress into a pustular or exfoliative dermatitis. There is lymphadenopathy and involvement of at least one other organ system, usually the liver, identified by abnormal blood liver function tests. Over 90 per cent of patients have eosinophilia. Involvement of other organ systems can lead to nephritis, pneumonitis, myocarditis, pericarditis, encephalitis, pancreatitis, and thyroid disease. Reactivation of herpes viruses, in particular HHV-6 and HHV-7, is associated with this condition. Skin biopsy shows a dense lymphocytic infiltrate. Management includes identification and withdrawal of the culprit drug, and the use of topical and, if required, systemic steroids. It is associated with 10 per cent mortality, often due to liver complications, and can progress to SJS or TEN.

Pseudolymphomatous drug hypersensitivity syndrome

This reaction is most commonly due to AEDs. Onset typically occurs within eight weeks of commencing the medication, but can occur as late as five years afterwards. As the name suggests, this reaction clinically mimics lymphoma, typically cutaneous T-cell lymphoma (also known as mycosis fungoides). It can present as an isolated plaque, nodule, or papule, or as erythematous patches, or with widespread erythroderma. Histology of lesions can help differentiate this condition from lymphoma. It runs a benign course and management is to withdraw the suspected drug.

> **Clinical tip** Sepsis or drug rash
>
> DRESS can easily be mistaken for sepsis. Although it is prudent to consider and investigate for sepsis, possible drug reaction should always be considered.

Other common cutaneous reactions secondary to AEDs

Other common cutaneous reactions to AEDs are listed in Table 22.7. This is not an exhaustive list, and there have been case reports of other cutaneous reactions. In addition many of these reactions occur with other drugs as well. Skin biopsy can be

Table 22.6 DRESS diagnostic criteria*

Fever >38°C
Acute rash
Lymphadenopathy at two sites
Involvement of at least one internal organ system
Blood count abnormalities (raised or reduced lymphocyte or elevated eosinophil counts or low platelets)
Hospitalization
Reaction suspected to be drug-related

*At least three of the seven criteria must be present for diagnosis of DRESS.
Source data from RegiSCAR Group inclusion criteria: http://www.regiscar.org/Diseases_HSS_DRESS.html

useful to distinguish different eruptions as well as the cause. If the causative drug cannot be withdrawn, supportive management to deal with symptoms is given for mild rashes.

Table 22.7 Other common cutaneous reactions secondary to AEDs

Skin reaction	Skin signs	Management
Exanthems	This is the most common type of reaction and its clinical features vary greatly. There may be a maculopapular, morbilliform (measles-like) or erythematous rash. The trunk is usually affected. It is associated with pruritus, fever, and eosinophilia. If the offending drug is continued the rash may subside or it may progress into an exfoliative dermatitis (see below). In contrast viral rashes tend to begin on the face and often there is conjunctivitis as well.	Resolves within weeks of stopping culprit drug Regular emollient Soap substitute (e.g. aqueous cream) Regular topical steroid Oral steroids (if severe and unresponsive to above treatment)
Exfoliative dermatitis (Figure 22.6)	There is erythema, scaling, and exudation in the flexures. This can rapidly become generalized. It may occur as a progression of an exanthem.	
Fixed drug eruption	Round or oval itchy erythematous plaques develop within 8 hours of drug administration and recur at the same site with each subsequent exposure. New lesions can also develop elsewhere. As the lesions fade there is post-inflammatory hyperpigmentation where the lesions were. Common sites affected are hands, feet, and genitalia.	
Vasculitis (Figure 22.7)	Pruritic non-blanching dusky red lesions often over dependent areas. There may be associated systemic involvement, especially renal disease.	Investigations to rule out other causes of vasculitis (bloods including autoantibody screen, HIV, hepatitis, TB serology, urine dipstick for renal involvement) Skin biopsy Topical steroids Compression bandaging if oedema in lower limbs
Lichenoid drug eruption (Figure 22.8)	Features are consistent with idiopathic lichen planus. There are psorasiform violaceous well-demarcated pruritic lesions which are often widespread. Unlike idiopathic lichen planus, oral involvement is rare. Distribution may be in a photo-exposed areas. This reaction can occur many months after initiation of the drug and can take up to four months before improving, even after cessation of the culprit drug.	Resolves within months of stopping culprit drug Regular emollient Soap substitute (e.g. aqueous cream) Regular topical steroid Oral steroids (if severe and unresponsive to above treatment) Sun protection
Lupus-erythematosus-like syndrome	Only 5% of lupus erythematosus cases are due to drugs and cutaneous findings are uncommon. When present they include photosensitivity and pruritic discoid lesions. There are usually systemic features of lupus as well. Positive ANA and anti-histone antibodies are characteristic. Antibodies against double-stranded DNA are usually negative and complement levels are normal. Unlike idiopathic lupus, there is no female or African Caribbean preponderance. Subacute lupus is associated with positive anti-Ro and anti-SSA antibodies	Resolves within weeks of stopping culprit drug Regular emollient Soap substitute (e.g. aqueous cream) Regular topical steroid
Acne	Comedones, papules, nodulo-cystic lesions develop over the face and upper trunk. Acne fulminans, a severe acute onset, inflammatory acne associated with fever and joint pains can rarely develop.	Topical benzoyl peroxide antibiotic or retinoid Oral antibiotics Oral retinoids (specialists only) Oral steroids (for acne fulminans)
Purpura	Non-blanching purpura related to platelet dysfunction	No specific treatment required unless symptomatic
Photosensitivity	This is noticed in sun-exposed areas and sunburn occurs easily	Sun protection
Hair changes: hypertrichosis and hirsutism or alopecia	Phenytoin is associated with hypertrichosis (a change in early vellus hair into thick terminal hair) as well as excess hirsutism (hair growth in a male-pattern distribution). This usually occurs within three months of commencing the drug, affects approximately half of users, and usually resolves on discontinuation of the drug. Transient hair loss has been reported with valproic acid.	Self-care with shaving, waxing, depilatory creams Laser or electrolysis treatment Anti-androgen treatment (e.g. combined contraceptive pill)

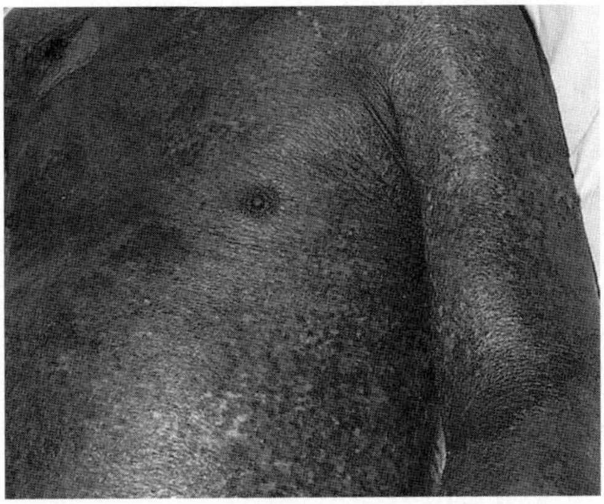

Figure 22.6 Exfoliative dermatitis. Please see colour plate section.

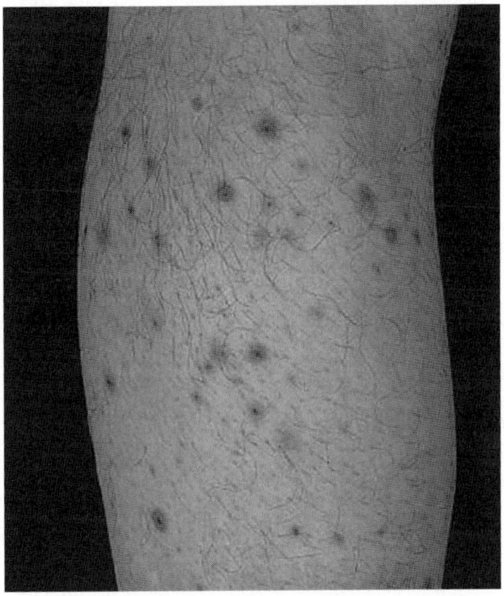

Figure 22.7 Vasculitis. Please see colour plate section.

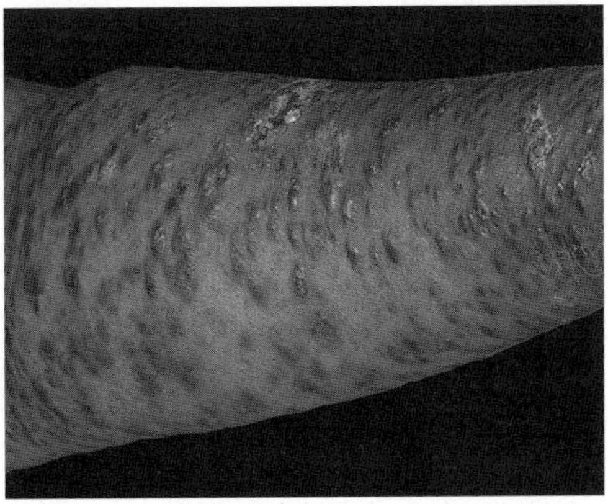

Figure 22.8 Lichenoid drug eruption. Please see colour plate section.

Final comment from the expert

Cutaneous reactions are very common with AEDs. The reactions can be frequent and mild, such as exanthematic rashes, or life-threatening such as with TEN. Measures should be taken to minimize risk, including performing genetic HLA screening in high-risk groups, commencing AEDs at low doses and titrating the dose up slowly, and educating patients about the risks of cutaneous eruptions, particularly within the first couple of month of starting the medication. Further understanding of the immunology and genetics of severe drug reactions will allow personalized prescribing in the future.

Acknowledgements

We are immensely grateful to Professor Rino Cerio, Queen Mary University of London, for providing images and advice in the writing of this case.

References

1. Gueudry J, Roujeau JC, Binaghi M, et al. Risk factors for the development of ocular complications of Stevens–Johnson syndrome and toxic epidermal necrolysis. *Arch Dermatol* 2009; 145: 157–62.
2. Gregory D. Treatment of acute Stevens–Johnson syndrome and toxic epidermal necrolysis using amniotic membrane: a review of 10 consecutive cases. *Ophthalmology* 2011; 118(5): 908–14.
3. Huang YC, Li YC, Chen TJ, et al. The efficacy of intravenous immunoglobulin for the treatment of toxic epidermal necrolysis: a systematic review and meta-analysis. *Br J Dermatol*. 2012; 167(2): 424–32.
4. Sekula P, Dunant A, Mockenhaupt M, et al. Comprehensive survival analysis of a cohort of patients with Stevens–Johnson syndrome and toxic epidermal necrolysis. *J Invest Dermatol* 2013; 133: 1197–1204.
5. Bastuji-Garin S, Fouchard N, Bertocchi M, et al. SCORTEN: a severity-of-illness score for toxic epidermal necrolysis. *J Invest Dermatol* 2000; 115: 149–53.
6. Arif H, Buchsbaum R, Weintraub D, *et al*. Comparison and predictors of rash associated with 15 antiepileptic drugs. *Neurology* 2007; 68: 1701–9.
7. Rzany B, Osvaldo C, Kelly J. Risk of Stevens–Johnson syndrome and toxic epidermal necrolysis during first weeks of antiepileptic therapy: a case control study. *Lancet* 1999; 353: 2190–4.
8. Chung WH, Hung SI, Hong HS, et al. Medical genetics: a marker for Stevens–Johnson syndrome. *Nature* 2004; 428: 486.
9. Chadwick D, Shaw MD, Foy P, et al. Serum anticonvulsant concentrations and the risk of drug induced skin eruptions. *J Neurol Neurosurg Psychiatry* 1984; 47: 642–4.
10. Zaccara G, Franciotta D, Perucca E. Idiosyncratic adverse reactions to antiepileptic drugs. *Epilepsia* 2007; 48(7): 1223–44.
11. Wang X, Lang S, Shi X, et al. Cross reactivity of skin rashes with current antiepileptic drugs in Chinese population. *Seizure* 2010; 19(9): 562–6.
12. Handoko KB, van Puijenbroek EP, Bijl AH, et al. Influence of chemical structure on hypersensitivity reactions induced by antiepileptic drugs: the role of the aromatic ring. *Drug Saf* 2008; 31(8): 695–702.
13. Hyson C, Sadler M. Cross sensitivity of skin rashes with antiepileptic drugs. *Can J Neurol Sci* 1997; 24(3): 245–9.

14. Hung SI, Chung WH, Jee SH, et al. Genetic susceptibility to carbamazepine-induced cutaneous adverse drug reactions. *Pharmacogenet Genomics* 2006; 16: 297–306.
15. Chen P, Lin JJ, Lu CS, et al. Carbamazepine-induced toxic effects and HLA-B*1502 screening in Taiwan. *N Engl J Med* 2011; 364: 1126–33.
16. Tangamornsuksan W, Chaiyakunapruk N, Somkrua R, et al. Relationship between the HLA-B*1502 allele and carbamazepine-induced Stevens–Johnson syndrome and toxic epidermal necrolysis: a systematic review and meta-analysis. *JAMA Dermatol* 2013; 149: 1025–32.
17. Ferrell PB Jr, McLeod HL. Carbamazepine, HLA-B*1502 and risk of Stevens–Johnson syndrome and toxic epidermal necrolysis: US FDA recommendations. *Pharmacogenomics* 2008; 9(10): 1543–1546.
18. McCormack M, Alfirevic A, Bourgeois S, et al. HLA-A*3101 and carbamazepine-induced hypersensitivity reactions in Europeans. *N Engl J Med.* 2011; 364; 1134-43.
19. Amstutz U, Shear NH, Rieder MJ, et al. Recommendations for HLA-B*15:02 and HLA-A*31:01 genetic testing to reduce the risk of carbamazepine-induced hypersensitivity reactions. *Epilepsia* 2014; 55(4): 496–506
20. Mockenhaupt M, Messenheimer J, Tennis P, et al. Risk of Stevens–Johnson syndrome and toxic epidermal necrolysis in new users of antiepileptics. *Neurology* 2005; 64: 1134–8.
21. Sassolas B, Haddad C, Mockenhaupt M, et al. ALDEN, an algorithm for assessment of drug causality in Stevens–Johnson syndrome and toxic epidermal necrolysis: comparison with case–control analysis. *Clin Pharmacol Ther* 2010; 88: 60–8.

INDEX

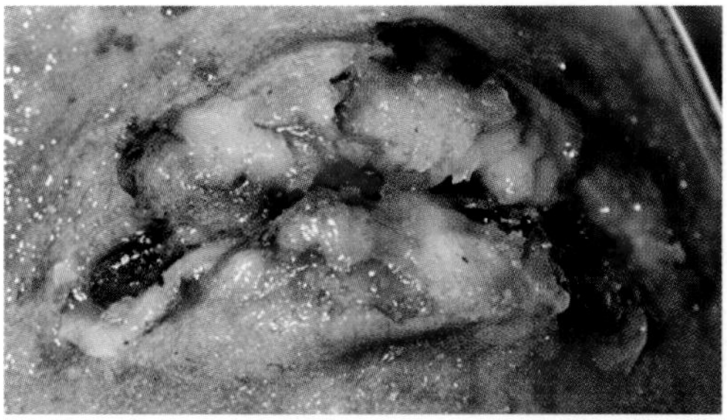

Figure 22.2 Clinical features of toxic epidermal necrolysis: oral mucosal involvement with sloughing and crusting of the lips.

Image courtesy of Professor Rino Cerio, Queen Mary University of London.

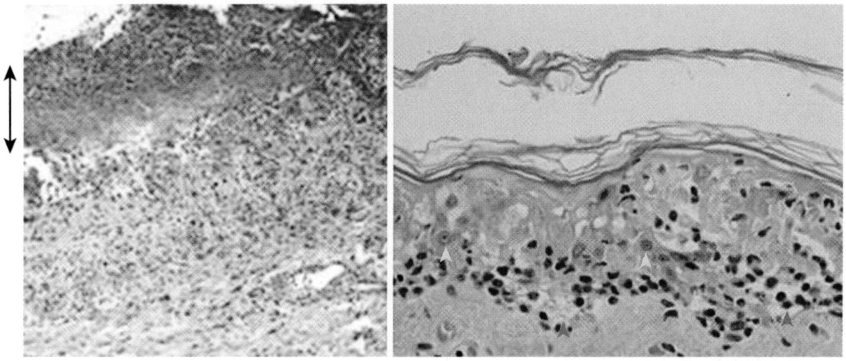

Figure 22.3 Histology of toxic epidermal necrolysis. Left panel: low-power view of skin biopsy with H&E staining showing full-thickness epidermal necrosis (double-headed arrow) with separation of epidermis and in some areas complete loss of epidermis. There is oedema in the underlying dermis with an inflammatory infiltrate. Right panel: medium-power view of early TEN lesional skin. There are scattered apoptotic keratinocytes (green arrowheads) and basal layer clefting (yellow arrowheads) with an inflammatory infiltrate in the upper dermis. Immunofluorescence was negative.

Images courtesy of Professor Rino Cerio, Queen Mary University of London.

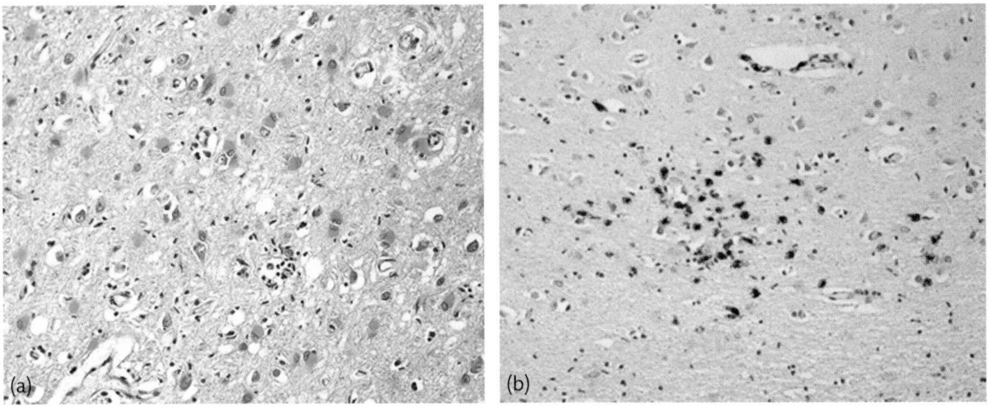

Figure 21.4 (a) Histology of the cerebral cortex (cingulate gyrus) showing neuronal loss, reactive gliosis, and lymphocytic infiltrate (H&E, 200x); (b) immunohistochemistry showing that the lymphocytic infiltrates are composed mostly of CD8 T cells (CD8, 100x).

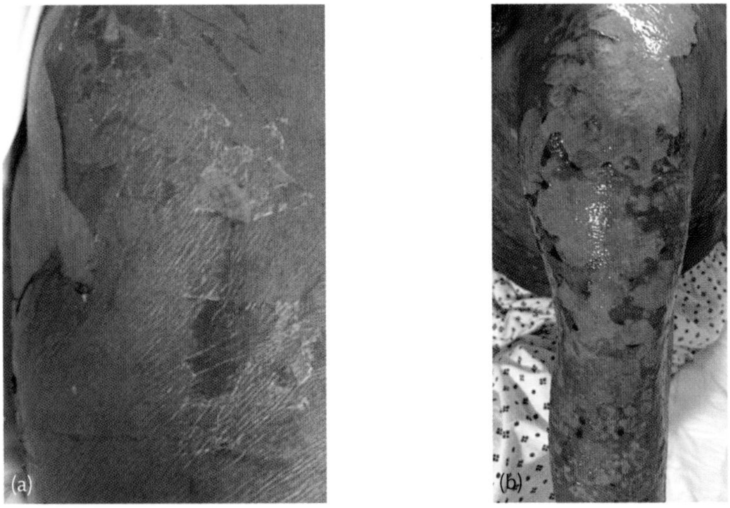

Figure 22.1 Clinical features of toxic epidermal necrolysis: (a) peeling skin; (b) denuded areas of skin.

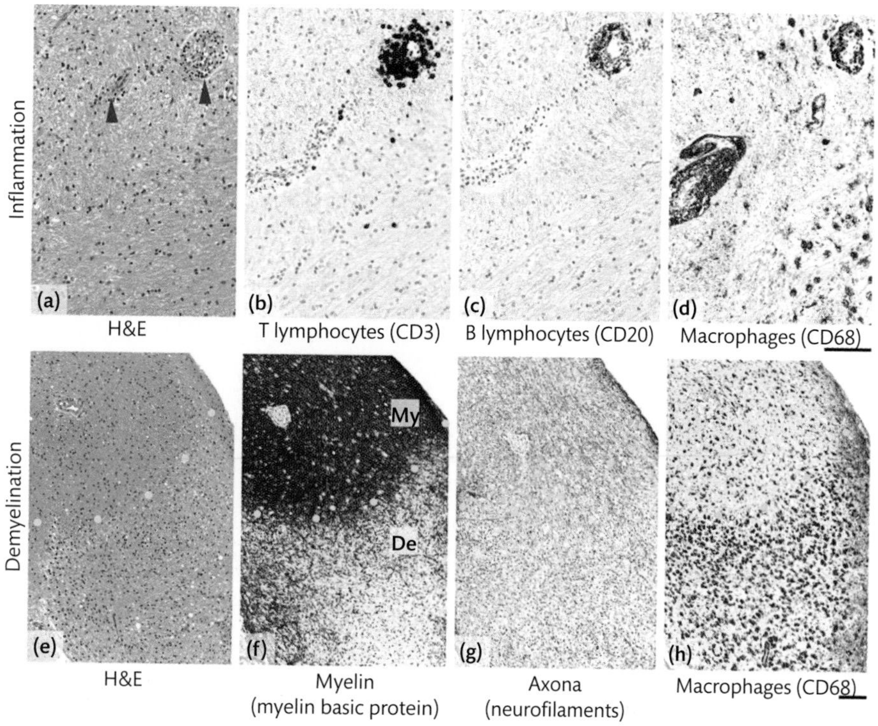

Figure 12.2 Brain biopsy specimen with stains specific for inflammation ((a)–(d)), demyelination ((e)–(h)), axonal integrity (g) and macrophages (h). (a)–(d) Inflammation: the haematoxylin-eosin (H&E) stained section (a) shows widespread perivascular infiltrates of mononuclear inflammatory cells; the majority of the lymphocytes are CD3+ T cells (b) with fewer CD20+ B cells (c); there are also numerous macrophages around the blood vessels and diffusely in the neural parenchyma (d). Demyelination ((e)–(h)): the H&E stained section (e) reveals a relatively sharp margin between the lesion and the surrounding neural parenchyma; immunostaining for myelin (f) with antibody for myelin basic protein (SMI94) accentuates the almost complete loss of myelin in the affected regions, while axons (g) immunostained with antibody for hyperphosphorylated neurofilaments (SMI31) are relatively preserved in the same areas. Immunostaining for CD68 (h) reveals numerous foamy macrophages in the demyelinated foci. Arrows indicate the perivascular inflammation. The dotted line indicates the border between myelinated (My) and demyelinated (De) regions. Scale bar: 100μm

Reproduced with thanks to Dr Zane Jaunmuktane, UCL Institute of Neurology, UK.

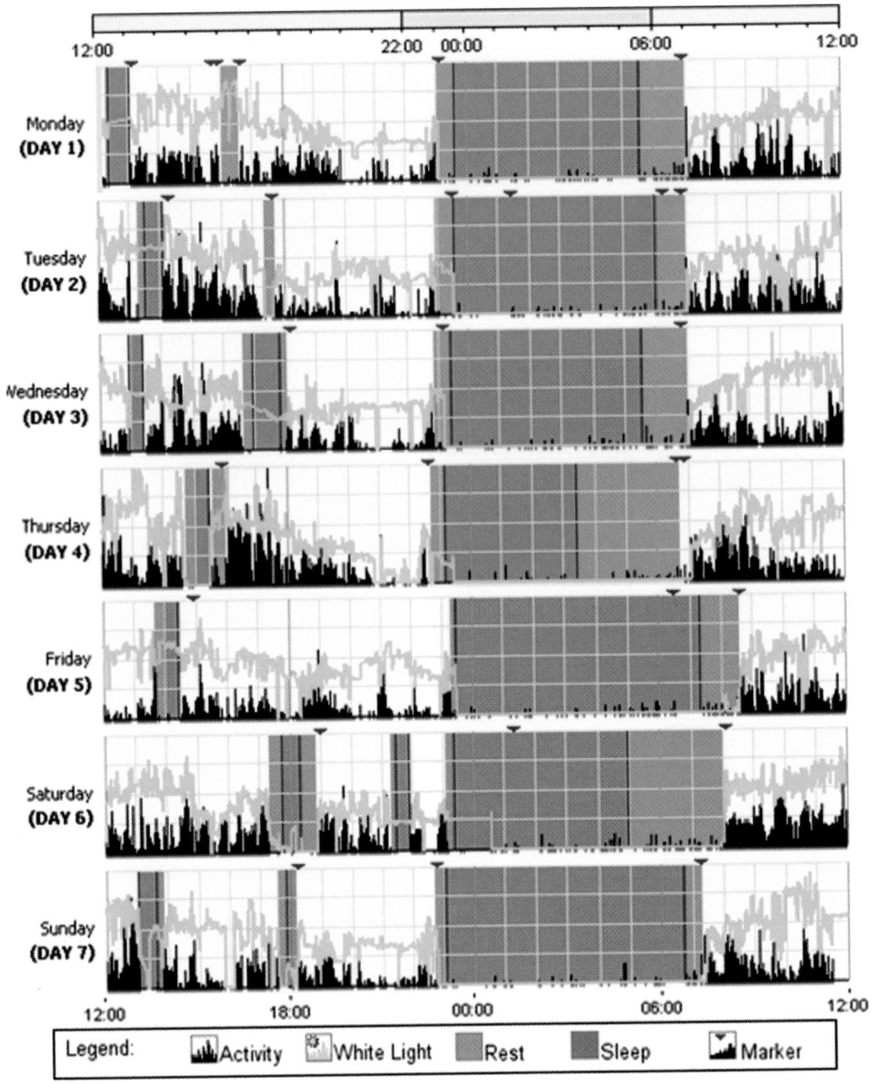

Figure 11.1 Actigraphy. The patient is asked to wear a watch ('actigraph') daily for a period of seven consecutive days. The watch contains an accelerometer which records low-frequency motion consistent with normal movement. Patients with narcolepsy show elevated and fragmented nocturnal motor activity and increased periods of sustained immobility during the day [1], which can be quantitatively assessed from the actogram.

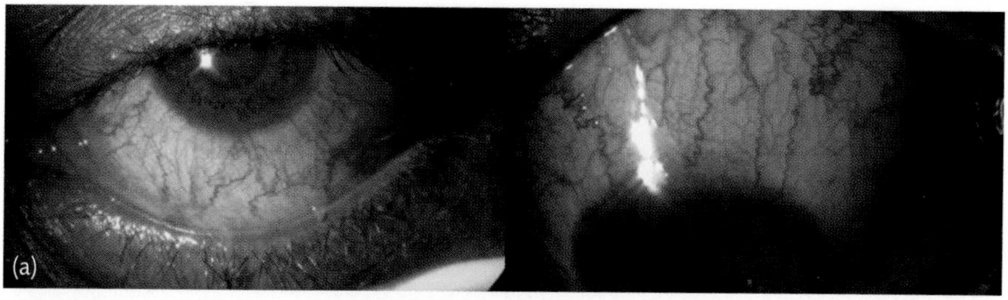

Figure 7.1a Examination findings at the time of presentation. (a) Slit-lamp biomicroscopy images show 'corkscrew' injected episcleral and conjunctival vessels with mild chemosis.

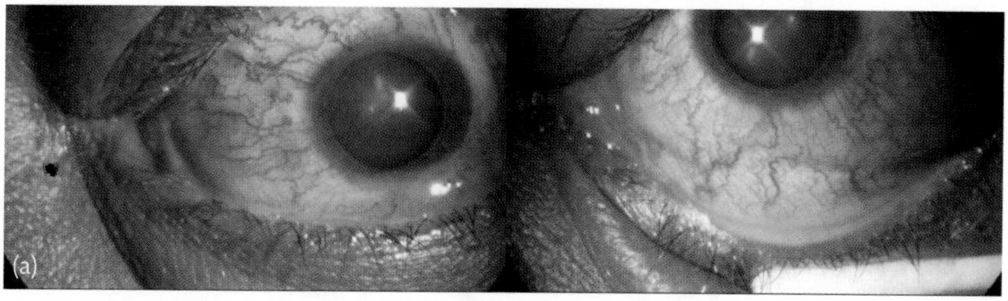

Figure 7.2a Examination findings at the time of admission to hospital 33 days after presentation. (a) Slit-lamp biomicroscopy images show 'corkscrew' injected episcleral and conjunctival vessels with chemosis and lid swelling.

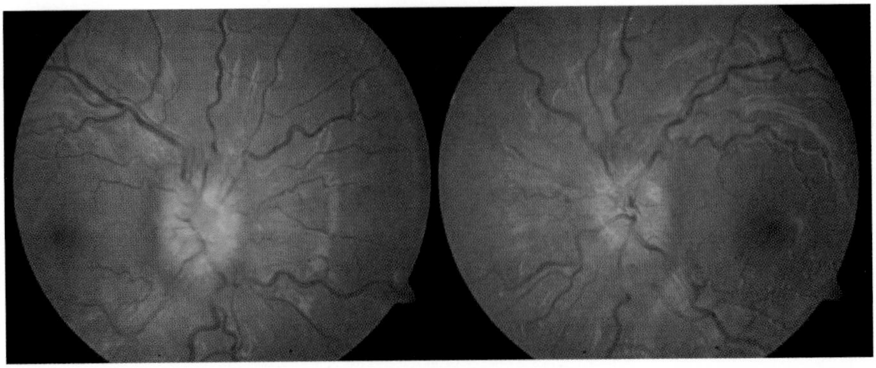

Figure 2.3 Fundus photographs showing bilateral optic disc swelling.

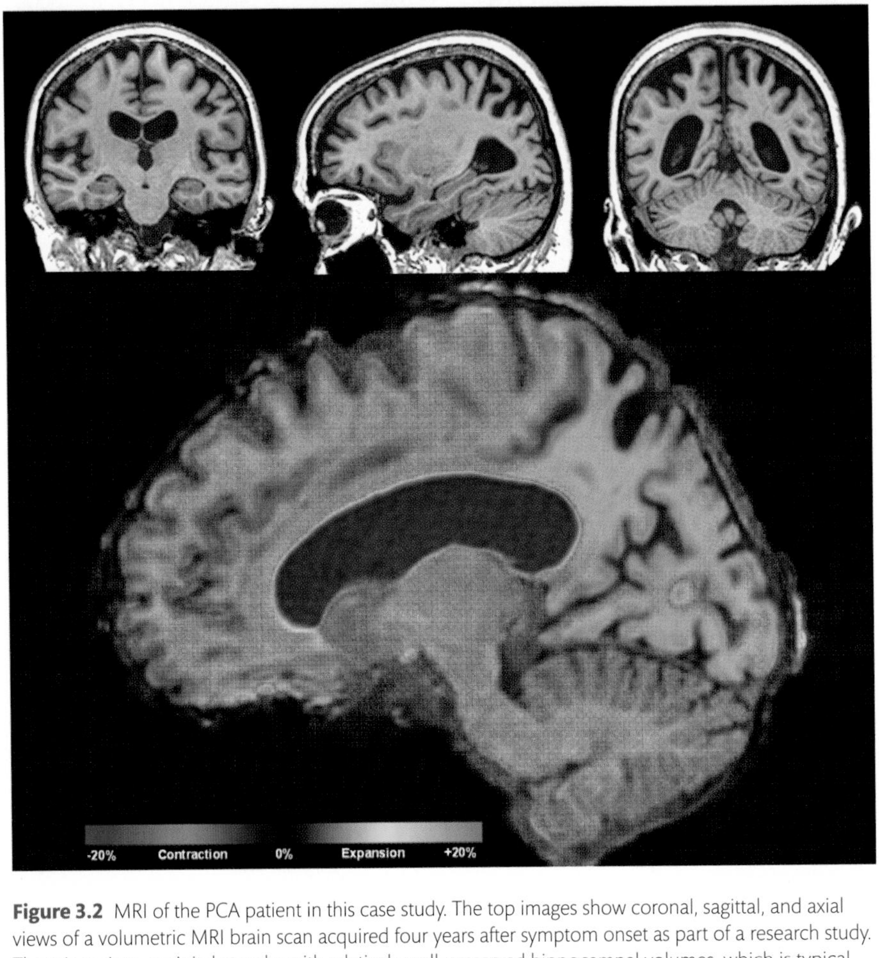

Figure 3.2 MRI of the PCA patient in this case study. The top images show coronal, sagittal, and axial views of a volumetric MRI brain scan acquired four years after symptom onset as part of a research study. There is parieto-occipital atrophy with relatively well-preserved hippocampal volumes, which is typical of PCA. A repeat scan two years later has been fluid registered to the baseline scan to produce the voxel compression map shown in the bottom image. The scale shows the percentage volume change per voxel (−20–20%) with green and blue representing contraction and yellow and red representing expansion. Atrophy over this interval is greatest in the parietal and occipital regions.

Image courtesy of Tim Shakespeare and Shona Clegg.